Field Epidemiology

Field Epidemiology

Second Edition

Edited by

Michael B. Gregg

OXFORD
UNIVERSITY PRESS

2002

OXFORD
UNIVERSITY PRESS

Oxford   New York
Auckland   Bangkok   Buenos Aires   Cape Town   Chennai
Dar es Salaam   Delhi   Hong Kong   Istanbul   Karachi   Kolkata
Kuala Lumpur   Madrid   Melbourne   Mexico City   Mumbai   Nairobi
São Paulo   Shanghai   Singapore   Taipei   Tokyo   Toronto

and an associated company in Berlin

Copyright © 1996, 2002 by Michael B. Gregg

Published by Oxford University Press Inc.,
198 Madison Avenue, New York, New York 10016
http://www.oup-usa.org

Library of Congress Cataloging-in-Publication Data
Field epidemiology / edited by Michael B. Gregg
p. cm.   Includes bibliographical references and index.
ISBN 0-19-514259-4
1. Epidemiology.   2. Epidemics
I. Gregg, Michael B.
RA651 .F495 2001   614.4—dc21   2001133067

9 8 7 6 5 4

Printed in the United States of America
on acid-free paper.

This book is dedicated to the memory of

Alexander D. Langmuir,

Originator, teacher, and practitioner of field epidemiology,
whose wisdom, vision, and inspiration have profoundly
strengthened the practice of public health
throughout the world.

PREFACE

Since the first edition of *Field Epidemiology* was published in 1996, it became apparent that it should be expanded to cover a wider variety of scenarios where the field epidemiologist may be called upon to investigate. In keeping with the motivation, purposes, and presentation of the book, as outlined in the preface of the first edition; several new chapters have been added. Included now in Part III are chapters covering (*1*) investigations in the workplace; (*2*) the practice of field epidemiology from the perspective of state and local health departments; (*3*) the role of the field epidemiologist in the arena of bioterrorism; and (*4*) the epidemiologist's response to and role in natural disasters. An appendix has also been added consisting of a "walk-through" exercise detailing a step-by-step method of how to investigate an outbreak of a food-borne disease. Finally, all chapters have been reviewed and updated, expanded, or modified where needed.

Over the past two decades it has become abundantly clear that the teaching and application of field epidemiology have spread widely throughout the world. The first edition of this book has been translated into Chinese, and epidemiologists from several other countries have shown similar interest. Such programs as the Global Health Leadership Officer Programme of the World Health Organization; the Public Health Schools Without Walls, supported by the Rockefeller Foundation; and the Field Epidemiology Training Programs (FETP) started by CDC all attest to the importance and application of field epidemiology in the practice of public health.

While *Field Epidemiology* does, indeed, cater to public health epidemiologists practicing in the United States, it is the hope of the editor and the contributors to this book that our collective efforts will contribute significantly to the understanding and practice of field epidemiology worldwide.

Guilford, Vermont   M.B.G.

PREFACE TO THE FIRST EDITION

Carl W. Tyler, Jr., M.D.

Epidemiology is becoming increasingly complex, theoretical, and specialized. While many epidemiologists are still engaged in the investigation of infectious disease problems, others are addressing new challenges such as homicides and unplanned pregnancy. Computers make it practical to calculate in seconds what might otherwise take months to complete. Whole new textbooks have appeared in such areas as pharmacoepidemiology, perinatal epidemiology, and occupational epidemiology.

Because of the advances in the real world of contemporary health problems, there is a need for a clearly written, highly usable book devoted to field epidemiology—the timely use of epidemiology in solving public health problems. This process involves the application of basic epidemiologic principles in real time, place, and person to solve health problems of an urgent or emergency nature.

This book, intended to meet this need, is based upon both science and experience. It deals with real problems, real places, and real people: nature's experiments, if you will, rather than carefully designed studies in a laboratory or clinical setting. So, in the lexicon of the epidemiologist, the book will be addressing issues relating to observational epidemiology—not experimental epidemiology.

To a great extent, this book takes it roots from the experience of the Centers for Disease Control and Prevention (CDC) over more than 40 years of training health professionals in the science and art of field epidemiology. In 1951,

ix

Alexander D. Langmuir, M.D., CDC's chief epidemiologist, founded the Epidemic Intelligence Service (EIS), and its 2-year on-the-job training program in practical, applied epidemiology. On call 24 hours a day, the trainee, called an EIS Officer, has been available upon request to go into the field to help state and local health officials investigate urgent health problems. Before going into the field, however, EIS Officers receive training at CDC in basic epidemiology, biostatistics, and public health practice. The 3-week, 8-hour-a-day course is designed to equip them with the essentials of how to mount a field investigation; how to investigate an epidemic; how to start a surveillance system; and how to apply science, technology, and common sense to meet real-life problems at the grass roots level of experience.

Based on the collective experience of EIS Officers and their CDC mentors, this book thus attempts to describe for the field investigator the relevant and appropriate operations necessary to solve urgent health problems at local, state, provincial, federal, and international levels.

Part I contains a definition of field epidemiology; a brief review of epidemiologic principles and methods, under the assumption that the reader has some knowledge of basic epidemiologic methods; and the concepts of surveillance. Part II covers the components of field epidemiology: (1) operational aspects of field investigations; (2) conducting a field investigation—a practical step-by-step description of what to do in the field; (3) describing the data—the elements of time, place, and person; (4) designing studies; (5) analyzing and interpreting data; (6) developing interventions; and (7) communicating the findings. Part III covers special issues such as (1) surveys and sampling; (2) use of microcomputers in the field; (3) dealing with the public and the press; (4) legal aspects of field investigations; (5) field investigations in institutional, day-care, and international settings, and (6) the collection and handling of laboratory specimens in association with a field investigation.

Copies of this book should be found more often in the briefcases of field epidemiologists than on the shelves of libraries. It is intended to be a close companion during the preparation and conduct of field investigations; it should be helpful during data analysis; and it should be a ready reference when the final epidemiologic report is being written. It is not intended to replace the detailed, hardbound, specialized reference works found on the shelves of libraries in medical centers and schools of public health. Rather, it is meant to be readily accessible and to serve as an important tool for any health professional responsible for investigating epidemiologic problems in the field.

ACKNOWLEDGMENTS

I wish to acknowledge the dedicated and helpful assistance of Marianne G. Lawrence, B.S., in the preparation of this book, and the patience and understanding of my wife, Lila W. Gregg.

CONTENTS

Contributors, xvii

I.   BACKGROUND

1. Field Epidemiology Defined, 3
   Richard A. Goodman and James W. Buehler

2. A Brief Review of the Basic Principles of Epidemiology, 8
   Richard C. Dicker

3. Surveillance, 26
   Stephen B. Thacker and Guthrie S. Birkhead

II.   THE FIELD INVESTIGATION

4. Operational Aspects of Epidemiologic Field Investigations, 53
   Richard A. Goodman, Michael B. Gregg, and Jeffrey J. Sacks

5. Conducting a Field Investigation, 62
   Michael B. Gregg

6. Describing the Findings, 78
   Robert E. Fontaine and Richard A. Goodman

7. Designing Studies in the Field, 117
   Richard C. Dicker

8. Analyzing and Interpreting Data, 132
   Richard C. Dicker

9. Developing Interventions, 173
   Richard A. Goodman, James W. Buehler, Jeffrey P. Koplan, and Duc J. Vugia

10. Communicating Epidemiologic Findings, 183
    Michael B. Gregg

11. Surveys and Sampling, 196
    Joan M. Herold and J. Virgil Peavy

12. Using a Computer for Field Investigations, 217
    Andrew G. Dean

13. Dealing with the Public and the Media, 236
    Bruce B. Dan

III.   SPECIAL CONSIDERATIONS

14. Legal Considerations in a Field Investigation, 255
    Verla S. Neslund

15. Investigations in Health-Care Settings, 268
    William R. Jarvis and Stephanie Zaza

16. Investigations in Out-of-Home Child Care Settings, 290
    Ralph L. Cordell and Margaret Swartz

17. Field Investigations of Occupational Disease and Injury, 306
    William E. Halperin

18. Field Investigations from the State and Local
    Health Department Perspective, 324
    Jeffrey P. Davis and Guthrie S. Birkhead

19. Epidemiologic Investigations in International Settings, 345
    Stanley O. Foster

20. Bioterrorism Preparedness and Response: Issues for Public Health, 354
    Scott R. Lillibridge and Kristy Murray-Lillibridge

21. Field Investigations of Natural Disasters, 365
    Eric K. Noji and Michael B. Gregg

22. Laboratory Support for the Epidemiologist in the Field, 384
    Janet K. A. Nicholson and Elaine W. Gunter

    Appendix A Walk-through Exercise, 413
    Michael B. Gregg

    Index, 435

CONTRIBUTORS

GUTHRIE S. BIRKHEAD, M.D., M.P.H.
Director
AIDS Institute and Center for Community
   Health
New York State Department of Health
Associate Professor of Epidemiology
School of Public Health
University at Albany
Albany, New York

JAMES W. BUEHLER, M.D.
Associate Director for Science
National Center for HIV, Sexually
   Transmitted Disease, and Tuberculosis
   Prevention
Centers for Disease Control and
   Prevention
Atlanta, Georgia

RALPH L. CORDELL, PH.D.
Acting Chief, Quality Research Section,
   Health Outcomes Branch,
Division of Healthcare Quality Promotion

National Center for Infectious
   Diseases
Centers for Disease Control and
   Prevention
Atlanta, Georgia

BRUCE B. DAN, M.D.
Adjunct Assistant Professor
Department of Preventive Medicine
Vanderbilt University School of
   Medicine
Nashville, Tennessee

JEFFREY P. DAVIS, M.D.
Chief Medical Officer and State
   Epidemiologist for Communicable
   Diseases
Wisconsin Division of Public Health
Adjunct Professor
Departments of Preventive Medicine and
   Pediatrics
University of Wisconsin Medical School
Madison, Wisconsin

ANDREW G. DEAN, M.D., M.P.H.
Chief
Software Development Activity
Division of Public Health Surveillance
    and Informatics
Epidemiology Program Office
Centers for Disease Control and
    Prevention
Atlanta, Georgia

RICHARD C. DICKER, M.D., M.S.
Supervisory Epidemiologist
Epidemiology Program Office
Centers for Disease Control and
    Prevention
Atlanta, Georgia

ROBERT E. FONTAINE, M.D., MSc.
Medical Epidemiologist
Division of International Health
Epidemiology Program Office
Centers for Disease Control and
    Prevention
Atlanta, Georgia

STANLEY O. FOSTER, M.D., M.P.H.
Visiting Professor for International Health
Rollins School of Public Health
Emory University
Atlanta, Georgia

RICHARD A. GOODMAN, M.D., J.D.
Senior Advisor for Science and Policy
Financial Management Office
Centers for Disease Control and
    Prevention
Atlanta, Georgia

MICHAEL B. GREGG, M.D.
Private Consultant in Epidemiology,
Epidemiologic Training, and
Disease Surveillance
Guilford, Vermont

ELAINE W. GUNTER, B.S., M.T.
Deputy Director for Management and
    Operations
Division of Laboratory Sciences
National Center for Environmental Health

Centers for Disease Control and
    Prevention
Atlanta, Georgia

WILLIAM E. HALPERIN, M.D., DR.P.H.
Chairman and Professor
Department of Preventive Medicine and
    Community Health
New Jersey Medical School
University of Medicine and Dentistry of
    New Jersey
Newark, New Jersey

JOAN M. HEROLD, PH.D.
Associate Professor
Rollins School of Public Health
Emory University
Atlanta, Georgia

WILLIAM R. JARVIS, M.D.
Associate Director for Program
    Development
Division of Healthcare Quality
    Promotion
Centers for Disease Control and
    Prevention
Atlanta, Georgia

JEFFREY P. KOPLAN, M.D., M.P.H.
Director
Centers for Disease Control and
    Prevention
Atlanta, Georgia

SCOTT R. LILLIBRIDGE, M.D.
Centers for Disease Control and
    Prevention
Atlanta, Georgia

KRISTY MURRAY-LILLIBRIDGE, D.V.M.
National Center for Infectious Diseases
Centers for Disease Control and
    Prevention
Atlanta, Georgia

VERLA S. NESLUND, J.D.
Deputy Legal Advisor to the
Centers for Disease Control and Prevention
Atlanta, Georgia

JANET K. A. NICHOLSON, PH.D.
Associate Director for Laboratory Science
National Center for Infectious Diseases
Centers for Disease Control and
  Prevention
Atlanta, Georgia

ERIC K. NOJI, M.D., M.P.H.
Associate Director for Bio-Emergency
  Preparedness and Response
Bioterrorism Preparedness and Response
  Program
National Center for Infectious Diseases
Centers for Disease Control and
  Prevention
Atlanta, Georgia

J. VIRGIL PEAVY, M.S.
Former Senior Training Consultant
Public Health Practice Program Office
Centers for Disease Control and
  Prevention
Atlanta, Georgia

JEFFREY J. SACKS, M.D., M.P.H.
Medical Epidemiologist
Health Care and Aging Studies Branch
Division of Adult and Community Health
National Center for Chronic Disease
  Prevention and Health Promotion
Centers for Disease Control and
  Prevention
Atlanta, Georgia

MARGARET SWARTZ, R.N.
Nurse Consultant
Illinois Department of Public Health
West Chicago, Illinois

STEPHEN B. THACKER, M.D.
Director, Epidemiology Program Office
Centers for Disease Control and
  Prevention
Atlanta, Georgia

CARL W. TYLER, JR., M.D.
Former Director, Epidemiology Program
  Office
Centers for Disease Control and
  Prevention
Atlanta, Georgia

DUC J. VUGIA, M.D., M.P.H.
Chief, Disease Investigations and
  Surveillance Branch
Division of Communicable Disease
  Control
California Department of Health
  Services
Berkeley, California

STEPHANIE ZAZA, M.D., M.P.H.
Chief, Community Guide Branch
Epidemiology Program Office
Centers for Disease Control and
  Prevention
Atlanta, Georgia

I

BACKGROUND

1

FIELD EPIDEMIOLOGY DEFINED

Richard A. Goodman
James W. Buehler

Despite the actual practice of "field epidemiology" in the United States and abroad for well over a century, it has not been defined in professional (i.e., epidemiologic and medical) dictionaries.[1] Therefore, the purpose of this chapter is to provide both a definition of the term and a framework for the concept of field epidemiology as it is used throughout this book.

The constellation of problems faced by epidemiologists who are called upon to investigate urgent public health problems gives shape to the definition of field epidemiology. For example, consider the following scenario: At 8:30 a.m. on Monday, August 2, 1976, Dr. Robert B. Craven, an Epidemic Intelligence Service Officer assigned to CDC's Viral Diseases Division, received a telephone call from a nurse at a veterans' hospital in Philadelphia, Pennsylvania. The nurse called to report two cases of severe respiratory illness (including one death) in persons who had attended the American Legion Convention in Philadelphia between July 21 and July 24. Subsequent conversations with local and state public health officials revealed that, from July 26 to August 2, 18 conventioneers had died, primarily from pneumonia. By the evening of August 2, an additional 71 cases had been identified among legionnaires. As a consequence of this information, a massive epidemiologic investigation was immediately initiated that involved public health agencies at the local, state, and federal levels. This problem became known as the outbreak of legionnaires' disease, and the investigation of the problem led directly to the discovery of the gram-negative pathogen, *Legionella pneumophila*.[2]

The legionnaires' disease outbreak and the public health response it triggered illustrate the raison d'être for field epidemiology. Using this epidemic as an example, we can define field epidemiology as the application of epidemiology under the following set of general conditions:

- The problem is unexpected.
- A timely response may be demanded.
- Public health epidemiologists must travel to and work in the field to solve the problem.
- The extent of the investigation is likely to be limited because of the imperative for timely intervention.

While field investigations of acute problems share many characteristics with prospectively planned epidemiologic studies, they may differ in at least three important aspects. First, because field investigations often start without clear hypotheses, they may require the use of descriptive studies to generate hypotheses before analytic studies are conducted to test these hypotheses. Second, as noted previously, when acute problems occur, there is an immediate need to protect the community's health and address its concerns. These responsibilities drive the epidemiologic field investigation beyond the confines of data collection and analysis and into the realm of public health action. Finally, field epidemiology requires one to consider when the data are sufficient to take action rather than to ask what additional questions might be answered by the data.

The concepts and methods used in field investigations derive from clinical medicine, epidemiology, laboratory science, decision theory, skill in communications, and common sense. In this book, the guidelines and approaches for conducting epidemiologic field investigations reflect the urgency of discovering causative factors, the use of multifaceted methods, and the need to make practical recommendations.

UNIQUE CHALLENGES TO EPIDEMIOLOGISTS IN FIELD INVESTIGATIONS

An epidemiologist investigating problems in the field is faced by unique challenges that sometimes constrain the ideal use of scientific methods. In contrast to prospectively planned studies, which are based on carefully developed and refined protocols, field investigations must rely on data sources that are less readily controlled and that may literally change with each successive hour or day. In addition to potential limitations in data sources, other factors that pose challenges for epidemiologists during field investigations include sampling considerations, the availability of specimens, the impact of publicity, the reluctance of subjects to participate, and the conflicting pressures to intervene.

Data Sources

Field investigations often use information abstracted from a variety of sources, such as hospital, outpatient medical, or school health records. These records vary dramatically in completeness and accuracy among patients, health care providers, and facilities, since entries are made for purposes other than conducting epidemiologic studies. Thus, the quality of such records as sources of data for epidemiologic investigations may be substantially less than the quality of information obtained, for example, from standard, pretested questionnaires.

Small Numbers

In a planned prospective study, the epidemiologist determines appropriate sample sizes based on statistical requirements for power. In contrast, outbreaks can involve a relatively small number of persons, thereby imposing substantial restrictions on study design, statistical power, and other aspects of analysis. These restrictions, in turn, place limitations on the inferences and conclusions that can be drawn from a field investigation.

Specimen Collection

Because the field investigator usually arrives on the scene "after the fact," collection of necessary environmental or biological specimens is not always possible. For example, suspect food items may have been entirely consumed or discarded, a suspect water system may have been flushed, or ill persons may have recovered, thereby precluding collection of acute specimens. Under these conditions the epidemiologist depends on the diligence of health care providers who first see the affected persons and on the recall of affected persons, their relatives, or other members of the affected community.

Publicity

Acute disease outbreaks often generate considerable local attention and publicity. In this regard, press coverage can assist the investigation by helping to develop information, to identify cases, or to promote and help implement control measures. On the other hand, such publicity may cause affected persons and others in the community to develop preconceptions about the source or cause of an outbreak, which in turn lead to potential biases in comparative studies or failure to fully explore alternate hypotheses. Parenthetically, media representatives in pursuit of the most current information on the investigation may demand a considerable amount of time to the detriment of the field investigation itself.

Reluctance to Participate

While health departments are empowered to conduct investigations and gain access to records, voluntary and willing participation of involved parties is more conducive to successful investigations than forced participation. In addition, persons whose livelihoods or related interests are at risk may be reluctant to cooperate voluntarily. This reluctance may often be the case for common source outbreaks associated with restaurants and other public establishments, in environmental or occupational hazard investigations, or among health care providers suspected as being sources for transmission of infectious diseases such as hepatitis B. When involved parties do not willingly cooperate, delays may compromise access to and quality of information (e.g., by introducing bias and decreasing statistical power).

Conflicting Pressures to Intervene

Epidemiologists conducting field investigations must weigh the need for further investigation against the need for immediate intervention. However, the strong and varying opinions of affected persons and others in the community can interfere with the optimal scientific approach.

Although not truly unique challenges as such to the field epidemiologist, two situations may occur during a field investigation that merit noting. First, on occasion, what appears to be a small, geographically well-defined epidemic turns out to be much larger in scope than originally appreciated. This has been particularly true with food-borne disease epidemics that initially seem localized, only soon to be recognized regionally or nationally after reports appear in the media. Second, rarely field investigations will turn up no evidence of an epidemic. Despite initial local concern, cries of epidemic, and a reasonable request by the local health officials, the field team may find no health problem at all.

STANDARDS FOR EPIDEMIOLOGIC FIELD INVESTIGATIONS

Field investigations are sometimes perceived to represent "quick and dirty" epidemiology. This perception may reflect the inherent nature of circumstances for which rapid responses are required. However, these requirements for action do not provide a rationalization for epidemiologic shortcuts. Rather, they underscore for the field epidemiologist the importance of combining good science with prudent judgment. A better description of a good epidemiologic field investigation would be "quick and appropriate."

In judging an epidemiologic field investigation, paramount consideration should be given to the quality of the science. This should not be the sole standard, however, for the full range of limitations, pressures, and responsibilities imposed on the investigator must also be taken into account. The goal should be to maximize the scientific quality of the field investigation in the face of these limitations and competing interests.

The epidemiologist in the public sector must reconcile the multiple competing and/or conflicting interests and develop the most scientifically optimal study design possible under the circumstances. Sound judgment combined with a rigorous scientific effort will lead to a field investigation that meets the public's needs and also provides scientific data of the highest quality. Thus, the standards for an epidemiologic field investigation are that it: (*1*) is timely; (*2*) addresses an important public health problem in the community, as defined by standard public health measures (e.g., attack rates, serious morbidity, or mortality) or community concern; (*3*) examines resource needs early and deploys them appropriately; (*4*) employs appropriate methods of descriptive and/or analytic epidemiology; (*5*) probes causality to the degree sufficient to enable identification of the source and/or etiology of the problem; and (*6*) establishes immediate control and long-term interventions.

REFERENCES

1. Last, J.M. (1988) (Ed.). *Dictionary of Epidemiology*, 2nd ed., Oxford University Press, New York.
2. Fraser, D.W., Tsai, T.R., Orenstein, W., et al. (1977). Legionnaires' disease: description of an epidemic of pneumonia. *N Engl J Med* 297, 1189–97.

2

A BRIEF REVIEW OF THE BASIC PRINCIPLES OF EPIDEMIOLOGY

Richard C. Dicker

Epidemiology is considered the basic science of public health for good reason. First, epidemiology is a quantitative basic science built on a working knowledge of probability, statistics, and sound research methods. Second, epidemiology is a method of causal reasoning based on developing and testing biologically plausible hypotheses about health states and events. Third, as a discipline within public health, epidemiology provides a foundation for directing public health action based on this science and causal reasoning, along with an understanding of what is practical and capable of being accomplished.[1]

The word *epidemiology* comes from the Greek words *epi*, meaning on or upon, *demos*, meaning people, and *logos*, meaning the study of. In other words, the word epidemiology has its roots in the study of what befalls the population. Many definitions have been proposed, but the following definition captures the underlying principles and the public health spirit of epidemiology: "Epidemiology is the study of the distribution and determinants of health-related states or events in specified populations, and the application of this study to the control of health problems."[2]

Key terms in this definition reflect some of the important principles of the practice of epidemiology.

Study. Epidemiology is a scientific discipline with sound methods of scientific inquiry at its foundation. These methods rely on careful observation and the use of valid comparison groups to determine whether the observed health events differ from what might be expected.

Distribution. Epidemiologists study the frequency and pattern of health events in a population. *Frequency* means not only the number of health events in a population but the relationship of that number to the size of the population, that is, the number of events divided by the study population. The resulting rate allows epidemiologists to compare disease occurrence between different populations.

Pattern refers to the description of health-related events by time, place, and personal characteristics. Time characteristics include annual occurrence, seasonal occurrence, and daily or even hourly occurrence during an epidemic. Place characteristics include geographic variation, urban–rural differences, and location of work sites or schools, as examples. Personal characteristics include demographic factors such as age, gender, marital status, and socioeconomic status, as well as behaviors and environmental exposures.

The above characterization of the distribution of health-related states or events comprises one broad aspect of epidemiology called *descriptive epidemiology*, described further in Chapter 6. Descriptive epidemiology provides the What, Who, When, and Where of health-related events.

Determinants. Epidemiologists also search for causes and other factors that influence the occurrence of health-related events. By attempting to provide the Why and How, the field epidemiologist performs *analytic epidemiology*—the process of assessing whether groups with different rates of disease have differences in demographic characteristics, genetic or immunologic makeup, behaviors, environmental exposures, and other so-called potential risk factors. Epidemiologic studies, such as cohort and case-control studies and the analytic methods used by epidemiologists to identify factors associated with the increased risk of disease, are discussed in Chapters 7 and 8. Often, these analyses provide sufficient evidence to direct prompt and effective public health control and prevention measures.

Health-related states or events. Originally, epidemiology was concerned with epidemics of communicable diseases. Then, it was extended to endemic communicable diseases and noncommunicable infectious diseases. By the middle of the twentieth century additional epidemiologic methods had been developed and applied to chronic diseases, injuries, birth defects, maternal–child health, occupational health, and environmental health. Within the past 20 years, epidemiologists began to look "upstream" at behaviors related to health and well-being such as amount of exercise and seat-belt use. Now, with the recent explosion in molecular methods, they can even examine genetic markers of disease risk.

Specified populations. Although epidemiologists and direct health care providers are both concerned with disease and the control of disease, they differ greatly in how they view "the patient." The clinician has concern for the health of an individual, while the epidemiologist has concern for the collective health of the people in a community or population under study. For example, when faced with a patient with diarrheal disease, the clinician and the epidemiologist have different responsibilities. Although both are interested in establishing the correct diagnosis, the clinician usually focuses on treating and caring for the individual. The epidemiologist focuses on the source or exposure that caused the illness, the number of other persons who may have been similarly exposed, the potential for further spread in the community, and interventions to prevent additional cases or recurrences.

Application. The definition given above moves epidemiology beyond merely "the study of. . . ." Field epidemiology, in particular, also embodies the practice of the discipline in real time and real place, which in turn involves both science and art. Consider again the medical model. To treat a patient, the clinician applies scientific knowledge, experience, and clinical judgment. Similarly, the field epidemiologist will use the scientific methods of descriptive and analytic epidemiology as well as experience and epidemiologic judgment in "diagnosing" the health of a group of people or a community. Your findings and recommendations will ultimately help determine appropriate public health action to control and prevent disease.

USES OF EPIDEMIOLOGY

Epidemiology and the information generated by epidemiologic methods have been put to innumerable uses. These uses can be grouped into the following categories.

Population or Community Health Assessment

Public health officials responsible for policy development, implementation, and evaluation use epidemiologic information as a factual framework for decision making. To assess the health of a population or community, relevant sources of data must be identified and analyzed by time, place, and person (descriptive epidemiology). What are the actual and potential health problems in the community? Where are they occurring? Who is at risk? Which problems are declining over time? Which ones are increasing or have the potential to increase? How do these patterns relate to the level and distribution of services available? More detailed data may need to be collected and analyzed to determine whether the health services are available, accessible, effective, and efficient. For example, public health officials used epidemiologic data and methods to identify baselines, to set health goals for the nation in 2000 and 2010, and to monitor progress toward those goals.[3–5]

Individual Decisions

Many individuals may not realize that they use epidemiologic information in their daily decisions. When persons decide to quit smoking, climb the stairs rather than wait for the elevator, eat a salad rather than a cheeseburger with fries for lunch, or use a condom, they may be influenced, consciously or unconsciously, by epidemiologists' assessment of risk. Since World War II, epidemiologists have provided information related to all those decisions. In the 1950s epidemiologists reported the increased risk of lung cancer among smokers; in the 1970s epidemiologists documented the role of exercise and proper diet in reducing the risk of heart disease, and in the mid-1980s epidemiologists identified the increased risk of human immunodeficiency virus (HIV) infection associated with certain sexual and drug-related behaviors. These and hundreds of other epidemiologic findings are directly relevant to the choices that people make every day, choices that affect their health over a lifetime.

Completing the Clinical Picture

When studying a disease outbreak, field epidemiologists will rely on health care providers and laboratory workers to help establish the proper diagnosis of individual patients. But their findings will also contribute to physicians' understanding of the clinical picture and natural history of disease. For example, in late 1989 three patients with unexplained eosinophilia (an increase in the number of white blood cells called eosinophils) and myalgias (severe muscle pains) were seen by a physician. The physician could not make a definitive diagnosis, but he did notify public health authorities. Within weeks, field epidemiologists had identified enough other cases to characterize the spectrum and course of the disease, as well as to identify the vehicle of the agent causing the disease—a condition that came to be known as eosinophilia–myalgia syndrome.[6] Similarly, epidemiologists have documented the course of HIV infection from the initial exposure to the development of a wide variety of clinical syndromes that include acquired immunodeficiency syndrome (AIDS). They have also documented the numerous conditions that are associated with cigarette smoking, from pulmonary and heart disease to lung and cervical cancer.

Search for Causes

Much of epidemiologic research is devoted to searching for causes or factors that influence one's risk of disease. Sometimes this is an academic pursuit, but in field epidemiology the goal is to identify a cause so that appropriate public health action can be taken. It has been said that epidemiology can never prove a causal relationship between an exposure and a disease. Nevertheless, epidemiology often provides enough information to support effective action. Examples date from the removal of the handle from the Broad Street pump following John Snow's investigation of cholera in the Golden Square area of London in 1854[7] to the withdrawal of a vaccine against rotavirus found by epidemiologists to be associated with an increased risk of intussusception.[8] Just as often, epidemiology and laboratory science converge to provide the evidence needed to establish causation. For example, field epidemiologists were able to identify a variety of risk factors during an outbreak of a pneumonia among persons attending the American Legion Convention in Philadelphia in 1976, but the outbreak was not "solved"' until the legionnaires' bacillus was identified in the laboratory from lung tissue of a fatal case of legionnaires' disease almost 6 months later.[9]

CORE EPIDEMIOLOGIC FUNCTIONS

Five tasks have been proposed as defining the field epidemiologist—public health surveillance, field investigation, data analysis, evaluation, and communication.[10] Recently, the Council of State and Territorial Epidemiologists has proposed a set of core functions that constitute the minimum recommended capacity of a state health department's epidemiology unit. Among these functions are public health surveillance, investigation (including analysis) and consultation, policy development, training, and linkages.[11] These tasks are described below.

Public Health Surveillance

Public health surveillance is the ongoing, systematic collection, analysis, interpretation and dissemination of health data to help guide public health decision making and action. Surveillance is equivalent to monitoring the pulse of the community. The purpose of public health surveillance, which is sometimes called "information for action,"[12] is to portray the ongoing patterns of disease occurrence and disease potential so that investigation, control, and prevention measures can be applied efficiently and effectively. This is accomplished through the systematic collection and evaluation of morbidity and mortality reports and other relevant health information, and the dissemination of these data and their interpretation to those involved in disease control and public health decision making (see Chapter 3). Since epidemiologists are likely to be called upon to design these and other new surveillance systems, an epidemiologist's core competencies must include design of data collection instruments, data management, descriptive methods and graphing, interpretation of data, and skills in scientific writing and presentation.

Field Investigation and Analytic Studies

Surveillance provides information for action, such as an investigation by the public health department following a report of a single case or multiple cases of a specific disease or event. The investigation may be as limited as a phone call to the health care provider to confirm or clarify the circumstances of the reported case, or it may involve a field investigation requiring the coordinated efforts of dozens of people to characterize the extent of an epidemic and to identify its cause.

The objectives of such field investigations also vary. They often lead to the identification of additional unreported or unrecognized cases who might otherwise continue to spread infection to others. For example, one of the hallmarks of investigations of persons with sexually transmitted disease is the identification of sexual contacts of cases. When investigated by local health staff, many of these contacts are often found to have asymptomatic infections and to require treatment for infections they did not know they had.

For some diseases, investigations may identify a source or vehicle of infection that can be controlled or eliminated. For example, the investigation of a case of botulism usually focuses on trying to identify the vehicle, such as improperly canned food. By identifying the vehicle, investigators can determine how many other persons might have already been exposed and how many continue to be at risk.

In some instances, the objective of an investigation may be to learn more about the natural history, clinical spectrum, descriptive epidemiology, and risk factors of an unknown or previously unrecognized condition. Early investigations of the nationwide outbreak of toxic shock syndrome in 1980 were needed to establish a case definition based on the clinical presentation and to characterize the populations at risk by time, place, and person. The descriptive epidemiology suggested hypotheses that could be tested with analytic studies. A series of studies was conducted to identify increasingly specific risk factors, from menstruating women, to tampon users, to users of a specific brand of tampon. This information prompted the withdrawal of that brand from the market, and also prompted sub-. sequent research to identify the specific composition and conditions necessary for the development of the syndrome.[13]

Field investigations of the type described above are sometimes referred to as "shoeleather epidemiology," conjuring up images of dedicated, if haggard, field epidemiologists beating the pavement in search of additional cases and clues regarding source and mode of transmission of a particular disease. This approach is commemorated in the symbol of the Epidemic Intelligence Service, CDC's training program of field epidemiologists—a shoe with a hole in the sole.

Surveillance and field investigations sometimes are sufficient to identify causes, modes of transmission, and appropriate control and prevention measures.

Sometimes they provide clues or hypotheses that must be assessed with *analytic techniques*.

Clusters or outbreaks of disease frequently are investigated initially with descriptive epidemiology. The descriptive approach involves the study of disease incidence and distribution by time, place, and person. It includes the calculation of rates and identification of parts of the population at higher risk than others. Occasionally, particularly when the association between exposure and disease is quite strong, the investigation may stop there and control measures may be implemented immediately. More frequently, descriptive studies, like case investigations, generate hypotheses that can be tested by analytic studies. While some field investigations are conducted in response to acute health problems such as outbreaks, many others are planned studies.

The hallmark of an epidemiologic study is the use of a valid comparison group. Epidemiologists must be familiar with all aspects of the epidemiologic study, including its design, conduct, analysis, interpretation, and communication of the findings.

- *Design* includes determining the appropriate study design, writing justifications and protocols, calculating sample sizes, deciding on criteria for subject selection (e.g., choosing controls), and designing questionnaires.
- *Conduct* involves securing appropriate clearances and approvals, abstracting records, tracking down and interviewing subjects, collecting and handling specimens, and managing the data.
- *Analysis* begins with describing the characteristics of the subjects. It progresses to calculation of rates, creating of comparative tables (e.g., two-by-two tables), and computation of measures of association (e.g., risk ratios or odds ratios), tests of significance (e.g., chi-square test), confidence intervals, and the like. Many epidemiologic studies require more advanced analytic techniques such as stratified analysis, regression, and modeling.
- Finally, you must be familiar enough with the subject matter to *interpret* the findings of the study, put them into proper perspective, and *communicate* them effectively (see Chapters 8 and 10).

Policy Development

While some academically minded epidemiologists have eschewed the link between epidemiology and policy,[14] public health epidemiologists have no such luxury. Indeed, epidemiologists who understand the problem and the population in which it occurs are often in a uniquely qualified position to recommend appropriate interventions. For example, epidemiologists regularly provide input, testimony, and recommendations regarding disease control strategies, reportable disease regulations, and immunization policy.

Linkages

Field epidemiologists rarely work in isolation. In fact, field epidemiology has sometimes been referred to as a "team sport." During a field investigation, you will usually participate as either a member of or the leader of a multidisciplinary team. Other members may be laboratory workers, sanitarians, infection control personnel, and nurses or other clinical staff. They may be from local, state, or federal levels of government, from academic institutions, from clinical facilities, or, increasingly, from the private sector. Epidemiologists are expected to maintain linkages with the agencies and institutions, whether through official linkages or through publication of periodic bulletins for public health audiences and outside partners.

THE BASIC OPERATIONS OF THE EPIDEMIOLOGIST OR WHAT DOES THE FIELD EPIDEMIOLOGIST REALLY DO

It should be clear by now what epidemiology is, how it is used, and what the focus of investigation is: a population of people, large or small, who share some health event, such as an illness. So your task will be to find out why they became ill, that is, what was the agent, where did it come from, how was it transmitted, who was at risk of getting sick, and what was the critical exposure. In most instances, particularly in infectious diseases, you will know the disease and its usual clinical and epidemiologic features, but you will be challenged to determine who was at risk and what the critical exposure was.

It is at this juncture that at least five separate operations are performed in virtually all epidemiologic studies:

- You will *count* cases (events).
- You will *describe* the cases in terms of time, place, and person.
- You will extract from these descriptions a plausible idea of who were probably at risk of illness and why and how they became sick. In other words you will pose a *hypothesis* that will explain all the facets of the epidemic or event.
- You will then perform long division; that is, you will *determine rates* of illness or rates of exposure.
- You will *compare these rates* to see what they mean.

The most critical operation is to compare rates: the sine qua non of epidemiology. You will compare either illness rates of persons exposed and persons not exposed to some agent or exposure rates among ill persons and well persons. Such comparisons may show significant differences in rates, different enough to suggest (but not prove) what exposure caused disease.

These operations truly constitute the universe of epidemiologic practice, and performing them is not that difficult. It only gets complicated when epidemiologists argue over what a case is, who is at risk, what comparisons are valid, and what the differences in rates really mean.

CONCEPTS OF DISEASE OCCURRENCE

Epidemiology is premised on the fact that disease and other health events do not occur randomly in a population—that disease is more likely to occur in some members of the population than others. As noted earlier, one important use of epidemiology is to identify the reasons (risk factors) that increase some members' risk of disease above others'.

Causation

A number of models of disease causation have been proposed. Among the simplest of these is the epidemiologic triad or triangle, the traditional model for infectious disease. The triad comprises an external *agent*, a susceptible *host*, and an *environment* that brings the host and agent together. In this model, disease results from the interaction between the agent and the susceptible host in an environment that supports transmission of the agent from a source to that host.

Agent factors

The word "agent" originally referred to an infectious microorganism—a virus, bacterium, parasite, or other microbe. Generally, these agents must be present for disease to occur, that is, they are necessary but not always sufficient to cause disease. A variety of factors influence whether exposure to an organism will result in disease, including the organism's pathogenicity (ability to cause disease) and dose.

Over time, the concept of agent has been broadened to include chemical and physical causes of disease. These include chemical contaminants such as the L-tryptophan contaminant responsible for eosinophilia–myalgia syndrome as well as physical movements such as repetitive mechanical forces associated with carpal tunnel syndrome. While the epidemiologic triad serves as a useful model for many diseases, it has proven inadequate for cardiovascular disease, cancer, and other diseases that appear to have multiple contributing causes without a single necessary one.

Host factors

Host factors are intrinsic factors that influence an individual's exposure, susceptibility, or response to a causative agent. Age, gender, and behaviors (smoking, drug abuse, lifestyle, sexual practices, contraception, and eating habits) are just some of the many host factors that affect a person's likelihood of exposure. Age, genetic composition, nutritional and immunologic status, anatomic structure, presence of disease or medications, and psychological makeup are some of the host factors that affect a person's susceptibility and response to an agent.

Environmental factors

Environmental factors are extrinsic factors that affect the agent and host and the opportunity for exposure. Generally, environmental factors include physical factors such as geology and climate; biologic factors such as insect vectors that transmit the agent; and socioeconomic factors such as crowding, sanitation, and the availability of health services.

Agent, host, and environmental factors interrelate in a variety of complex ways to produce disease in humans. Different diseases require different balances and interactions of these three components. Development of appropriate, practical, and effective public health measures to control or prevent disease usually requires assessment of these three components of disease occurrence and, in particular, their interactions.

The Natural History and Spectrum of Disease

The natural history of disease refers to the progression of a disease process in an individual over time, in the absence of intervention. Many, if not most, diseases have a characteristic natural history, although the time frame and specific manifestations of disease may vary from individual to individual and will be influenced by preventive and therapeutic measures.

The process begins with the appropriate exposure to or accumulation of factors sufficient to begin the disease process in a susceptible host. For an infectious disease, the exposure usually is a microorganism. For cancer, the critical factors may require both cancer initiators such as asbestos fibers or components in tobacco smoke (for lung cancer), and cancer promoters such as estrogen (for endometrial cancer).

Following the start of the disease process, pathological changes then occur that are usually not apparent to the individual. This stage of subclinical disease, extending from the time of exposure to onset of disease symptoms, is usually called the incubation period for infectious diseases and the latency period for chronic diseases. This period may be as brief as seconds for hypersensitivity and toxic reactions to as long as decades for certain chronic diseases. Even for a single disease, the characteristic incubation period has a range. For example, the typical incubation period for hepatitis A is about 4 weeks, but may be as brief as 2 weeks or as long as 6 weeks.

The onset of symptoms marks the transition from subclinical to clinical disease. Most diagnoses are made during the stage of clinical disease. In some people, however, the disease process may never progress to clinically apparent illness. In others, the disease process may result in a wide spectrum of clinical illness, ranging from mild to severe or fatal. Ultimately, the disease process ends either in recovery, disability, or death.

For an infectious agent, *infectivity* refers to the proportion of exposed persons who become infected. *Pathogenicity* refers to the proportion of infected individuals who develop clinically apparent disease. *Virulence* refers to the proportion of clinically apparent cases that are severe or fatal.

The natural history and spectrum of disease present challenges to the clinician and to the field epidemiologist. Because the clinical spectrum of many diseases ranges from asymptomatic to severe illness, cases of illness diagnosed by clinicians in the community often represent only the tip of the iceberg. Many additional cases may be too early to diagnose or may remain inapparent. For the public health practioner, the challenge is that persons with inapparent or undiagnosed infections may nonetheless be able to transmit infection to others. Such persons who are infectious but have subclinical disease are called *carriers*. Frequently, carriers are persons incubating disease or with inapparent infection. Persons with measles, hepatitis A, and several other diseases become infectious a few days before the onset of symptoms. However, carriers may also be persons who appear to have recovered from their clinical illness, such as chronic carriers of hepatitis B virus, or persons who never exhibited symptoms at all, such as the famous Typhoid Mary.

Chain of Infection

The traditional epidemiologic triad model holds that infectious diseases result from the interaction of agent, host, and environment. More specifically, transmission occurs when the agent leaves its reservoir or host through a portal of exit, is conveyed by some mode of transmission, and enters through an appropriate portal of entry to infect a susceptible host. This sequence is sometimes called the chain of infection.

Reservoir

The *reservoir* of an infectious agent is the habitat in which the agent normally lives, grows, and multiplies. Reservoirs include humans, animals, and the environment. The reservoir may or may not be the source from which an agent is transferred to a host. For example, the reservoir of *Clostridium botulinum* spores is soil, but the source of most botulism intoxications is improperly canned food containing *C. botulinum* spores and a neurotoxin released by the bacteria.

Many of the common infectious diseases have human reservoirs. Diseases that are transmitted from person to person without intermediaries include the sexually transmitted diseases, measles, mumps, streptococcal infections, and many respiratory pathogens. Because humans were the only reservoir for the smallpox virus, smallpox was eradicated after the last human case was identified and isolated.

Humans are also subject to diseases that have animal reservoirs. Many of these diseases are transmitted from animal to animal, with humans as incidental hosts. The term *zoonosis* refers to an infectious disease that is transmissible under natural conditions from animals to humans. Such diseases include brucellosis (cows, goats, and pigs), anthrax (sheep, goats, and cattle), plague (rodents), trichinosis (swine), and rabies (bats, raccoons, dogs, and other mammals).

Plants, soil, and water in the environment are also reservoirs for some infectious agents. Many fungal agents, such as those causing histoplasmosis, live and multiply in the soil. The legionnaires' bacillus is often traced to pools of water such as those produced by cooling towers and evaporative condensers.

Modes of transmission

An agent may be transmitted from its natural reservoir to a susceptible host in a variety of ways. These modes of transmission may be classified as:

- Direct
  Direct contact
  Droplet spread
- Indirect
  Airborne
  Vehicle-borne
  Vector-borne
  Mechanical
  Biologic

In direct transmission, an agent is transferred from a reservoir to a susceptible host by direct contact or droplet spread. Direct contact occurs through kissing, skin-to-skin contact, and sexual intercourse. Direct contact also refers to contact with soil or vegetation harboring infectious organisms. Thus, infectious mononucleosis ("kissing disease") and gonorrhea are spread from person to person by direct contact. Hookworm is spread by direct contact with contaminated soil. Droplet spread refers to spray with relatively large, short-range aerosols produced by sneezing, coughing, or even talking. Droplet spread is classified as direct because transmission is by direct spray over a few feet, before the droplets fall to the ground.

Indirect transmission refers to the transfer of an agent from a reservoir to a host by suspended air particles, inanimate objects (vehicles), or animate intermediaries (vectors).

Airborne transmission occurs by dust or droplet nuclei suspended in air. Airborne dust includes material that has settled on surfaces and becomes resuspended by air currents as well as infectious particles blown from the soil by the wind. Droplet nuclei are dried residue of less than 5 microns in size. In contrast to droplets that fall to the ground within a few feet, droplet nuclei may remain suspended in the air for long periods of time and may be blown over great distances.

Vehicles that may indirectly transmit an agent include food, water, biologic products (blood), and fomites (inanimate objects such as handkerchiefs, bedding, or surgical scalpels). A vehicle may passively carry an agent—as food or water may carry hepatitis A virus—or may provide an environment in which the agent grows, multiplies, or produces toxin—as improperly canned foods provide an environment in which *C. botulinum* bacteria produce a toxin.

Vectors, such as mosquitoes, fleas, and ticks, may carry the agent through purely mechanical means or may support growth or changes in the agent. Examples of mechanical transmission are flies carrying shigella on their appendages and fleas carrying *Yersinia pestis*, the causative agent of plague, in their gut. In contrast, biological transmission occurs when the causative agent of malaria or guinea worm disease undergoes maturation in an intermediate host before it can be transmitted to humans.

Host

The final link in the chain of infection is a susceptible host. Susceptibility of a host depends on genetic or constitutional factors, other general factors that affect an individual's ability to resist infection or to limit pathogenicity, and specific acquired immunity. An individual's genetic makeup may either increase or decrease susceptibility. General factors that defend against infection include the skin, mucous membranes, gastric acidity, cilia in the respiratory tract, the cough reflex, and nonspecific immune responses. General factors that may increase susceptibility are malnutrition, alcoholism, and disease or therapy that impairs the nonspecific immune response. Specific acquired immunity refers to protective antibodies that are directed against a specific agent. These antibodies may develop in response to infection, vaccine, or toxoid (active immunity) or may be acquired by transplacental transfer from mother to fetus or by injection of antitoxin or immune globulin (passive immunity).

Implications for public health

Knowledge of the portals of exit and entry and modes of transmission provide a basis for determining appropriate control measures. In general, control measures are usually directed against the segment in the infection chain that is most susceptible to intervention, unless practical issues dictate otherwise. For some diseases, the most appropriate intervention may be directed at controlling or eliminating the agent at its source. In the hospital setting, patients may be treated and/ or isolated, with appropriate "contact precautions," "respiratory precautions," and the like for different exit pathways. In the community, soil may be decontaminated or covered to prevent escape of the agent.

Some interventions are directed at the mode of transmission. Direct transmission may require that the source host be treated or educated to avoid the specific type of contact associated with transmission. Vehicle-borne transmission may be interrupted by elimination or decontamination of the vehicle. For fecal–oral transmission, efforts often focus on changing behaviors such as promoting handwashing and on rearranging the environment to reduce the risk of contamination in the future. For airborne diseases, strategies may be directed at modifying ventilation or air pressure and filtering or treating the air. For vector-borne transmission, some measures are directed toward controlling the vector population. However, simple strategies to avoid or block exposure, such as wearing long pants and sleeves and/or use of insect repellant to reduce the risk of mosquito-borne infections, remain prudent as well.

Some strategies that protect portals of entry are simple and effective. For example, a dentist's mask and gloves are intended to protect the dentist from a patient's blood, secretions, and droplets, as well to protect the patient from the dentist. To reduce the risk of West Nile virus infection, persons have been advised to wear long pants and sleeves, and to use insect repellant.

Finally, some interventions aim to increase a host's defenses. Prophylactic antibiotics administered before surgery combat microorganisms and reduce the likelihood of post-surgical infections. Immunizations promote the development of specific antibodies.

Epidemic Disease Occurrence

Levels of disease

The amount of a particular disease that is usually present in a community may be referred to as the baseline or *endemic* level of the disease. This level is not necessarily the preferred level, which should in fact be zero; rather, it is the observed level. In the absence of intervention and assuming that the level is not high enough to deplete the pool of susceptible persons, the disease would likely continue to occur at this level indefinitely. Thus, the baseline level is often regarded as the expected level of the disease.

While some diseases are so rare in a given population that a single case warrants an epidemiologic investigation (poliomyelitis, rabies, plague in the United States), other diseases occur more commonly so that only deviations from the norm warrant investigation. *Sporadic* refers to a disease that occurs infrequently and irregularly. *Endemic* refers to the constant presence and/or usual prevalence of a disease or infectious agent in a population within a geographic area. *Hyperendemic* refers to persistent, high levels of disease occurrence.

Occasionally, the level of disease rises above the expected level. *Epidemic* refers to an increase, often sudden, in cases of the disease above what is normally expected in that population in that area. *Outbreak* carries the same definition as epidemic but is often used for a more limited geographic area. *Cluster* refers to an aggregation of cases grouped in place and time that are suspected to be greater than the expected number. Often, however, the expected number is not known. *Pandemic* refers to an epidemic that has spread over several countries or continents, usually affecting a large number of people.

Epidemics occur when an agent and susceptible hosts are present in adequate numbers, and the agent can be effectively conveyed from a source to the susceptible hosts because of a favorable environment. More specifically, an epidemic may result from:

- a recent increase in amount or virulence of the agent,
- the recent introduction of the agent into a setting where it has not been before,
- an enhanced mode of transmission so that more susceptible persons are exposed,
- an environment conducive to interaction between the host and the agent,
- a change in the susceptibility of the host response to the agent, and/or
- factors that increase host exposure or involve introduction through new portals of entry.[15]

Epidemic patterns

Epidemics can be classified according to their manner of spread through a population:

- Common source
  Point
  Intermittent
  Continuous

- Propagated
- Mixed
- Other

A common source outbreak is one in which persons are exposed to a common noxious influence such as an infectious agent or a toxin. If the group is exposed over a relatively brief period, so that everyone who becomes ill develops disease at the end of one incubation period, then the common source outbreak is further classified as a point source outbreak. The epidemic of leukemia cases in Hiroshima following the atomic bomb blast and the epidemic of hepatitis A among college football players who unknowingly drank contaminated water after practice one day each had a point source of exposure.[16,17] A graph of the number of cases over time, known as an *epidemic curve*, classically has a steep upslope and a more gradual downslope (a so-called log-normal distribution).

In some common source outbreaks, cases may be exposed over a period of days, weeks, or longer. In a continuous common source outbreak, the range of exposures and range of incubation periods tend to dampen and widen the peaks of the epidemic curve. The epidemic curve of an intermittent common source outbreak often has a pattern reflecting the intermittent nature of the exposure.

A propagated outbreak results from transmission from one person to another. Usually, transmission is by direct person-to-person contact, as with syphilis. Transmission may also be vehicle-borne, as the transmission of hepatitis B or HIV by sharing needles, or vector-borne, as the transmission of yellow fever by mosquitoes. In propagated outbreaks, cases occur over more than one incubation period. The epidemic usually wanes after a few generations, either because the number of susceptible persons falls below some critical level required to sustain transmission, or because intervention measures become effective.

Some epidemics have features of both common source epidemics and propagated epidemics. The pattern of a common source outbreak followed by secondary person-to-person spread is not uncommon. These are called mixed epidemics. For example, a common source epidemic of shigellosis occurred among a group of 3000 women attending a national music festival. Many developed symptoms after returning home. Over the next few weeks, several state health departments detected subsequent generations of shigella cases spread by person-to-person transmission from festival attendees.[18]

Finally, some epidemics are neither common source in its usual sense nor propagated from person to person. Outbreaks of zoonotic or vector-borne disease may result from sufficient prevalence of infection in host species, sufficient presence of vectors, and sufficient human–vector interaction. Examples include the epidemic of Lyme disease that affected several states in the northeastern United

States in the late 1980s and the epidemic of West Nile encephalitis in New York City in 1999.[19,20]

SUMMARY

As a discipline within public health, epidemiology includes the study of the frequency, patterns, and causes of health-related states or events in populations, and the application of that study to address public health issues. Epidemiologists use a systematic approach to assess the What, Who, Where, When, and the Why and How of these health states or events. Two essential aspects in this systematic approach entail studying populations and making comparisons. Differences in disease occurrence in different populations are assessed by generating and evaluating hypotheses about risk factors and causes. In carrying out these tasks, the field epidemiologist is part of the team of individuals in institutions dedicated to promoting and protecting the public's health.

REFERENCES

1. Centers for Disease Control and Prevention (1992) *Principles of Epidemiology*, 2nd ed. Centers for Disease Control and Prevention, Atlanta.
2. Last, J.M. (Ed.) (1988) *Dictionary of Epidemiology*, 2nd ed., p. 42. Oxford University Press, New York.
3. U.S. Department of Health and Human Services (1991). *Healthy People 2000: national health promotion and disease prevention objectives.* U.S. Department of Health and Human Services , Public Health Service, Washington, D.C.
4. U.S. Department of Health and Human Services (2000). *Healthy People 2010*, 2nd ed. U.S. Government Printing Office, Washington, D.C.
5. U.S. Department of Health and Human Services (2000). *Tracking Healthy People 2010.* U.S. Government Printing Office, Washington, D.C.
6. Eidson, M., Philen, R.M., Sewell, C.M., et al. (1990). L-tryptophan and eosinophilia-myalgia syndrome in New Mexico. *Lancet* 335, 645–48.
7. Snow, J (1936). *Snow on Cholera.* Oxford University Press, London.
8. Murphy, T.V., Gargiullo, P.M., Massoudi, M.S., et al. (2001). Intussusception among infants given an oral rotavirus vaccine. *N Engl J Med* 344, 564–72.
9. Fraser, D.W., Tsai, T.R., Orenstein, W., et al. (1977). Legionnaires' disease: description of an epidemic of pneumonia. *N Engl J Med* 297, 1189–97.
10. Tyler, C.W., Last, J.M. (1992). Epidemiology. In J.M. Last, R.B. Wallace, eds., *Maxcy-Rosenau-Last Public Health and Preventive Medicine*, 13th ed., p. 11. Appleton & Lange, Norwalk, Connecticut / San Mateo, California.
11. Hopkins, R.S. (2000). Proposed core epidemiology functions of state health departments. CSTE Update, 00-4, 4–6.
12. Orenstein, W.A., Bernier, R.H. (1990). Surveillance: information for action. *Pediatr Clin North Am* 37, 709–34.

13. Centers for Disease Control (1990). Reduced incidence of menstrual toxic shock syndrome—United States, 1980–1990. *Morb Mortal Wkly Rep* 39,421–23.

14. Rothman, K.J. (1993). Policy recommendations in epidemiology research papers. *Epidemiology* 4, 94–95.

15. Kelsey, J.L., Thompson, W.D., Evans, A.S. (1986). *Methods in Observational Epidemiology*, p. 216. Oxford University Press, New York.

16. Cobb, S., Miller, M., Wald N. (1959). On the estimation of the incubation period in malignant disease. *J Chronic Dis* 9, 385–93.

17. Morse, L.J., Bryan, J.A., Hurley, J.P., et al. (1972). The Holy Cross College football team hepatitis outbreak. *JAMA* 219, 706–8.

18. Lee, L.A., Ostroff, S.M., McGee, H.B., et al. (1991). An outbreak of shigellosis at an outdoor music festival. *Am J Epidemiol* 133, 608–15.

19. White, D.J., Chang, H-G., Benach, J.L., et al. (1991). Geographic spread and temporal increase of the Lyme disease epidemic. *JAMA* 266, 1230–36.

20. Centers for Disease Control and Prevention (1999). Outbreak of West Nile-like viral encephalitis—New York, 1999. *Morb Mortal Wkly Rep* 48, 845–49.

3

SURVEILLANCE

Stephen B. Thacker
Guthrie S. Birkhead

The two previous chapters reviewed the basic principles and practices of epidemiology and their use in a newly defined application of epidemiologic study, namely field epidemiology. With or without the urgency to investigate, make recommendations, or take specific action, all epidemiologic studies obtain data on a study population and capture facts to analyze. But for the public health epidemiologist and, in particular, the field investigator, getting timely health-related data, either in a hurry (e.g., in response to an obvious or suspected acute public health problem) or on an ongoing basis (e.g., to assess or monitor trends in major public health problems affecting a population), carries a distinct implication—the idea of information for action. So in this context the acquisition of information for use in the public health arena has been called surveillance.

DEFINITION

There is no standard, universally accepted definition of surveillance in public health practice. CDC, however, has promoted the following generally agreed-upon definition:

> Public health surveillance (sometimes called epidemiologic surveillance) is the ongoing systematic collection, analysis, and interpretation of outcome-specific

data essential to the planning, implementation, and evaluation of public health practice, closely integrated with the timely dissemination of these data to those who need to know. Outcomes may include disease, injury, and disability, as well as risk factors, vector exposures, environmental hazards, or other exposures. The final link of the surveillance chain is the application of these data to prevent and control human disease and injury.

Some have compared the surveillance system with a nerve cell that has an afferent arm that receives information, a cell body that analyzes the data, and an efferent arm that takes appropriate action. This analogy is particularly appropriate in the context of field investigations of acute public health problems, where, very often, surveillance must be started quickly to get necessary data so that the right action can be taken.[1,2] Using surveillance to guide immediate public health prevention and control measures is often a major goal of the field epidemiologist.

BACKGROUND

Following the discoveries of infectious disease agents in the late 1800s, the first use of scientifically based surveillance concepts in public health practice was monitoring contacts of persons with serious communicable diseases such as plague, smallpox, typhus, and yellow fever. A common feature of these diseases is the potential for explosive outbreaks with high case-fatality rates. One purpose of surveillance is to detect the first signs and symptoms of disease and to begin prompt isolation to prevent further spread. For many decades in the United States, early detection and isolation were functions of municipal and state health departments and of foreign quarantine stations—not only of the United States Public Health Service—but of quarantine agencies throughout the world.

In the late 1940s, Alexander D. Langmuir, M.D., then the chief epidemiologist of the Communicable Disease Center (now the Centers for Disease Control and Prevention [CDC]), began to broaden the concept of surveillance. Although surveillance of persons at risk for specific disease continued at quarantine stations, Langmuir and his colleagues changed the focus of attention to diseases, such as malaria and smallpox, rather than individuals. They emphasized rapid collection and analysis of data on a particular disease with quick dissemination of the findings to those who needed to know.[3]

Now this credo of rapid reporting, analysis, and action applies to nearly 100 infectious diseases and health events of noninfectious etiology at the local, state, and national levels. Many ongoing systems of reporting have resulted from local or national emergencies such as poliomyelitis resulting from contaminated lots of vaccine (the so-called Cutter incident of 1955), the Asian influenza epidemic of 1957, shellfish-associated hepatitis A in 1961, toxic shock syndrome in 1980, Hantavirus pulmonary syndrome in 1994 in the Four Corners area, widespread outbreaks of *E. coli* O157:H7 from 1994 to 1999, and an outbreak of West Nile encephalitis in the Northeast in 1999. Within days following the investigation of L-tryptophan-associated eosinophilia–myalgia syndrome (EMS) in 1990, a national reporting system was established for a previously rare and nonreportable condition.

TYPES OF SURVEILLANCE

Surveillance has been classified historically as either active or passive. Passive surveillance (i.e., initiated by the source of the data, often a health care provider or clinical laboratory rather than the health department) refers to data supplied to a health department based on a known set of rules or regulations that require such reporting. For example, in the United States, certain diseases (mostly communicable diseases but also cancers and certain injuries in some areas) are required by state law or regulation to be reported by practicing physicians to a local health department. In turn, these reports might be sent to state health departments and forwarded to the federal government's CDC. Most surveillance systems throughout the world are passive, because they are cheaper and easier for health departments to operate. However, in general, they also substantially undercount the occurrence of most reportable diseases.

On the other hand, in active surveillance (i.e., surveillance initiated by a health department), which is also based on certain regulations, the health agency regularly or routinely solicits reports from various providers. Active surveillance is most commonly implemented in an epidemic setting such as the 1976 epidemic of legionnaires' disease in Philadelphia or the 1990 epidemic of EMS in the United States. A modification of passive and active surveillance is an enhanced passive surveillance system where active follow-up of each case is used to pursue other possible cases, (e.g., contact tracing of sexually transmitted disease performed by investigators in local health departments). Thus, the system of surveillance will vary by disease, source of report, need for complete case counting, and sense of urgency, because public health measures often need to be taken in response to each case (e.g., prophylaxis of contacts of cases of meningitis).

The principles and practices relating to surveillance that are discussed in this chapter apply broadly to all surveillance efforts, but because of the time frame involved, some practices are more appropriate when acute disease problems occur in the field: the primary focus of our attention. Other systems are more adaptable to what we refer to as "ongoing" or long-term surveillance practices where there often is no real sense of urgency. Obviously, there is a gray area, but the basic differences will remain clear and logical.

PURPOSES OF SURVEILLANCE

Whether investigating an epidemic in the field or implementing a statewide program of prevention, surveillance is a basic tool for the field epidemiologist; it is the cornerstone and the management tool for public health practice. Just as businesses manage their day-to-day affairs by well-recognized precepts and actions, so must those of us in the practice of public health. Good surveillance, like good business practice, provides the data needed to give

- an accurate *assessment* of the status of health in a given population,
- an early warning of disease problems to guide immediate *control measures*,
- a quantitative base to define *objectives* for action,
- measures to define specific *priorities*,
- information to *design and plan* public health programs,
- measures to *evaluate* interventions and programs, and
- information to plan and conduct *research*.

In short, surveillance data provide a scientific and factual basis for appropriate policy and disease control decisions in public health practice as well as an evaluation of public health efforts and allocation of resources.

DATA SOURCES

Before discussing how to start a surveillance system, let us look at some of the kinds of data that are often readily available in the field and where they can be found. Depending on the problem, the epidemiologist will have to choose which data are most appropriate to collect and understand the strengths and weaknesses of different data sources. If certain information is not available, you might have to get it by conducting surveys or administering questionnaires (see Chapter 11).

In any event, every effort should be made to follow a simple, standardized method at the beginning, knowing that as the health problem becomes more clearly understood or circumstances change during the investigation, you might have to modify the surveillance system accordingly. The growth and acceptance of personal computers and the Internet have made a variety of morbidity and mortality data widely available and readily accessible to the field epidemiologist.[4]

Mortality Data

Mortality data are regularly available at the local and state level, and because of burial laws, mortality statistics can be used at the local level within a matter of days. Mortality data for selected causes of death are available on a weekly basis from 122 large United States cities as part of a national influenza surveillance system. Maintained and published weekly during the influenza season by CDC, in collaboration with local health jurisdictions, these mortality statistics come from cities that represent approximately 27% of the nation's population and give a useful, timely index of the extent and impact of influenza at local, state, and national levels.

Medical examiners and coroners are excellent sources for data concerning sudden or unexpected deaths. Data are available at the state or county level and include detailed information regarding the cause and the nature of death that is unavailable on the death certificate. For investigations of acute disease outbreaks, recent mortality data often have to be accessed by hand tally of death certificates, although electronically filed death certificates are becoming more widely available. These data are especially valuable for surveillance of intentional and unintentional injuries as well as sudden deaths of unknown cause. However, death certificate data have certain limitations: the lack of standardization in determining and listing the cause of death by physicians and the limited information on the circumstances of death (i.e., external causes). Nonetheless, for field investigations, death certificates can be used to contact the attending physician and to locate the patient medical record to obtain further information.

Another source is the National Mortality Followback Survey, which is conducted periodically by CDC on a sample of knowledgeable informants to ascertain social and health information on decedents. (*Note*: For this and many of the surveillance systems discussed in this chapter, more information and surveillance data are available on the Internet [see Appendix 3–1]). This data source might be useful to establish baseline expected rates of death for conditions of interest. Multiple cause of death data are generally available with a several year lag and might also serve as a useful source of expected rates of death against which to judge mortality data used for the surveillance of acute disease problems.

The quality of death certificate data might vary from location to location, state to state, and particularly from country to country. Physicians' assessments of cause(s) of death are divergent at times, and even definitions of death, time of death, and words like "infant" are subject to variation. Therefore, comparisons of mortality statistics between time frames and across geopolitical boundaries should be made with caution and only after obtaining in-depth knowledge regarding important considerations such as local customs, changes in coding of death certificates, and advances in medical knowledge. In some areas, computerized mortality data on underlying cause of death might not be available for many months after the period of interest; the availability of multiple cause of death listings often takes longer.

Morbidity Data

Most countries require the reporting of certain diseases (usually infectious) that are considered important to health authorities. In the United States, laws and regulations of each state health department list from 50 to 130 notifiable diseases (or conditions) that are reportable health events.[5] A complete listing of physician and laboratory disease reporting requirements by state is available at http//:www.cste.org. These data are used routinely and published for surveillance purposes at local, state, and national levels. Virtually all surveillance systems rely on physicians or other health care providers for these reports. Unfortunately, most infectious diseases are underreported by practicing physicians. Increasing reliance on reporting from clinical laboratories and use of computerized medical record, billing, or managed care data could improve the completeness of reporting diagnosed cases. Of course, unrecognized or undiagnosed illnesses never enter the reporting loop. However, the sensitivity and specificity of reports of both infectious and noninfectious conditions tend to increase the more severe and more rare the disease. In these cases, physicians might be more likely to report because they see the direct benefit of reporting, not only for the sake of public health but also for the benefit of obtaining the assistance and expertise of the health department in confirming the diagnosis and gaining access to appropriate treatment. A good example is surveillance of botulism when the health department laboratory can help to confirm the diagnosis and the epidemiologist can assist in obtaining botulism antitoxin from the U.S. Public Health Service. Reporting diseases under intensive surveillance (e.g., measles and AIDS in the United States) can reach a sensitivity of more than 90%. However, such levels of reporting are uncommon and depend heavily on resource-intensive active surveillance.

Other sources of morbidity data can prove useful in both ongoing systems of surveillance and in field situations. Private physicians are contacted by several survey groups. The National Ambulatory Medical Care Survey (NAMCS) is a national probability sample of visits to office-based physicians, which began in 1974. Three thousand physicians have participated in the survey, which has been conducted annually since 1989; data are collected on diagnosis, symptoms, drugs, and referrals. The National Drug and Therapeutic Index, a similar sample, is conducted by a private company, IMS Health. Diagnostic, specialty, therapeutic, and disposition data are available from both of these samples. The Ambulatory Sentinel Practice Network, initiated in 1978 by the North American Primary Care Research Group, is an example of a voluntary office-based system that looks at particular health problems selected on a periodic basis. These surveys provide a useful source of baseline data on several conditions but lack timeliness and full geographic coverage to be useful in most local field investigations. Recently, networks of sentinel emergency rooms and travel physicians have collected data on emerging infectious disease threats. These systems provide more rapid data, although they do not cover all geographic areas; they have the advantage of the flexibility to look for new diseases of interest on short notice. One example is the 1999 outbreak of West Nile encephalitis in the northeastern United States where these networks were mobilized to look for cases of unexplained encephalitis nationwide to gauge the extent of the outbreak.

Health Maintenance Organizations and other forms of managed care have become a substantial component of health services in the United States. Both managed care organizations and public health practitioners need population-based data on disease, injury, and risk for assessment and planning. This common interest has stimulated collaboration between managed care and public health officials at both the local and national levels for research purposes as well as health promotion and disease prevention. At the local level, such alliances should prove especially useful to the field epidemiologist.

Hospital data are another useful source of surveillance information. The National Hospital Discharge Survey and the National Hospital Ambulatory Medical Care Survey, conducted by the National Center for Health Statistics (NCHS), provide data abstracted from hospital records. State-specific hospital discharge data are available in many areas. Information typically includes diagnosis, length of stay, operative procedures, laboratory findings, and costs. However, hospital discharge data might be of limited use in detecting or evaluating acute disease outbreaks, because of the lack of timeliness of data collection and the lack of accuracy of diagnostic coding.

The National Birth Defects Prevention Network was established in the 1990s to form a national surveillance system based on reports from hospitals and physicians to state health department congenital malformation registries. These data have been used recently by some states to look for potential birth defects in infants of HIV-infected mothers who took antiretroviral therapy during pregnancy. Natality (birth certificate data) is used to monitor prenatal care practices and adverse birth outcomes. Electronically recorded birth certificates make such information available within a few days of birth, allowing immediate public health questions to be addressed. The National Nosocomial Infection Surveillance System consists of a group of hospitals that voluntarily reports hospital-acquired infections to CDC. These data provide useful baseline rates of infection and an early warning system of regional trends (e.g., hospital-acquired infections that are resistant to antibiotics).

Laboratory Data

Whether serving the interests of a single hospital, local or state health department, or national or international health agency, the laboratory has given the field epidemiologist invaluable information, particularly during infectious disease outbreaks. Now, at the beginning of the twenty-first century, the consolidation of many laboratories into regional ones and the near-universal computerization of laboratory data have substantially increased the usefulness of the laboratory in surveillance efforts. Establishment of regular, even daily, reporting from large clinical laboratories to state and local health departments, essentially a form of active surveillance, holds promise to provide complete reporting of laboratory diagnosed cases. Increases in microbial isolates, recognition of rare or unusual sero- or biotypes, or even simply an increase in demands for laboratory facilities provide essential data for the detection and investigation of epidemics caused by agents such as salmonella, shigella, *E. coli,* and staphylococcus. New molecular fingerprinting techniques, such as pulsed-field gel electrophoresis, can identify clusters of related cases and can link human isolates to isolates from food, water, or other sources.[6] Ongoing laboratory surveillance of influenza and poliomyelitis isolates as well as laboratory studies of lead and other environmental hazards continue to provide pivotal information for prevention and control. With the rapid sophistication of laboratory tools in environmental health, the laboratory is playing an increasingly important role in field investigations of toxicants such as lead, mercury, pesticides, and volatile organic compounds.

Individual Case Reports

Because some infectious diseases have high ratios of inapparent-to-apparent disease, a single case should be considered a sentinel health event and should be investigated immediately. A single case of paralytic poliomyelitis or aseptic meningitis represents 100 to 200 other cases of mild to subclinical disease elsewhere in the community. One full-blown case of arthropod-borne encephalitis or dengue reflects tens, if not hundreds, of other cases yet unrecognized or unreported. Also, recall the variability of individual response to toxic exposures. A single clinical case of intoxication should alert you to the possibility of unrecognized exposures in the family or in the neighborhood. Similarly, a single case of some chemical or heavy metal poisoning, such as mercury-induced acrodynia, could be an indication of a potentially widespread risk.

Epidemic Reporting

Sometimes it is easier, more practical, and more useful to count epidemics rather than single cases of disease. This is particularly true for common diseases that have epidemic potential and for which there is limited public health action in response to individual cases; diseases that are poorly reported; and, in some instances, diseases with a wide clinical spectrum. Probably the best example is influenza.

One of the time-honored methods of tracking influenza by CDC includes several degrees of involvement, assessed by each state, that describe influenza levels as isolated cases, sporadic outbreaks, outbreaks affecting less than one-half of the counties in the state, and outbreaks affecting over one-half of the state's counties. This method is not rigorous science but extremely useful, nonetheless. Rubella, rubeola, varicella, and dengue, can be grossly assessed in this fashion—primarily to inform the public—but also to determine where control or prevention efforts should be directed. In fact, during the successful smallpox eradication program of West Africa in the early 1970s, the field teams stopped counting cases and counted only epidemics, which were defined as one or more cases. Focusing most of the effort on control, much time and effort were saved.

Sentinel Systems

Existing systems of morbidity reporting should be sensitive and specific enough to detect early the appearance of an outbreak. For many reasons, however, not all such systems are that effective. Also, some diseases of public health importance are not reportable conditions. Regardless of the reason for inadequate reporting, there might be times to consider starting a sentinel system—a simple, relatively sensitive way of early detection and monitoring.

Again, probably the best example of this kind of surveillance has been influenza. Many states do not require that physicians report influenza, so when epidemics are impending and it is considered important to know when they arrive, the state will ask or even pay selected physicians to report influenza cases on a daily basis. Usually, these kinds of voluntary systems are not statistically valid. Selection is usually based on willingness of the physician to cooperate and geographic location, both very practical and compelling reasons. In some countries, because diagnostic capabilities in remote areas barely exist, the sentinel system will merely require reports of "unusual events"; nonetheless, such systems still can be useful.

Knowledge of Vertebrate and Arthropod Vector Species

In any assessment of zoonotic disease, you should be aware that an important adjunct to or surrogate for human disease surveillance is the monitoring of non-human vertebrate hosts and species. For example, in many arboviral infections, generally with high inapparent-to-apparent disease ratios, humans represent an incidental or dead-end host. Human disease contributes insignificantly to disease in zoonotic species, and human surveillance of these diseases is usually poor or nonexistent. Eastern equine encephalitis (EEE) is a mosquito-borne viral disease that has a reservoir in birds and infects horses and other vertebrates, including humans, as a dead-end host. A comprehensive surveillance system for EEE involves integrating data from viral culture of captured mosquitoes, regular serologic testing of sentinel flocks of chickens or pheasants kept outdoors, surveillance by veterinarians for EEE-like illness in horses, and surveillance of encephalitis cases and deaths in humans. In the 1999 outbreak of West Nile encephalitis, another mosquito-borne viral infection, in New York City, all these surveillance methods were used once the outbreak was recognized. In addition, since this infection resulted in increased mortality of crows and other birds, surveillance of dead birds was very helpful in measuring the geographic extent of the outbreak and in reassuring persons in the areas that were not affected.

Similarly, illness in vertebrate or nonvertebrate animals might reflect exposure to environmental toxins before clinical disease appears in human populations. In circumstances where toxic exposures are thought to be increased, regular communication should be established between health officers, the veterinary community, and agencies responsible for monitoring other animal and insect populations.

Surveys of Health in General Populations and Special Databases

Although databases are not frequently used in field investigation settings, several provide baseline or background incidence and prevalence information that might help assess the magnitude of a problem under study. The Behavioral Risk Factor Surveillance System (BRFSS) is a representative telephone survey of health promotion and risk behaviors in the population, which is conducted annually by all states. These data are used to gauge the magnitude and trends of behaviors of public health interest (e.g., smoking) and to measure the impact of public health programs (e.g., programs to reduce sexual activity that places persons at risk for HIV and other sexually transmitted diseases). The survey can be expanded to ask questions of local interest (e.g., insurance coverage for childhood immunizations in New York). BRFSS is used so extensively that some states are now funding county-level versions of BRFSS to provide surveillance data for targeting and evaluating local public health programs.

You can access several other useful databases for surveillance purposes; three are available from CDC. The National Health and Nutrition Examination Survey (NHANES) is a periodic survey that includes clinical examinations and collection of laboratory specimens as well as demographic data and medical histories. NHANES has been conducted three times since 1971 and became an ongoing activity in 1999. The National Health Interview Survey is a continuing survey of about 45,000 civilian households that collects information on illness, disability, health service utilization, and activity restriction.

Before you create a system or perform a field study, you should know several other national surveillance systems with distinctive features that might be useful. The National Cancer Institute funds the Surveillance Epidemiology and End Results (SEER) system, a group of cancer registries in 11 geographic areas of the United States (states and large metropolitan areas) that collects information on cancer, histologic type, site, residence, and relevant demographic information. This information is particularly useful to investigate clusters of cancer in the field. The National Electronic Injury Surveillance System (NEISS), sponsored by the Consumer Product Safety Commission (CPSC), is a stratified, random sample of hospital emergency rooms. NEISS collects continuous reports on product-related injuries and has conducted special studies on problems such as fire-related injuries and injuries caused by motor vehicle crashes. In 2000, CPSC and CDC initiated a collaborative effort to include all injuries in the NEISS system. The Fatality Analysis Reporting System (FARS), initiated by the National Highway Traffic Safety Administration (NHTSA), collects information on fatal crashes occurring on public roadways. The National Automotive Sampling System (NASS) is another NHTSA program that includes a random sample of traffic crashes reported by the police in the United States. The Environmental Protection Agency compiles air monitoring data from 51 U.S. areas regarding seven selected air pollutants to monitor compliance with the Clean Air Act. Finally, the National Fire Administration compiles the National Fire Incident Reporting System from local fire departments that report both fire incidents and casualties. These various data sources have been used to combine health event and risk factor data for surveillance purposes.

Medical school researchers, university hospitals, and voluntary organizations such as the Cystic Fibrosis Foundation collect and maintain incidence and prevalence data on several health conditions that could be sources of valuable information during an investigation in the field.

Demographic and Environmental Factors

As in all epidemiologic investigations, basic demographic characteristics of the population at risk (i.e., number, age, and gender distribution) are among the many important variables that should be available. Without these data, no rates can be determined. In other words, there must be a denominator to calculate rates of illness or exposure. The U.S. Bureau of the Census is an important source of data from which denominators can be calculated for any analysis of surveillance data http:\\www.census.gov. These data are collected once every decade, but intercensile estimates are available. In some instances, particularly in developing countries, these data are not readily available, and you must get them yourself during the field investigation. However time consuming and expensive to acquire, demographic data are indispensable; without them valid comparisons of populations and exposures are impossible.

You might also need to document such characteristics as heat, cold, airflow, humidity, rainfall, and other environmental determinants that predispose to disease or injury during the investigations. Weather data and data concerning air pollutants are available from the U.S. Weather Service for many areas of the country.

LEGAL CONCERNS

Before establishing any surveillance system—whether it is an emergency system during a field investigation or a process of continued monitoring for months or years to come—you should first be very clear about the legal aspects of such a plan (see Chapter 14). In most instances, surveillance is conducted under the aegis of state health laws passed by state legislatures or regulations developed by health departments or boards of health through an administrative process. So be careful to avoid any activities that violate such requirements.[7] State health commissioners and local health officers are often empowered by these laws and regulations to determine which conditions should be under surveillance and what data may be collected. They are also often empowered to respond to emergency situations with broad powers to collect data and authorize preventive actions. Nongovernmental entities may conduct surveillance, but they should determine the legal basis for such activity and discuss the plan with the appropriate health department before proceeding. In epidemic investigations, the field team is usually given oral approval for setting up emergency surveillance systems, but when long-term programs of surveillance are being considered, it might be necessary to obtain written clearance from the appropriate authorities.

Issues such as confidentiality and the public's right to know can be in conflict with each other, and you must consider these issues carefully at all steps in the surveillance process. In many cases, health care providers can be required, by law or regulation, to provide data to a new surveillance system. However, data collection from individual citizens is done on a voluntary basis and cannot be compelled. Consent should be obtained at least orally (even in an outbreak setting) to collect data directly from individuals. Any authorization to conduct surveillance should contain strong confidentiality protections, so that data cannot be released in a form that could identify an individual and that data cannot be used for purposes other than the original intent. Similarly, you must recognize who will be affected at each level of surveillance, including individuals in the community such as patients (both in and outside of institutions); physicians, nurses, and others involved in the health-care delivery system; members of the local health department; and, of course, members of your immediate staff. Failure to recognize potential conflicts of interest or lack of acceptability to any of these persons could derail the surveillance process. Policies concerning the release of personal data should be in place for all surveillance data. These policies should specify that individuals cannot be identified without their consent.

HOW TO ESTABLISH A SURVEILLANCE SYSTEM

Goals

At the beginning, you need to state clearly the purpose of establishing or maintaining a surveillance program. You should know which surveillance data are necessary and how and when they are to be used. A particular surveillance system may have more than one goal, including monitoring the occurrence of fatal and non-fatal disease, evaluating the effect of a public health program, or detecting epidemics for control and prevention activities. These needs might require multiple surveillance systems to monitor a single condition such as data to track morbidity, mortality, laboratory tests, exposures, and risk factors. Regardless of the goal, you must ask (*1*) "What action will be taken?" and (*2*) "What will you or others do with the data and the analyses?" There must be a specific action-oriented commitment; otherwise, do not bother.

Case Study: The West Nile Encephalitis Outbreak.   On August 23, 1999, the communicable disease epidemiologist at the New York City Department of Health (NYCDOH) was contacted by a hospital-based infectious disease physician who had two patients with undiagnosed encephalitis of apparently infectious etiology. In addition to the usual symptoms of encephalitis, one patient had profound muscle weakness, possibly Guillain-Barré syndrome, or less likely, botulism. Viral encephalitis and botulism are reportable conditions in New York State, including New York City, and the legal basis for reporting human cases was the New York State Sanitary Code and New York City Health Code. However, the main reason the physician called was to request assistance in diagnosing botulism and to obtain botulinum antitoxin, if indicated. Because of the unusual nature of the reported illnesses, telephone calls were made by the local health department to several other hospitals in the area, a form of active surveillance (case finding). These calls identified a total of eight patients ill with similar symptoms. Most of the initial patients lived in a 2-by-2 mile area in northeastern New York City.

The initial surveillance goals were to confirm a diagnosis in the initially reported cases and to determine if other cases were occurring. Laboratory specimens were sent via NYCDOH to the New York State public health laboratory and CDC. On September 2, testing revealed evidence of viral encephalitis, first thought to be St. Louis encephalitis, but later determined to be West Nile encephalitis

(WNE). WNE is a mosquito-borne viral infection that can be fatal and that had not been seen previously in the Western Hemisphere.

With this initial information, the surveillance goals were expanded to define the geographic extent and time course of the outbreak, to ascertain the populations and areas (including neighboring counties and states) at risk, and to determine the source of the outbreak. This information ultimately led to targeting mosquito-control activities and notifying the public in these areas to avoid mosquito exposure. Mammal and bird surveillance was initiated in response to reports of a die-off of crows, other birds, and possible disease in horses.

Personnel

You must know not only who is responsible for overseeing the surveillance activities but also who will be providing the data, collecting and tabulating the data, analyzing and preparing the data for display, and finally, who will be interpreting these data and disseminating them to those who need to know. In the field, you will likely personally know who these persons are; in longer-range systems implemented or orchestrated from some distance, these key persons will probably be names only.

The entire surveillance system in a small area might have only one person doing essentially all these tasks. At the state and national levels, several persons will likely be involved in the surveillance of specific health events. In an acute outbreak setting, a large number of persons at various professional levels might be involved in starting and conducting the necessary active surveillance. As time progresses and the epidemic becomes better understood, the participants will likely assume a more well defined role.

Case Study.   Because of the potential magnitude of the West Nile outbreak, a number of public health agencies and public health specialities were involved. The New York City Department of Health and the New York State Department of Health worked jointly on surveillance activities, with the state health department coordinating surveillance efforts with neighboring counties and states. The state agriculture department became involved in surveillance of domestic animals. CDC also provided technical assistance on zoonotic and vector surveillance, vector control, and laboratory support. Those with "a need to know" who would use information derived from surveillance included state and city environmental and emergency management agencies as well as political leaders.

Case Definition

A case definition should be as clear and as simple as possible. Ideally, it should be practical and include quantifiable and, when possible, explicit criteria. Minimal criteria for definition of a case must be made clear and exact, including the essential clinical and laboratory information. During an epidemic investigation, when laboratory data are often not available, the case definition is usually broad, sometimes depending only on clinical and epidemiologic criteria. As understanding of the disease process increases, a more refined definition may be used. In this context, you should consider classifying cases by levels of probability (e.g., confirmed case, probable case, or possible case). This method gives you more informative case categories to analyze.

Case Study.   Early in the expanded surveillance for WNE, clinical and laboratory case definitions for probable and confirmed cases were developed and transmitted by fax to health care providers in all acute health-care settings. Probable cases had symptoms clinically compatible with encephalitis; confirmed cases required laboratory confirmation. Because public interest was high, many physicians and individuals reported mild, nonspecific illness. To increase the specificity of surveillance, the investigators focused on collection of epidemiologic and laboratory data from patients with the most pronounced symptoms. Clinicians were encouraged to call the health department if they had a suspect case of WNE. In this way, the health department was able to coordinate collection and submission of appropriate clinical specimens for laboratory testing. Positive laboratory tests for WNE were necessary to confirm a case. In addition, laboratory criteria were established for the confirmation of West Nile virus in mammal, bird, and arthropod specimens. After the primary geographic area of the outbreak was defined, surveillance methods were used to determine the impact of control measures in these areas. In addition, suspect cases reported from outside the primary geographic area were prioritized for follow-up to determine if the outbreak was spreading to new areas. After the outbreak was under control, retrospective surveillance of hospital records was conducted in an attempt to determine if there was a missed "source" case, for example, someone who might have acquired disease through foreign travel.

The "Human Element" in Surveillance

After you have designed and developed the surveillance system and are prepared to start, consider the human element involved. The system should be acceptable to everyone who plays a part in collection, analysis, dissemination, and use of the data. Be sure to make some personal contact—not only with those who supply the data—but also with those who collect and analyze the data. Successful systems almost always have included personal contact as an essential ingredient. An occasional visit, particularly to persons who provide the data, enhances interest and a sense of purpose; gives faces and names to remember; "humanizes" an otherwise often impersonal activity; gives the participants visibility and recognizes their importance; and makes people glad they belong. In short, all of these ingredients build and support a team, which is absolutely essential in any field investigation. At the beginning, if possible, you should also make contact with potential users of surveillance data to incorporate their needs into the collection, analysis, and dissemination process. From a strict management viewpoint, this means planning for travel costs in the budget.

Case Study.   During the outbreak of WNE, which had such potential importance and magnitude, the human element in surveillance was critical. From the end of August through September 1999, the New York City Department of Health assigned staff to maintain regular contact by fax with all hospitals in the city to inform physicians of the current situation, the criteria for diagnosis, the process of specimen submission, and advice on supportive therapy for patients. This communication helped ensure the appropriate diagnosis and reporting of true WNE cases and minimize overdiagnosis. Furthermore, the ability to communicate regularly with other members of the team created a comprehensive and coordinated approach for assessment and control efforts.

Teams for human, mammal, bird, and mosquito surveillance were formed with members from the local, state, and federal levels. Communication within and among these groups was key to successful coordination of surveillance efforts and integration of surveillance data. This communication was achieved by daily, or more frequent, conference calls and e-mail and fax communication. Dissemination of surveillance data was carried out by daily briefings for policy makers and daily press releases for the general public. Three articles in CDC's *Morbidity and Mortality Weekly Report* (*MMWR*) provided authoritative information and interpretation to health-care and public health officials in the region and around the country.

Early in an epidemic investigation, an important part of the human element is to keep an open mind; do not narrow the range of surveillance approaches prematurely. Make certain that you have a solid understanding of the epidemic processes before curtailing particular elements of the surveillance activities.

Get the System Started

A final element in establishing a surveillance system is the need to get the system going. During an epidemic, this need is obvious. When reports of toxic shock syndrome began to appear in unprecedented numbers in early 1980, it became clear that a surveillance system was essential to assess the magnitude of the epidemic as well as the nature and distribution of cases. The same was true, of course, with AIDS the following year and the eosinophilia–myalgia syndrome 10 years later. In any setting, however, try to engender a sense of the health event's importance to stimulate and maintain interest in studying it.

In establishing a long-term or ongoing system, a natural tendency at the start will be to make the system as specific and sensitive as humanly possible. Logical and defensible though this may be, do not let it stand in the way of getting the system off the ground. Many systems have languished for months, even years, because of needless worry over missing or misclassifying a case or two; thus, interest, cooperation, and potential impact were diminished. Get the system moving; get the team energized and committed. You can always refine the system as it progresses. Remember, surveillance is a fluid process: as populations or health problems change, the surveillance system must adapt. If you know this, you will overcome a tendency to wait or postpone starting the system until everything is academically perfect. Finally, because surveillance needs always change, you should also establish some type of ongoing mechanism to monitor and evaluate the surveillance process.

Case Study.   In the WNE outbreak, the need to get the surveillance system up and running efficiently and effectively was obvious to everyone involved. Use of modern electronic and computer technologies such as telephone, fax, and electronic mail enabled surveillance activities to be initiated quickly and to involve almost the entire medical community. A combination of sensitive and specific case definitions was established quickly and modified as needed to ensure comprehensive, yet manageable surveillance. The main participants in the public health system (the New York City Department of Health, the New York State Department of Health, and CDC) had a long history of collaboration and understood the roles of the various players. However, the ground rules and agreement on the responsibilities for each component of the system still needed ongoing reinforcement. The surveillance systems relied upon during the outbreak were a combination of current, revived, and new systems. Human surveillance for encephalitis in New York City and New York State had been in place for many years, but detection of an event such as WNE highlighted the importance of direct personal connections between state and city health department epidemiologists and practicing physicians. The detection of WNE was an opportunity to reemphasize to the clinical community the importance of reporting clinical syndromes such as encephalitis. This outbreak would not have been recognized by laboratory reporting alone because testing for WNE was not available in New York. However, the role of the New York State and CDC public health laboratories became essential for recognizing and tracking a pathogen not previously known in the western hemisphere.

A combination of local, state, and federal public health laboratory resources is critical for successful surveillance for new and emerging diseases as well as diseases of traditional public health importance. The 1999 WNE outbreak in New York also underscored the importance of mosquito, mammal, and bird surveillance. Surveillance of these species had been done in New York City previously but had been stopped for many years because of an apparent lack of any detected disease. As a result, additional local, state, and federal resources are now being directed to maintain these surveillance activities in the Northeast.

ANALYSIS AND DISSEMINATION OF SURVEILLANCE DATA

If you are responsible for a surveillance system, be sure to analyze the data appropriately and disseminate them in a timely manner. Programmed data analysis packages are a first step to data analysis, but you should review the results of these analyses and further "customize" the analysis as needed. As with all descriptive epidemiologic data, surveillance information must be analyzed in terms of time, place, and person. Apply simple tabular and graphic techniques for display and analysis (see Chapter 6). More sophisticated methods such as cluster and time-series analyses and computer mapping techniques might be appropriate at some point, but concentrate initially on simple analyses and presentations.

Critical to the usefulness of surveillance systems is the timely dissemination of surveillance data to those who need to know. Publish the data and the analyses together with your interpretation on a regular basis. Whatever format is chosen, be sure to define your audience clearly. The composition of your readers might dictate data collection, interpretation, and the dissemination processes. Distribute the data in a regular and timely manner so that control and prevention measures can be implemented. Because some of those who need to know include policy makers and administrators, people with little epidemiologic knowledge or background, make the reports simple and easy to understand. Finally, in print, recognize persons who have contributed to the surveillance effort. People like to see their names in print and people like to belong; it helps justify their role in the prevention process. Recognizing people by name not only gives them credit, but it gives them a degree of responsibility as well.

Dissemination of Findings during a Field Investigation

In the field setting, particularly in epidemics with large numbers of cases or cases covering large geographic areas, it is often extremely useful to make a surveillance report available daily or semiweekly. The benefits include informing all interested parties; avoiding misinformation and misunderstanding; identifying the players; giving credit to persons who deserve it; identifying who is responsible for what; and serving as an extremely useful diary of what was done, why, and what was found. Finally, making a surveillance report available daily or semiweekly is useful for distribution to the media (thus minimizing interviews) and allows them to better inform the public and the medical community. In short, a regular surveillance report serves as an extremely important management and public information tool. Again, however, keep it simple, emphasizing tables, charts, and figures with minimal text. To some degree, let the facts speak for themselves.

Dissemination of Findings from Ongoing Surveillance Systems

Virtually all states and many local health departments publish their own reports at least once per year and disseminate them to health care providers and other interested persons in their respective locales. CDC also gives information to persons who need to know through the *Morbidity and Mortality Weekly Report* and through the *CDC Surveillance Summaries*, *MMWR Recommendations and Reports*, the *Summary of Notifiable Diseases* and special condition-specific reports. All of these publications are available on the Internet at http://www.cdc.gov/mmwr. When personal identifiers are protected appropriately, customized data analyses requested by investigators or the public could be conducted over the Internet. Also, surveillance data are analyzed and published in the medical literature, although the timeliness of these papers might often leave a good deal to be desired.

ADDITIONAL USES OF SURVEILLANCE DATA

Although we have previously discussed, in general, the purposes of surveillance activities, perhaps it would be useful to outline some additional uses of such systems, particularly those that are long range.

Portrayal of Natural History of Disease

Surveillance data are often used to identify or verify perceived trends in health problems. For example, the reported occurrence of malaria in the United States during the previous 50 years has documented the impact of improved diagnosis, importation of cases from foreign wars, and the impact of both increased international travel by U. S. citizens and foreign immigrants (Fig. 3–1). At the local level (and to a lesser degree national level) surveillance data are used to detect epidemics that lead to control and prevention activities.

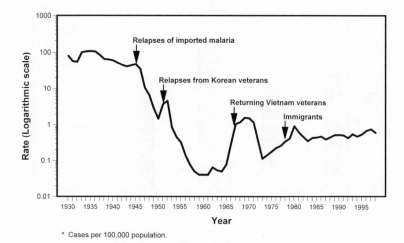

Figure 3-1. Rate (cases per 100,000 population) of malaria, by year—United States, 1930–1998. [*Source:* CDC, 1999.]

Test Hypotheses

In the day-to-day monitoring of health problems in a community, you often cannot wait to do special studies. The data that are available must be analyzed. Although the information might not be ideal for analysis, it can often be used to test certain hypotheses. For example, the impact of laws specifying when children enter school in the United States was expected to change the patterns of reported cases of certain diseases by age. Indeed, the peak incidence of measles changed. Before the widespread adoption of these laws in 1980, the peak incidence occurred among children 10–14 years of age. Within 2 years, the peak incidence occurred among children less than 5 years of age (Fig. 3–2).

Identify and Evaluate Control Measures

Surveillance data are used to quantify the impact of intervention programs. For example, decreases in poliomyelitis rates occurred following the introduction of both the inactivated and oral polio vaccines (Fig. 3–3). Also, broad-based community interventions such as increased legal age of driving and seat-belt laws have had demonstrable effects on mortality.

Monitor Changes in Infectious Agents

In hospital and health department laboratories, various infectious agents are monitored for changes in bacterial resistance to antibiotics or antigenic composition.

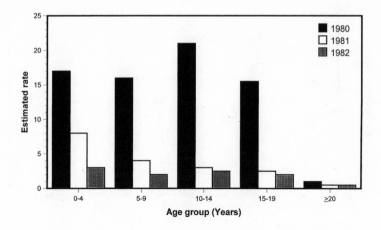

Note: Rates were estimated by extrapolating age from the records of case-patients with known age.

Figure 3–2. Estimated rate (cases per 100,000 population) of measles, by age group—United States, 1980–1982. Rates were estimated by extrapolating age from the records of case-patients. [*Source:* CDC, 1983.]

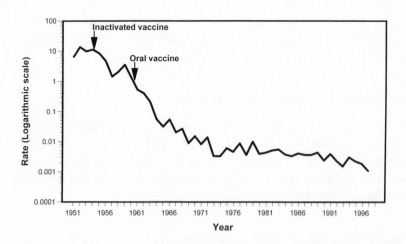

Figure 3–3. Rate (reported cases per 100,000 population) of paralytic poliomyelitis—United States, 1951–1998. [*Source:* CDC, 1999.]

The detection of penicillinase-producing *Neisseria gonorrhoeae* in the United States has provided critical information for the proper treatment of gonorrhea (Fig. 3–4). The National Nosocomial Infection Surveillance System monitors the occurrence of hospital-acquired infections, including changes in antibiotic resistance. Another example has been the detection of the continual change in the influenza virus structure, information vital to vaccine formulation.

Monitor Isolation Activities

The traditional use of surveillance was to quarantine persons infected with or exposed to a particular disease and to monitor their health status. Although this measure is used rarely today, isolation and surveillance are performed on patients with multidrug-resistant tuberculosis and those suspected of having serious, imported diseases such as the hemorrhagic fevers.

Detect Changes in Health Practices

Surveillance has been used to monitor health practices such as hysterectomy, cesarean delivery, mammography, and tubal sterilization. The surveillance of such practices and health-care technologies has been increasing in public health practice in recent years.[12]

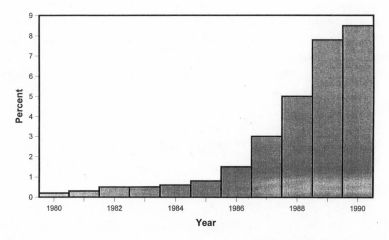

Figure 3–4. Percentage of reported cases of gonorrhea caused by antibiotic-resistant strains of *Neisseria gonorrhoeae*—United States, 1980–1990. [*Source:* CDC, 1990.]

EVALUATION OF A SURVEILLANCE SYSTEM

This chapter describes the essentials of a surveillance system and how to start and maintain one. It is important to understand the basic levels of evaluation of such systems. They should be evaluated at three levels: (*1*) the public health importance of the health event; (*2*) the usefulness and cost of the surveillance system (e.g., whether it is meeting its goals and at what cost); and (*3*) the explicit attributes of the quality of the surveillance system, including sensitivity, specificity, representativeness, timeliness, simplicity, flexibility, and acceptability.[13]

The decision to establish, maintain, or deemphasize a surveillance system should be guided by assessments based on these criteria. Ultimately, the decision rests on whether a health event under surveillance is a public health priority and whether the surveillance system is useful and cost effective.

SUMMARY

Public health surveillance is a basic tool of the field epidemiologist, providing the scientific and factual database essential to informed decision making and to the conduct of public health prevention and control programs. Surveillance is based on morbidity, mortality, and risk factor data, often from multiple sources. Some data, such as vital statistics, are collected primarily for other uses; other data, such as behavioral risk factors, are collected specifically for the surveillance system.

Surveillance systems are established by the field epidemiologist for specific outcomes, such as a disease or injury, and must have clearly expressed goals. Explicit case definitions are at the core of a surveillance system. The initiation and maintenance of any successful surveillance system will reflect recognition of the human element in surveillance practice: data collection, analysis, and data dissemination. Insensitivity to the persons involved in such a system dooms it to failure.

Surveillance data have many uses but, in general, are needed to assess the health status of a population, to set public health priorities, and to determine appropriate actions. Effective systems of public health surveillance are evaluated regularly on the basis of their usefulness in public health practice.

REFERENCES

1. Thacker, S.B., Berkelman, R.L. (1988). Public health surveillance in the United States. *Epidemiol Rev* 10, 164–90.
2. Thacker, S.B., Stroup, D.F. (1992). Future directions for comprehensive public health surveillance and health information systems in the United States. *Am J Epidemiol* 140, 383–97.

3. Langmuir, A.D. (1963). The surveillance of communicable diseases of national importance. *N Engl J Med* 268, 182–92.
4. Koo, D., Parrish, R.G., II. (2000). The changing health-care information infrastructure in the United States: opportunities for a new approach to public health surveillance. In S.M. Teutsch, R. E. Churchill (Eds.), *Principles and Practice of Public Health Surveillance*, vol. 1, pp. 76–94. Oxford University Press, New York.
5. Centers for Disease Control and Prevention (1997). Case definitions for public health surveillance. *Morb Mortal Wkly Rep* 46, (RR-10) 1–55.
6. Bender, J.B., Hedberg, C.W., Besser, J.M., et al. (1997). Surveillance for Escherichia coli O157:H7 infections in Minnesota by molecular subtyping. *N Engl J Med* 337(6), 338–94.
7. Roush, S., Birkhead, G., Koo, D., et al. (1999). Mandatory reporting of diseases and conditions by healthcare professionals and laboratories. *J Am Med Assoc,* 282, 164–70.
8. Centers for Disease Control and Prevention (1999). Summary of notifiable disease, United States, 1998. *Morb Mortal Wkly Rep* 47, 47.
9. Centers for Disease Control and Prevention (1983). Annual Summary 1983: Reported morbidity and mortality in the United States. *Morb Mortal Wkly Rep* 32, 33.
10. Centers for Disease Control and Prevention (1999). Summary of notifiable diseases, United States, 1998. *Morb Mortal Wkly Rep* 47, 54.
11. Centers for Disease Control and Prevention (1990). Sexually Transmitted Disease Surveillance Morbidity Report.
12. Thacker, S.B., Berkelman, R.L. (1986). Surveillance of medical technologies. *J Public Health Policy* 7, 353–77.
13. Romaguera, R.A., German, R.R., Klaucke, D.N. (2000). Evaluating public health surveillance. In S.M.Teutsch, RE. Churchill, *Principles and Practice of Public Health Surveillance*, 2nd ed., pp. 176–93. Oxford University Press, New York.

APPENDIX 3-1 WEB SITES FOR THE FIELD EPIDEMIOLOGIST

DATA SETS

- Behavioral Risk Factor Surveillance System (BRFSS)
  Available: http://www2.cdc.gov/nccdphp/brfss2/publications/index.asp#search
- National Mortality Follow-back Survey
  Available: http://www.cdc.gov/nchs/about/major/nmfs/nmfs.htm
- National Ambulatory Medical Care Survey (NAMCS)
  Available: http://www.cdc.gov/nchs/about/major/ahcd/ahcd1.htm
- National Hospital Ambulatory Medical Care Survey: 1997 Outpatient Department Summary
  Link to PDF file: http://www.cdc.gov/nchs/products/pubs/pubd/ad/301–310/301– 310.htm#ad304
- National Health and Nutrition Examination Survey (NHANES/NCHS)
  Available: http:www.cdc.gov/nchs/nhanes.htm

- National Health Interview Survey (NHIS/NCHS)
  Available: http://www.cdc.gov/nchs/nhis.htm
- 1997 Summary: National Hospital Discharge Survey
  Link to PDF file: 310.htm#ad304
- National Nosocomial Infections Surveillance (NNIS)System
  Available: http://www.cdc.gov/ncidod/hip/nnis/@nnis.htm
- National Nosocomial Infections Surveillance (NNIS) report, Data
  summary June 1999
  Available: National Disease and Therapeutic Index (IMS Health) Not
  Available on the Internet. This item is available for purchase through
  IMS Health North America
  (http://us.imshealth.com/intersite/default.asp) No price listed.
- Ambulatory Sentinel Practice Network
  Available: http://www.aspn.denver.co.us/index.html
- National Birth Defects Prevention Network
  Available: http://www.nbdpn.org/
- Surveillance Epidemiology and End Results (SEER) System- National
  Cancer Institute
  Available: http://www-seer.ims.nci.nih.gov/Publications/CSR7393/
  index.html
- National Electronic Injury Surveillance System (NEISS) —CPSC
  Not Available Online
- Fatality Analysis Reporting System (FARS)— NHTSA
  Available: http://www.nhtsa.dot.gov/people/ncsa/fars.html
- National Automotive Sampling System—NHTSA
  Available: http://www.nhtsa.dot.gov/people/ncsa/nass_ges.html
- National Fire Incident Reporting System USFA/FEMA
  Available: http://www.nfirs.fema.gov/
- National Weather Service
  Available: http://www.nws.noaa.gov/

INSTITUTIONS AND OTHER ORGANIZATIONS

- Centers for Disease Control and Prevention http://www.cdc.gov
- Morbidity and Mortality Weekly Report (MMWR)
  Available: http://www.cdc.gov/mmwr/
- Council of State and Territorial Epidemiologists
  Available: http:/www.cste.org
  Bureau of the Census
  Available: http://www.census.gov

II

THE FIELD INVESTIGATION

4

OPERATIONAL ASPECTS OF EPIDEMIOLOGIC FIELD INVESTIGATIONS

Richard A. Goodman
Michael B. Gregg
Jeffrey J. Sacks

An epidemiologic field investigation entails considerably more effort than simply following the recommended steps in Chapter 5. Besides the necessary collection, tabulation, and analyses of the data, there are numerous and at times overwhelming operational issues that must be addressed as well. This chapter describes certain critical operational and management principles that apply before, during, and after the field work. These principles include: evaluation of and response to an invitation to perform an investigation and the proper preparation—including collaboration and consultation; basic administrative instructions prior to departure to the field; and, finally, initiation, implementation, and aftermath of the field investigation. These considerations extend far beyond the scientific work of the investigators. However, if these considerations are not addressed, the field investigation can be done only with great difficulty, or may even fail.[1]

THE INVITATION

An essential consideration is the need to have a formal request for assistance from an official who is authorized to request help. In the United States, the responsibility for public health rests primarily in the state and local health agencies. In most instances, the state epidemiologist has the authority and responsibility for major epidemiologic field investigations that include whether to investigate independently or to seek help elsewhere. Other persons or authorities may also be involved in the generation of a request for epidemiologic assistance, including those in institutional hierarchies (e.g., nursing homes, hospitals, and businesses), as well as institutions with special jurisdiction, including prisons, military facilities, cruise ships, and reservations for Native Americans. For international problems, the determination of authority for a request may be considerably more complicated and may involve, for example, ministries of health and multinational organizations (e.g., the World Health Organization) (see Chapter 19).

The relationships between larger and smaller health jurisdictions vary not only from state to state (or province to province) within countries but also from country to country. In general, the larger health jurisdictions help serve the smaller in time of need. Yet the sensitivities between these two authorities are often delicate, particularly as they relate to perceived competence, local jurisdiction, and ultimate authority. The health officers of the jurisdiction providing assistance must decide—on the basis of prevailing local–state amenities and agreements, as well as their best judgment—what is the most appropriate response.

At the time of the initial request for assistance, the field epidemiologist should attempt to determine three factors. First, what is the purpose of the investigation? Is the health department simply requesting more help to perform or complete the investigation? Has the health department been unable to determine the nature or source of disease or the mode of spread? Perhaps the health department wants to share the responsibility of the investigation with a more seasoned and knowledgeable health authority in order to be relieved of political or scientific pressure. Occasionally, legal or ethical issues may have become prominent in the early investigation, and you should be aware of this possibility. Rarely, an epidemic may even be declared or announced by health authorities or citizens. Assistance is then requested to publicize perceived adverse health conditions, to awaken state or national health leaders, or even to secure funds. Second, and clearly related to the first, there is a need to determine specifically what the investigation is expected to accomplish. The team may be asked to confirm the findings already collected, collect new or different data for local analysis, or perform an entirely new investigation, including analysis and recommendations. And third, you should confirm that the requestor is authorized to invite assistance. Occasionally field studies have been aborted simply because those requesting assistance either had no authority to do so, or state or national teams were investigating without local permission.

THE RESPONSE AND THE RESPONSIBILITIES

There are several reasons why field investigations should be done, if not encouraged:

- To control and prevent further disease
- To provide agreed upon or statutorily-mandated services
- To derive more information about interaction among the human host, the agent, and the environment
- To strengthen surveillance at the local level through assessment of its quality and by direct and personal contact, or to determine the need to establish a new surveillance system
- To provide training opportunities in field epidemiology.[2]

If a decision is made to provide field assistance, the following points must be discussed with the local health official:

- What resources (including personnel) will be available locally?
- What resources will be provided by the visiting team?
- Who will direct the day-to-day investigation?
- Who will provide overall supervision and ultimately be responsible for the investigation?
- How will the data be shared and who will be responsible for their analysis?
- Will a report of the findings be written, who will write it, to whom will it go?
- Who will be the senior author of a scientific paper, should one be written?

These are extremely critical issues, some of which cannot be totally resolved before the investigative team arrives on the scene. However, they must be addressed, discussed openly, and agreed upon as soon as possible.

PREPARATION

Collaboration and Consultation

Many field investigations require support of a competent laboratory. Even if local laboratories are capable of processing and identifying specimens, you should immediately, upon being informed of the proposed investigation, contact your counterparts within your support laboratory. The laboratory scientists should be requested to provide any needed guidance and laboratory assistance. Now is the time to obtain assurance of cooperation and commitment rather than during the field investigation or near the end when specimens have already been collected. Not only must the laboratory staff schedule the processing of specimens, but they should be asked to recommend what kinds of specimens should be collected and how they should be collected and processed (see Chapter 22). There also may be substantive basic or applied research questions that could be appropriately addressed and answered during the field investigation. Discuss these issues in detail with these professionals, and make every effort to enlist their interest and support.

Advice on statistical methods may also be sought at this time as well. The same consideration applies to contacting other health professionals, such as veterinarians, mammalogists, entomologists, and environmental experts, whose expertise can be crucial to a successful field investigation. Moreover, give serious consideration to include such professionals on the investigative team. Determine whether they should be part of the initial team so that appropriate data and, particularly, specimens can be collected at the same time as other relevant epidemiologic information. Information specialists can also be extremely important in the overall management of a field investigation (see Chapter 13). Because large outbreaks will likely attract moderate local or regional attention in the media, the presence of an experienced and knowledgeable information officer who can respond to public inquiries and meet the media on a regular basis can be invaluable. Consider including secretarial and/or administrative personnel on the investigating team—not only to use their services but to expose them to a real-life situation. They will return home with a better understanding of field work and with an increased ability to support future field investigations.

Basic Administrative Instructions and Notification

Once the field team has been chosen, certain key measures should be taken:
- Identify the team leader and the person to whom the leader should report regularly at the "home base."
- Try to arrange in advance an initial meeting with the requestor or persons either designated or identified by the requestor. This will ensure that local authorities are not surprised by an unexpected arrival. In addition, this step underscores for all parties the need for advance planning and orderliness in the investigation—in essence, it sets a tone for the conduct of the investigation.
- Before leaving for the field, a senior member of the team should write a memorandum. It should summarize how and when the request was made, what information was provided by the local health department, what is the agreed upon purpose of the investigation, what are the commitments of both the visiting team and the local health authorities, who is on the field team, and when the latter is expected to arrive in the field.

This memorandum should be distributed to key personnel in the health offices of the visiting team and the offices of the host health department, and to others who need to know. This kind of communication will serve not only as notification to all concerned but as a method to prevent redundant responses (i.e., to avoid "crossing wires"). It will also identify expertise and resources from other programs that may contribute to the investigation.

Basic programmatic jurisdictions and interests must also be respected, and some programs and staff simply want to or need to know as a courtesy. Even when a problem does not directly involve a state (e.g., as in the case of a prison or a military facility), state and local officials are generally notified because of possible ramifications to populations in surrounding communities.

• Lastly, before departing for the field, each member of the investigative team should review a basic checklist to be sure they have materials and aids, essential for field operations, and have covered fundamental travel and logistic considerations. Such items include, for example, background journal articles, statistical references, portable microcomputers, cameras and film, portable tape recorders and tape, credit cards, and travel and lodging reservations.

INITIATION OF THE INVESTIGATION

A key concept and philosophy for the epidemiologist and the team to keep in mind is the importance of the role, "consultant/collaborator," and what that implies. In general, the guiding principle should be that you are there to provide help, not simply to "take charge." Equally important, try to balance the focus of the investigation with the competing priorities in the local jurisdiction. While the immediate problem is your sole concern, the local people must continue to address a myriad of other priorities and ongoing problems. This dichotomy can be appreciated if you and your team try to take the local point of view early in the investigation.

Once on site, you should meet promptly with the authority who requested assistance—usually the state, provincial, or local epidemiologist or program director. Essential steps at this initial meeting include:

• Review and update the status of the problem
• Identification/review of who are the primary contacts
• Identification of a principal collaborator who can also serve as a "guardian angel" during the investigation
• Identification of local resources (e.g., office space, clerical support, assistance for surveys, and laboratory support)
• Creation of a method and schedule for providing updates to local authorities and headquarters
• A review of sensitivities, including potential problems with institutions and individuals (e.g., hospitals, administrators, practitioners, and local public health staff) likely to be encountered during the investigation. Ideally, you should take the day or so needed to meet the requesting authority initially—

so that key "doors" will be opened—rather than spend valuable time later in the investigation mending bridges.

During the initial meeting, you also should identify the appropriate local person to speak for the entire investigative team, when necessary. In general, you and your team should try to avoid direct contact with the news media and should always defer to local health officials (see Chapter 13). The field team is essentially working at the request and under the aegis of the local health authorities. Therefore, it is the local officials who not only know and appreciate the local situation but also are the appropriate persons to comment on the investigation. In the most practical sense, the less the media make contact with you and your associates, the more you can do at your own pace and discretion.

The work required to organize an investigation through this stage (i.e., starting travel and convening the initial meeting) is relatively straightforward and uncomplicated. In contrast, however, at least three factors will likely complicate the start of your scientific investigation: (1) the effects of a new setting (i.e., you are an outsider and unfamiliar with the environment); (2) the often intense pressure to solve the problem immediately and end the outbreak; and (3) the queries of the media and other demands for your time. Thus, in short order, circumstances may change from tranquillity and orderliness to a situation of pressure and confusion. To overcome the myriad of potential distractions, you must maintain the proper perspective by adhering to the basics: focus the mission to collect data systematically; verify the diagnosis; and then proceed through case identification, orientation of data, and development and testing of hypotheses (see Chapter 5). Therefore, at the conclusion of the initial meeting, you should try to visit patients to verify the diagnosis through interviews and, if necessary, physical examination and review of laboratory data.

MANAGEMENT

Because of the potential complexity of field investigations, as well as the distracting circumstances under which they are typically conducted, you may want to take the following approaches to ensure the systematic and orderly progression of events. First, maintain lists of necessary tasks, check off those actions that have been completed, and update the list at least twice daily. Second, communicate frequently with coworkers, the requesting authority, and the person designated to be the media contact. A team meeting should be held each day at a regularly scheduled time. Third, never hesitate to request additional help if required by the circumstances. Fourth, to ensure the investigation will be completed, avoid setting a departure date in advance or succumbing to the pressure of family members to return earlier.

Investigations of large and complex problems may be particularly challenging for field teams and require even more rigorous organization of field operations. The following framework, reflected by the mnemonic "SLACK OFF," was developed in 1986 by one of the authors (J.S.) during a complicated and protracted epidemiologic field investigation of a cluster of unexplained cardiopulmonary arrests. The methods and techniques used during the investigation were encompassed by this acronym to help organize and manage the activities of a large field team that worked with multiple data sets.

S—Shells (i.e., Table Shells)

- Begin at the end. In other words, ask, What are the questions to answer? Think in terms of who is at risk and what was the exposure that led to disease.
- Create the table shells (two × two tables) needed to answer your questions. These shells help define what data you need and how to get them.
- Collect sufficient data to classify subsequently or to stratify levels of exposure and outcome.
- Think quantitatively, for example:
  How much (food or water)
  How long (outdoors, in a room)
  How sick (died, hospitalized, ambulatory)
- Remember that you may need to consult a statistician before collecting data.

L—Log Decisions

Record your decisions as you make them—it will ensure consistency and will make the study reproducible. This is particularly important in regard to case definitions and why certain criteria were used.

A—Accuracy

Remember the need for quality control measures such as training and monitoring of data collectors and abstractors; conducting error checks and validating data independently; and evaluating nonrespondents and missing records.

C—Communication

As mentioned above, there are different, but necessary, approaches to both internal (i.e., with colleagues and field team members) and external (i.e., the press) communications.

K—KISS (Keep It Simple, Stupid)

- Try to reduce the problem to one two × two table.
- Resist collecting more data than are needed (e.g., excessive clinical details).

O—Ongoing Writing

- Write down the reason you went to investigate and what was there when you arrived (i.e., a background section).
- Write while the investigation is ongoing—months later you will have forgotten what you did.
- Write the methods while you are defining them—a decision log helps.

F—Filing

- Maintain and retain an inventory of data files.
- Protect the confidentiality of subjects.

F—Friendship

- Because field investigations are difficult—associated with long hours and great stress—make a special effort to maintain morale.
- Provide encouragement, positive reinforcement, and appreciation to those who participate.

DEPARTURE

Upon concluding the on-site field investigation, organize a departure meeting to include the requestor, other key officials, and members of the investigative team. In addition to helping conclude formally the on-site work, the departure meeting enables you to debrief the requestor on the findings of the investigation, review preliminary recommendations, provide acknowledgments, and express appreciation to local hosts and collaborators. Obtain any additional names, titles, and addresses for follow-up letters and correspondence. If at all possible, leave on site a preliminary written report, label it as such, and be certain to make a commitment to provide a complete written report within an agreed upon, specified time period.

The departure meeting also may be the most appropriate occasion for planning follow-up activities with the local organization. Such activities include the needs for additional studies, evaluation of control measures, analysis and maintenance of data collected during the investigation, plans for final reports and manuscripts (including discussion of authorship), and determination of who is responsible for each of these different follow-up activities.

REPORTS

Written summaries of the investigation include both preliminary and final reports. The preliminary report fulfills the immediate obligation to the requesting authority. It should include a summary of methods used to conduct the investigation, preliminary epidemiologic and laboratory findings, recommendations, a clear delineation of tasks and activities that must be completed, and appropriate "thank yous." In addition to the preliminary report, which optimally should be delivered to the requestor on departure from the field or certainly within 1–2 weeks of completion of the investigation, you should prepare follow-up letters to other principals (e.g., local health officials, co-investigators) to inform them and to reinforce long-term relations.

The final reports should be written as quickly as possible—before you are called out to another field investigation! The final report should include complete and final data. In addition to a written final report, you should consider other methods or forums for communicating the findings of the investigation. Options include formal seminars where an oral presentation will promote critical feedback; reports for public health bulletins intended for public health practitioners; comprehensive articles for peer-reviewed journals; and presentations at professional meetings.

REFERENCES

1. Vaughan, J.P., Morrow, R.D. (1989) (Eds.). *Manual of Epidemiology for District Health Management*, World Health Organization, Geneva.
2. Gregg, M.B. (1997). The principles of an epidemic field investigation. In Detels, R., Holland, W., McEwen, J. (Eds.) *Oxford Textbook of Public Health*, vol 2, 3rd ed., Oxford University Press, London.

5

CONDUCTING A FIELD INVESTIGATION

Michael B. Gregg

This chapter explains how to perform an epidemiologic field investigation. It focuses on a presumed point source (common source) epidemic, recognized and reported by local health authorities to a state (provincial) health department. This is a typical setting that highlights the tasks that need to be performed. Although the context is one of an acute infectious disease epidemic in a community, the epidemiologic and public health principles apply equally well to noninfectious disease investigations.

BACKGROUND CONSIDERATIONS

Overall Purposes and Methods

Some purposes of epidemiology include determining the cause(s) of a disease, its source, its mode of transmission, who is at risk of developing the disease, and what exposure(s) predispose to the disease. Fortunately, in many outbreak investigations the clinical syndromes are easily identifiable; the agents can be readily isolated and characterized; and the source, mode of transmission, and risk factors of the disease are usually well known and understood. Therefore, one is often well prepared for the field investigation. However, when the clinical diagnosis and/or laboratory findings are unclear, the task becomes much more difficult. It requires more careful consideration of the clinical presentation of disease in an effort to determine the source, mode of spread, and population(s) at risk. For example, bacterial contamination of food or water is usually manifested by signs and symptoms referable to the gastrointestinal tract. Pathogenic agents transmitted in air often affect the respiratory tract and sometimes the skin, eyes, or mucous membranes. Skin abrasions or lesions may suggest animal or insect transmission. So the clinical manifestations of disease may serve as critical leads.

Regardless of how secure the clinical diagnosis may be, the thought process must include clinical, laboratory, and epidemiologic evidence. Together these provide leads and pathways to take or reject to discover the natural history of the epidemic.

Although field epidemiologists will perform several separate operations, in broad strokes they will really do two things. First, they will collect information that describes the setting of the outbreak, namely: when people became sick, where they acquired disease, and what the characteristics of the ill people were. These are the descriptive aspects of the investigation. Often, simply by knowing these facts (and the diagnosis), you can determine the source and mode of spread of the agent and can identify those primarily at risk of developing disease. Common sense will often give you these answers, and relatively little, if any, further analysis is required.

On occasion, however, it will not be readily apparent where the agent resided, how it was transmitted, who was at risk of disease, and what the exposure was. Under these circumstances, a second operation, analytic epidemiology, must be used to provide the answers. And the critical operations here include determining rates and comparing these rates. Virtually all epidemiologic analyses require comparisons, usually groups of persons—ill and well or exposed and not exposed (see Chapter 7). In epidemic situations you will usually compare ill and well people— both believed at risk of disease—to determine what exposures ill people had that well people did not have. These comparisons are made by using appropriate statistical techniques (see Chapters 7 and 8). If the differences between ill and well persons are greater than one would expect by chance, you can draw certain inferences about why the epidemic occurred. In some situations, comparisons can be made between exposed persons and those not exposed to see if there are significant differences in rates of illness between the two groups.

The Pace and Commitment of a Field Investigation

An underlying theme throughout this chapter is the need to act quickly, establish clear operational priorities, and perform the investigation responsibly. This should not imply haphazard collection and inappropriate analysis of data, but rather the use of simple and workable case definitions, case-finding methods, and analyses (see Chapters 4 and 9).

Data collection, analyses, and recommendations should be performed in the field. There is a strong tendency to collect what you think is the essential information in the field and then retreat to "home base" for analysis—particularly now with the availability of personal computers. Avoid this reflex at all costs. Such action will likely be viewed as lack of interest or concern or even possessiveness by the local constituency. A premature departure also makes any further collection of data or direct contact with study populations and local health officials difficult, if not impossible. Once home, you lose the urgency and momentum to perform, the sense of relevancy of the epidemic, and, most of all, the totally committed time for the investigation. Every field investigation should be completed not only to the field team's satisfaction, but particularly to that of the local health department as well.

THE INVESTIGATION

Introduction

Ten basic tasks will be described in a logical order (Table 5–1). However, you may perform several of these functions simultaneously or in different order during the investigation. Control and prevention measures may even be recommended soon after beginning the investigation simply on the basis of intuitive reasoning and/or common sense. Sometimes the local officials know why the epidemic occurred, and you are there simply to supply a scientific basis for their conclusion.

No two epidemiologists will take the exact pathway of investigation. Yet, in general, the data they collect, the analyses they apply, and the control and prevention measures they recommend will likely be similar.

Since, by definition, our example epidemic has resulted from a point source and may be nearly over before the field team arrives, the investigation will in all likelihood be retrospective in nature. This should alert you to some fundamental aspects of any investigation that occurs "after the fact." First of all, because many illnesses and critical events have already occurred, virtually all information acquired and related to the epidemic will be based upon memory. Health officers, physicians, and patients will likely have different recollections, views, or perceptions of what transpired. Information may conflict, may not be accurate, and certainly cannot be expected to reflect the precise occurrence of past events. Like the clinician, you may have to ask patients what they think made them sick, what they think caused the epidemic. Most critically, in parallel with medical practice, action may have to be taken without the benefit of all the desired data (see Chapter 9).

Table 5–1. The Ten Steps of a Field Investigation

1. Determine the existence of the epidemic
2. Confirm the diagnosis
3. Define a case and count cases
4. Orient the data in terms of time, place, and person
5. Determine who is at risk of becoming ill
6. Develop a hypothesis that explains the specific exposure that caused disease and test this hypothesis by appropriate statistical methods
7. Compare the hypothesis with the established facts
8. Plan a more systematic study
9. Prepare a written report
10. Execute control and prevention measures

For the young, inexperienced medical epidemiologist steeped in the tradition of molecule and millimole determinations, the "more-or-less" measurements of the field epidemiologist can initially be major hurdles to a successful field investigation. However lacking in accuracy these data may be, they are often the only data you have; and they must be collected, analyzed, and interpreted with care, imagination, and caution. Furthermore, you have not seen the epidemiologic method work in real life. Unlike clinical medicine when in a matter of minutes to a few hours the physical examination usually reinforces the history, and the laboratory results usually reinforce both, there often is no immediate reinforcement of the thought processes and activities in the field. It usually takes several days or a week before data start coming in that begin to reassure you that you are on the right track.

Determine the Existence of an Epidemic

Local health officials usually will know if more disease is occurring than would normally be expected. Since most local health departments have ongoing records of communicable diseases and certain noninfectious conditions, by comparing weekly, monthly, or yearly data, you can easily determine if the observed numbers exceed the expected level. Although there may not be laboratory confirmation at this time, an increase in reported cases by local physicians is enough evidence to investigate. However, at this time avoid the use of the terms "epidemic" or "outbreak." These words are quite subjective. Local health officials take different views of the normal rise and fall in cases, and whether changes in the pattern merit investigation.

You must be aware of artifactual causes of increases or decreases in reported cases such as changes in local reporting practices, increased interest in certain diseases because of local or national awareness, a new physician or clinic in town, or changes in diagnostic methods. An excellent example of artifactual reporting occurred in southwest Florida in 1977 when a new physician in the community reported many cases of encephalitis in his practice. After extensive field work by local, state, and federal epidemiologists, it was clear there was no epidemic, but simply misdiagnoses by the physician.[1]

Sometimes, however, it may be difficult to document the existence of an epidemic rapidly. You may need to acquire absentee records from schools or factories, records of outpatient clinic visits, hospitalizations, laboratory records, or death certificates. A simple telephone survey of practicing physicians will strongly support the existence of an epidemic, as would a similar rapid survey of households in the community. In such quick assessments, you could ask about signs and symptoms rather than about specific diagnoses. Ask physicians or clinics if they are treating more people than usual with sore throats, gastroenteritis, or fever with rash, as examples, in order to obtain an index of disease incidence. Although not specific for any given disease, such surveys can often establish the existence of an epidemic. Sometimes it is extremely difficult to determine if there is an epidemic. Yet because of local pressures, the team may have to continue the investigation even if they believe no significant health problem exists.

Confirm the Diagnosis

Confirm the clinical diagnosis by standard laboratory techniques such as serology and/or isolation and characterization of the agent. Do not try to use newly introduced, experimental, or otherwise not broadly recognized confirmatory tests—at least not at this stage in the investigation. If at all possible, visit the laboratory and verify the laboratory findings in person. For example, talk to the technician, check the record books, and look at the gram stain yourself.

Not every reported case has to be confirmed in the laboratory. If most patients have signs and symptoms compatible with the working diagnosis, and, perhaps, 15% to 20% are laboratory confirmed, you do not need more confirmation at this time. This usually is ample confirmatory evidence. See and examine several representative cases of the disease as well, if at all possible. Clinical assumptions should not be made; the diagnosis should be verified by you or a qualified physician with you. Nothing convinces supervisors and health officers more than an eyewitness confirmation of clinical disease by you and the investigating team.

Define a Case and Count Cases

Now try to create a workable case definition, decide how to find cases, and count them. The simplest and most objective criteria for a case definition are usually the best (e.g., fever, X-ray evidence of pneumonia, white blood cells in the spinal fluid, number of bowel movements per day, blood in the stool, or skin rash). However, be guided by the accepted, usual presentation of the disease with or without standard laboratory confirmation in the case definition. Where time may be a critical factor in a rapidly unfolding field investigation, use a simple, easily applicable definition—recognizing that some cases will be missed and some non-cases included. For example, in an epidemic of hepatitis A, a history of jaundice, fever, and an abnormal liver enzyme test should be quite adequate to start with. Later you can refine the definition.

Some factors that can help determine the levels of sensitivity and specificity of the case definition are the following:

- What is the usual apparent-to-inapparent clinical case ratio?
- What are the important and obvious pathognomonic or strongly clinically suggestive signs and symptoms of the disease?
- What microbiologic or chemical isolations, identification, and serologic techniques are easy, practical, and reliable?
- How accessible are the patients or those at risk; can they be contacted again after the initial investigation for follow-up questions, examination, or serology?
- In the event that the investigation requires long-term follow-up, can the case definitions be applied easily and consistently by others not on the current investigating team?
- Is it absolutely necessary that all patients be identified during the initial investigation or would only those seen by physicians or hospitalized suffice?

No matter what criteria are used, you must apply the case definition equally and without bias to all persons under investigation.

Methods for case finding will vary considerably according to the disease in question and the community setting. Most outbreaks involve certain clearly identifiable groups at risk, therefore, finding cases will be relatively self-evident and easy. Active, direct contact with selected physicians, hospitals, laboratories, schools, or industries or using some form of public announcement will find most of the remaining, unreported cases. However, sometimes more intensive efforts—such as physician, telephone, door-to-door, or culture or serologic surveys—may be necessary to find cases. Regardless of the method, you must establish some system(s) of case finding during the investigation and perhaps afterwards (see Chapter 3).

Simply knowing the number of cases does not provide adequate information. Control and prevention measures depend upon knowing the source and mode of spread of an agent as well as the characteristics of ill patients. Therefore, case finding should include collecting pertinent information likely to provide clues or leads to the natural history of the epidemic and, particularly, relevant characteristics of the ill. First, collect basic information about each patient's age, gender, residence, occupation, date of onset, for example, to define the basic descriptive aspects of the epidemic. Next, get pertinent signs, symptoms, and laboratory data. If the disease under investigation is usually water- or food-borne, ask questions about exposure to various water and food sources; if transmitted by person-to-person contact, ask about the frequency, duration, and nature of personal contacts. If the nature of the disease is not known or cannot be comfortably presumed, you will need to ask a variety of questions covering all possible aspects of disease transmission and risk. Also be mentally prepared for the possibility of having to apply a second questionnaire if the first analysis does not help.

Orient the Data in Terms of Time, Place, and Person

Now the team should have a reasonably accurate number of cases to view descriptively. So it is time to characterize the epidemic in terms of when patients became ill, where they lived or became ill, and what special attributes the patients had (see Chapter 6 for greater detail). You may want to wait until the epidemic is over or until all likely cases have been reported before performing such an analysis. Don't. The earlier you develop ideas of why the epidemic started, the more pertinent data you can collect. The addition of a proportionately small number of cases later on will usually not affect the analysis or recommendations.

Time

Characterize the cases by plotting a graph that shows the number of cases (y axis) over the time of onset of illness using an appropriate time interval (x axis) (Fig. 5–1). This "epidemic curve" gives a considerably deep appreciation for the magnitude of the outbreak, its possible mode of spread, and the possible duration of the epidemic—much more than would a simple "line-listing" of cases. One can often infer a remarkable amount of information from a simple picture of times of onset of disease. If the incubation period of the disease is known, relatively firm inferences can be made regarding the likelihood of a point source exposure, person-to-person spread, or a mixture of the two. And just the opposite: if you know when the exposure occurred, you may be able to determine the incubation period. This is particularly important if you do not know what the disease is. Also, if the epidemic is still

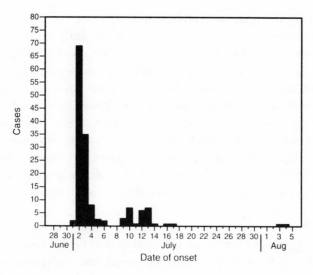

Figure 5-1. Cases of Pontiac fever, by date of onset—Michigan, June 28–August 5, 1968. [*Source:* Glick et al., 1978.[2]]

in progress and you have a good idea of the disease, you may be able to predict how many more cases are likely to occur. Finally, an epidemic curve provides an excellent "prop" for ready communication to nonepidemiologists, administrators, and the like who need to grasp in some fashion the nature and magnitude of the epidemic.

The epidemic curve in Figure 5–1 shows cases of Pontiac fever (subsequently confirmed as legionnaires' disease) that occurred in Pontiac, Michigan, July and August 1968, by day of onset.[2] The epidemic was explosive in onset suggesting (*1*) a virtually simultaneous point-source exposure of many persons; (*2*) a disease with a short incubation period (because of the very tight clustering of cases over a very narrow time frame; and (*3*) a continuing exposure spanning several weeks— all of which were subsequently verified.

Place

Sometimes diseases occur or are acquired in unique locations in the community, which, if you can visualize, may provide major clues or evidence regarding the source of the agent and/or the nature of exposure. Water supplies, milk distribution routes, sewage disposal outflows, prevailing wind currents, air-flow patterns in buildings, and ecologic habitats of vectors may play important roles in disseminating microbial or environmental pathogens and determining who is at risk of acquiring disease. If one plots cases geographically, a distribution pattern may appear that approximates these known sources and routes of potential exposure. This, in turn, may help identify the vehicle or mode of transmission.

Figure 5–2 illustrates the usefulness of a "spot map" in the investigation of an outbreak of shigellosis in Dubuque, Iowa, in 1974.[3] Early analysis showed that cases were not clustered by place of residence. A history of drinking water gave no useful clue as to a possible source and mode of transmission. However, it was later learned that many cases had been exposed to water by recent swimming in a camping park located on the Mississippi River. Figure 5–2 shows the river sites where 22 culture-positive cases swam within 3 days of onset of illness, strongly suggesting a common source of exposure. Ultimately, the epidemiologists incriminated Mississippi River water by documenting gross contamination by the city's sewage treatment plant 5 miles upstream and by isolating *Shigella sonnei* from a sample of river water taken from the camping park beach area.

Person

Lastly, you must examine the characteristics of the patients themselves in terms of a variety of attributes, such as age, gender, race, occupation, or virtually

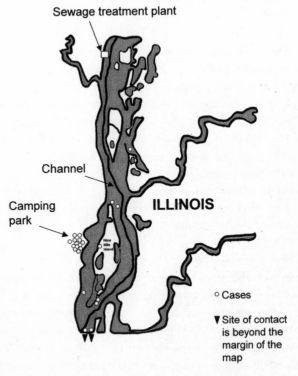

Figure 5–2. Culture-positive cases of Shigella, by sites along the Mississippi River where each case swam within 3 days of onset of illness. [*Source*: Rosenberg et al., 1976.[3]]

any other characteristic that may be useful in portraying the uniqueness of the case population. If a singular or special attribute emerges, this frequently suggests a strong lead as to the group at risk and even an idea of the specific exposure. Some diseases primarily affect certain age groups or races; frequently, occupation is the key attribute of people with certain diseases. The list of human characteristics— really potential risks and exposures—is nearly endless. However, the more you know about the disease in question (the agent's reservoir, mode(s) of spread, persons usually at greatest risk), the more specific and pertinent information you should seek to determine whether any of these risks or exposures predispose to illness.

Determine Who Is at Risk of Becoming Ill

You now know the number of people ill, when and where they were when they became ill, what their general characteristics are, and, usually, a firm diagnosis or a good "working" diagnosis. These data frequently provide enough information to determine with reasonable assurance how and why the epidemic started. For example, a time, place, and person description of the epidemic will strongly suggest that only people in a particular community supplied by a specific water system were at risk of getting sick, or that only certain students in a school or workers in a single factory became ill. Perhaps it was only a group of people who attended a local restaurant who reported illness. However, no matter how obvious it might appear that only a single group of persons was at risk, one should look carefully at the entire community to be sure there are not other affected persons.

Sometimes it is very difficult to know who is at risk, particularly in epidemics that cover large geographic areas and involve many age groups with initially no obvious unique characteristics. Under these circumstances the team may have to do a survey of some kind to get more specific information about the ill persons and some idea of who is at risk.

Develop a Hypothesis that Explains the Specific Exposure that Caused Disease and Test this Hypothesis by Appropriate Statistical Methods

This next step, the first real epidemiologic analysis of the field investigation, is often the most difficult one to perform. By now you should have an excellent grasp of the epidemic and an overall feel for the most likely source and mode of transmission. However, the exposure that caused disease must be determined.

A simple example was the 1989 investigation of an epidemic of nausea, vomiting, and diarrhea among 20 people who ate at a single pizzeria in McKeesport, Pennsylvania.[4] Since the disease was most likely acquired by eating something (because of the signs and symptoms) and because no other cluster of similar disease had occurred elsewhere in the community, the epidemiologists focused attention only on those who bought food from the pizzeria. The logical hypothesis then was that the exposure necessary to develop nausea, vomiting, and diarrhea was consumption of some food(s) contaminated with a microbial or chemical agent. Therefore, those who bought and ate food from the pizzeria on the presumed day of exposure were given a questionnaire asking what beverages and kinds of foods and pizza they had eaten, that is, what foods had they been exposed to. Early analysis showed that 100% of the ill persons (cases) had eaten mushrooms on pizza. Because so many ill people had eaten these pizzas, one might quickly assume it was the contaminated food. Yet the 100% simply represents how popular the mushroom pizza was among the ill attendees. Alone, the 100% does not give adequate valid support to the hypothesis that exposure to the pizza (i.e., eating the mushroom-topped pizza) caused illness. What had to be done was to determine the food histories of the well pizza eaters (controls) and compare their histories to the ill persons. When this comparison was done, the food histories were very similar between the two groups except for one food, the mushroom pizzas: only 33% of the well attendees ate the mushroom-topped pizza. The hypothesis, then, was that the difference in exposure rates—100% among the ill and 33% among the well— was because the mushroom pizza was contaminated. When these rates were tested statistically, it showed that, assuming that eating the particular pizza had no relation to getting ill, such a difference would occur less than one time in 10,000 such instances. Therefore, the statistical evidence as well as other information (isolation of *S. aureus* from cans of mushrooms) supported the hypothesis that eating the mushroom pizza was the exposure that caused the outbreak.

Again, this phase of the investigation clearly will pose the greatest challenge. Field epidemiologists must review the findings carefully, weigh the clinical, laboratory, and epidemiologic features of the disease, and hypothesize possible exposures that could plausibly cause disease. In other words, you must seek from the patients' histories exposures that could conceivably predispose to illness. If exposure histories for ill and well are not significantly different, a new hypothesis must be developed. This will require imagination, perseverance, and sometimes resurveying those at risk to obtain more pertinent information.

Compare the Hypothesis with the Established Facts

At this time in the investigation epidemiologic and statistical inferences have provided the most probable exposure responsible for the epidemic. Yet you must "square" the hypothesis with the clinical, laboratory, and other epidemiologic facts of the investigation. In other words, do the proposed exposure, mode of spread, and population affected fit well with the known facts of the disease? For example, if, in the gastroenteritis outbreak referred to above, the analysis incriminated a food of high protein and low acid content that supports growth of staphylococcal organisms and production of enterotoxin (as is the case with mushrooms), the hypothesis fits well with our understanding of staphylococcal food poisoning. However, if the analysis incriminated coffee or water—highly unlikely sources of staphylococcal enterotoxin—you must then reassess the findings, perhaps secure more information, reconsider the clinical diagnosis, and certainly pose and test new hypotheses. Unfortunately, on rare occasions this reassessment is necessary, and you should be prepared.

The following investigations illustrate the uses of simple descriptive and analytic epidemiology, how some analyses may not prove helpful, how posing new hypotheses may be necessary, how the facts must fit logically, and how important persistence is in arriving at a defensible conclusion.

Thirty-four cases of perinatal listeriosis and seven cases of adult disease occurred between March 1 and September 1, 1981, in several maritime provinces of Canada.[5] These cases represented a severalfold increase over the number of cases diagnosed in previous years, suggesting some common exposure. Although *L. monocytogenes* is a common cause of abortion and nervous system disease in cattle, sheep, and goats, the source of human infection has been obscure. Cases could not be linked together by person-to-person contact; they shared no common water source; and food exposures, as determined from a general food history, were not different between cases and controls. However, a second, more detailed food history and subsequent intensive interrogation of cases and controls revealed that there was a statistically significant difference between cases and controls regarding exposure to coleslaw. Even though this food had never been previously incriminated as a source of listeria, it was the only food item positively associated with disease and essentially the only lead the investigators had at the time. Armed with this clue, the team subsequently found a specimen of coleslaw in the refrigerator of one of the patients that grew out the same serotype of listeria isolated from the epidemic cases. No other food items in the refrigerator were positive for listeria.

The coleslaw had been prepared by a regional manufacturer who had obtained cabbages and carrots from several wholesale dealers and many local farmers. Although environmental cultures from the coleslaw plant failed to reveal listeria organisms, two unopened packages of coleslaw from the plant subsequently grew *L. monocytogenes* of the same epidemic serotype. A review of the sources of the vegetable ingredients was made, and a single farmer was identified who had grown cabbages and also maintained a flock of sheep. Two of his sheep had previously died of listeriosis in 1979 and 1981. Also, he was in the habit of using sheep manure to fertilize his cabbage.

This information does not prove this farm was the source of the listeria organisms that caused the epidemic. However, the hypothesis that coleslaw was the source and the statistical test that supported this hypothesis provided the necessary impetus to continue the investigation. And, ultimately, a single, highly likely source of the bacteria was discovered. These findings strongly suggest listeriosis is a zoonotic infection transmitted from infected animals via contaminated vegetables to humans.

In January and February 1980, an epidemic of 85 cases of salmonellosis in Ohio prompted an extensive field investigation by Taylor et al.[6] All cases were caused by an uncommon serotype of salmonella, *S. muenchen*. This finding plus the fact that all cases were among teenagers and young adults strongly suggested a common source of exposure. Knowing that the natural reservoirs for almost all serotypes are poultry, chicken eggs, and other domestic farm animals and that the majority of salmonella epidemics can be traced to eating meat or poultry products or having contact with these animals, Taylor and colleagues questioned the cases and appropriate controls. Their questions included food histories and contact with farm animals. Not too surprisingly the investigators found that significantly more cases than controls gave a history of eating ham. On the surface this evidence strongly incriminated ham as the vehicle of infection. However, in trying to define the source of the contaminated ham, Taylor learned that the ham eaten by the patients came from five different distributors. How likely would one uncommon serotype come from five different distributors who, in turn, secured their ham from different producers? The logic was overwhelming: despite a reasonable food source of the salmonella and persuasive statistics, the ham was not the source of the salmonella, and more questioning had to be done.

At this same time another identical epidemic of salmonella was reported in Michigan. Having more cases to work with and focusing on possible unique characteristics of the teenage/young adult population, the team asked many more questions of cases and controls including questions about the use of drugs. To their great surprise, they found a highly significant association between illness and smoking marijuana. Although this association seemed as equally implausible as that with ham, samples of marijuana smoked by the cases were culture positive for *S. muenchen*, strongly incriminating the marijuana as the vehicle of infection.

Plan a More Systematic Study

The actual field investigation and analyses have now been completed, requiring only a written report (see below). However, because there may be a need to find more cases, to define better the extent of the epidemic, or to evaluate a new laboratory method or case-finding technique, you may want to perform more detailed and carefully executed studies. With the pressure of the investigation somewhat removed, consider surveying the population at risk in a variety of ways to help improve the quality of data and answer particular questions.

Perhaps the most important reasons to perform such studies are to improve the sensitivity and specificity of the case definition and establish more accurately the true number of persons at risk, that is, to improve the quality of numerators and denominators. For example, serosurveys coupled with a more complete clinical history can often sharpen the accuracy of the case count and define more clearly those truly at risk of developing disease. Moreover, repeated interviews of patients with confirmed disease may allow for rough quantitation of degrees of exposure or dose responses—useful information in understanding the pathogenesis of certain diseases.

Prepare a Written Report

Frequently, your final responsibility is to prepare a written report to document the investigation, the findings, and the recommendations (see Chapter 10). There are several important reasons why a report should be written and as soon as possible:

A document for action

Sometimes control and prevention efforts will only be taken when a report of all relevant findings has been written. This can and should place a heavy, but necessary, burden on the field team to complete its work quickly. Even if all possible cases have not yet been found or some laboratory results are still pending, reasonable written assumptions and recommendations can usually be made without fear of retraction or subsequent major change.

A record of performance

In this day of input and output measurements, program planning, program justifications, and performance evaluations, there is often no better record of accomplishment than a well-written report of a completed field investigation. The number of investigations performed and the time and resources expended not only document the magnitude of health problems, changes in disease trends, and the results of control and prevention efforts but also serve as concrete evidence of program justification and needs.

A document for potential medical/legal issues

Presumably, epidemiologists investigate epidemics with objective, unbiased, and scientific purposes and similarly prepare written reports of their findings and conclusions objectively, honestly, and fairly. Such information may prove absolutely invaluable to consumers, practicing physicians, or local and state health department officials in any legal action regarding health responsibilities and jurisdictions (see Chapter 14). In the long run, the health of the public is best served by simple, careful, honest documentation of events and findings made available to all for interpretation and comment.

Enhancement of the quality of the investigation

Although not fully understood and rarely referred to, the actual process of writing and viewing data in written form often generates new and different thought processes and associations in one's mind (see Chapter 10). The discipline of committing to paper the clinical, laboratory, and epidemiologic findings of an epidemic investigation almost always will bring to light a better understanding of the natural unfolding of events and their importance in terms of the natural history and development of the epidemic. The actual process of creating scientific prose, summarizing data, and creating tables and figures representing the known established facts forces you to view the entire series of events in a balanced, rational, and explainable way. This process is considerably more demanding than preparing an oral report to give to the local health department the day of departure from the field. Occasionally, previously unrecognized associations will emerge from a careful, step-by-step written analysis that may be critically important in the final interpretation and recommendations. The exercise of writing what was done and what was found will sometimes uncover facts and events that were more or less assumed to be true, but not specifically sought for during the investigation. This, in turn, may stimulate further inquiry and fact finding in order to verify these assumptions.

An instrument for teaching epidemiology

There would hardly be disagreement among epidemiologists that the exercise of writing the results of an investigation constitutes an essential building block in learning epidemiology. Much the way a lawyer prepares a brief, the epidemiologist should know how to organize and present in logical sequence the important and pertinent findings of an investigation, their quality and validity, and the scientific inferences that can be made by their written presentation. The simple, direct, and orderly array of facts and inferences will not only reflect the quality of the investigation itself but also the writer's basic understanding and knowledge of the epidemiologic method.

Execute control and prevention measures

It is not the purpose of this chapter to discuss this aspect of a field investigation. Nevertheless, the underlying purposes of all epidemic investigations are to control and/or prevent further disease.

SUMMARY

The field investigation is a direct application of the epidemiologic method very often with an implied and relatively circumscribed timetable. This forces field epidemiologists to: (1) establish workable case finding techniques; (2) collect data rapidly but carefully; and (3) describe cases in a general sense regarding the time and place of occurrence and those primarily affected. Usually, you will know the agent and its sources and modes of transmission, which will allow you to identify the source and mode of spread rapidly. However, when the clinical disease is obscure and/or the origin of the agent ill-defined, you may be hard-pressed to create a hypothesis that will not only identify the critical exposure and show statistical significance but will logically explain the occurrence of the epidemic. Although you will not be able to prove, scientifically, causation in the strictest sense, in most instances the careful development of epidemiologic inferences, coupled with persuasive clinical and laboratory data, will almost always provide convincing evidence as to why the epidemic occurred. Lastly, a written report sharpens your communication and epidemiologic skills and provides the health community with permanent documentation of the investigation.

REFERENCES

1. Centers for Disease Control and Prevention (1977). Unpublished data.
2. Glick, T.H., Gregg, M.B., Berman, B., et al. (1978). Pontiac fever. An epidemic of unknown etiology in a health department. I. Clinical and epidemiological aspects. *Am J Epidemiol* 107, 149–60.
3. Rosenberg, M.D., Hazlet, K.K., Schaefer, J., et al. (1976). Shigellosis from swimming. *JAMA* 236, 1849–52.
4. Centers for Disease Control (1989). Multiple outbreaks of staphylococcal food poisoning caused by canned mushrooms. *MMWR* 38, 417–18.
5. Schlech, W.F. III, Lavigne, P.M., Bortobussi, R.A., et al. (1983). Epidemic listeriosis—evidence for transmission by food. *N Engl J Med* 308, 203–6.
6. Taylor, D.N., Wachsmith, K., Shangkuan, Y., et al. (1982). Salmonellosis associated marijuana. A multistate outbreak traced by plasmid fingerprinting. *N Engl J Med* 306, 1249–53.

6

DESCRIBING THE FINDINGS

Robert E. Fontaine
Richard A. Goodman

As a field epidemiologist, one of the first things you will do will be to collect or be presented with data from outbreak investigations, surveillance systems, vital statistics, or other sources of information—all for appropriate analysis. One of the fundamental "tasks" will be to orient and organize these data to construct useful and relevant presentations and interpretations. This task is called *descriptive epidemiology*. Descriptive epidemiology answers the following questions about disease occurrence: How much? When? Where? and among Whom? The first dimension, "How much?", is expressed as counts or rates, while the last three dimensions are usually referred to as time, place, and person. Time, place, and person have universally standardized units of measurement (e.g., years, longitude and latitude, county, or age group) that can be applied both to the cases or events under study and the underlying population. Once the data are organized and appropriately displayed, the practice of descriptive epidemiology then involves interpretation of these patterns that should allow the epidemiologist to construct ideas that explain why illness or adverse health events occurred—in other words, to generate hypotheses.

In epidemics and other health-related events, the causative agents and exposures to these agents are usually not distributed randomly with regard to the time, place, and person; but assume a unique profile of their own. In descriptive epidemiology these patterns are contrasted with the expected patterns or norms, and inferences are then made. Through this process of organization, inspection, and interpretation of data, descriptive epidemiology serves several purposes. It:

- Provides a systematic method for dissecting a health problem into its component parts.
- Ensures that you are fully versed in the basic dimensions of a health problem.
- Helps identify populations at increased risk of the health problem under investigation.
- Provides immediate information that may be given to decision makers, the media, the public, and others regarding the progress of investigations and the relative probabilities of different causative factors.
- Enables generation of testable hypotheses relevant to the etiology, mode of exposure, effectiveness of control, and other aspects of the health problem.
- Provides validation of eventual incriminated factors. Whether you use analytic epidemiology, microbiology, or experimental studies, these methods must explain the observed patterns by time, place, and person.

COUNTS—WHAT IS THE NUMERATOR?

The simplest way to determine the extent of a health problem is to count cases or events. Cases are customarily organized in a line-listing format as shown in Table 6–1),[1] or in Table A–2 in the Appendix at the end of the book. Whether on paper, index cards, or as a computerized database, this arrangement makes it easier to regroup and count cases by their characteristics. Cases may be either incident cases or prevalent cases. Incident cases or health events are changes in the status of an individual—from well to ill, from uninfected to infected, from alive to dead. Prevalent cases represent the existing status of an individual— well, ill, uninfected, infected, alive, deceased. Incident cases are determined by following individuals over time and counting those who change their status. If the change in status is overt, a population may be followed and incident cases identified through public health surveillance or other health information systems. On the other hand, prevalent cases are determined by taking a measurement on individuals usually at one point in time. Prevalence is determined by two factors:

- Incidence, which converts an individual from an unaffected state to an affected state, and
- Recovery (or death), which converts the affected state to another state.

Table 6–1. A Line Listing of Cases of Intussusception by State, Gender, Number of Doses of Rotavirus Vaccine Received, and Onset of Symptoms in Days Following Immunization

STATE	AGE [MOS]	SEX	NO. DOSES OF VACCINE RECEIVED	NO. DAYS FROM DOSE TO SYMPTOM ONSET
California	7	M	2	4
California	4	F	2	14
California	3	M	1	3
California	5	M	1	59
Colorado	4	F	1	4
Colorado	3	M	1	5
Kansas	2	F	1	5
Missouri	11	M	1	5
New York	3	F	1	5
New York	2	M	1	3
North Carolina	4	F	1	5
Pennsylvania	6	M	1	3
Pennsylvania	2	M	1	4
Pennsylvania	2	M	1	29
Pennsylvania	3	M	1	7

For diseases or conditions with a fairly long duration (years or decades) and negligible mortality, incident cases may be estimated by taking periodic measurements of the prevalent state of the individuals. Incident cases must be counted over a specified time period, whereas a count of prevalent cases has no dimension in time. Figure 6–1 shows time lines representing 10 illnesses among 20 individuals over 16 months.[2] Between October 1, 1990, and September 30, 1991, 4 had onset of disease and are, therefore, incident cases of illness during the year period. At a specific point in time, April 1, 1991, there are 7 persons with disease, and, therefore, they are prevalent cases. It is always critical to know if data sources you use are providing incident or prevalent cases. Similarly, you should not mix incident with prevalent cases in the analyses.

RATES

Once counted, either incident or prevalent cases may be compared to their historical norm, expressed as an expected value or distribution. For instance, we might expect that, based on the experience in the previous 5 years that 175 incident cases of hepatitis A would be expected in the current year for a specific urban area. If double that number were actually observed, we might conclude that the area is experiencing an increase in transmission of hepatitis A. However, these simple case counts are valid for epidemiologic comparisons only when they come from the same or nearly the same population. Suppose that in a large urban county twice the number of persons developed hepatitis A than in a small rural county. Is the urban dweller twice as likely to contract hepatitis than the rural dweller? Clearly, the hepatitis A count depends upon the number of persons available to acquire hepatitis A. In this example the excess number may simply reflect the far larger population of the urban area.

Therefore, to make valid comparisons of health events between population groups and to assess the issue of risk, cases must be assessed in light of the size of the population they came from. Rates, then, rather than simple numbers, must be determined by relating case counts to the population under study. Through the use of rates you may determine whether one group is at increased risk of disease and to what degree. From a population perspective, these so-called high-risk groups can be further targeted for special intervention. From an individual perspective, by comparing rates, you may also identify risk factors for disease. Identification of these risk factors may be used by individuals in their day-to-day decision making about behaviors that influence their health. A variety of rates, ratios, and derivatives thereof are used in epidemiology to quantify risk. In descriptive epidemiology only a few elementary rates are widely used and include incidence, cumulative incidence, prevalence, specific rates, and adjusted rates.

Incidence Rates

All incidence rates involve counts of incident cases over a defined time period in a defined population. The numerator is the number of incident cases in a time period and is called incidence. The denominator is normally the midpoint estimate of the population from which the cases arose. Returning to Figure 6–1, we see that the 4 incident cases occurred in a population of 20 persons at the beginning of the year. [Note: only sick persons are represented. The well (10 persons) are not shown.] Two persons died of the disease before the middle of the year, leaving a midpoint population of 18. Thus, the incidence rate for the year is 4/18 per year or 22 per 100 per year. Clearly, this is an artificial example, since in a natural population births, deaths, immigration, and emigration will affect the midyear population. However, normally, these are estimated from census data. A wide range of standard morbidity and mortality incidence rates are available for routine use in field epidemiology (Table 6–2).[2]

Attack Rates or Cumulative Incidence Rates

Whereas many morbidity and mortality rates use standard time periods, certain situations such as outbreaks, epidemics, or problems in limited populations re-

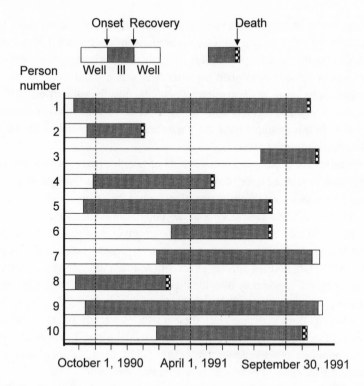

Figure 6–1. Ten episodes of an illness in a population of 20 [*Source*: CDC, 1992.[2]]

quire counting incident cases over limited periods of time. For these attack rates or cumulative incidence rates, the denominator is the population at risk at the beginning of the time period. Theoretically, persons who are not at risk, for example, because of previous disease or infection, are not included in this denominator. In the example (Fig. 6–1) between October 1, 1990 and September 30, 1991, 4 incident cases occurred. The population at risk was 20 at the beginning of the period yielding an attack rate of 4/20 or 20% for the 12-month period. If knowledge of preexisting disease were available, we would then also subtract previously affected persons from the denominator. You must be careful, when comparing attack rates to standard morbidity incidence rates, to adjust both rates to the same time period.

Secondary Attack Rates

A secondary attack rate is a measure of the frequency of new cases of a disease among contacts of cases. A secondary attack rate equals the number of cases among

Table 6–2. Frequently Used Measures of Morbidity

MEASURE	NUMERATOR (x)	DENOMINATOR (Y)	EXPRESSED PER NUMBER AT RISK (10^N)
Incidence rate	No. new cases of a specific disease reported during a given time interval	Average population during time interval	Varies: 10^n where $n = 2,3,4,5,6$
Attack rate	No. new cases of a specified disease reported during an epidemic period	Population at start of the epidemic period	Varies: 10^n where $n = 2,3,4,5,6$
Secondary attack rate	No. new cases of a specified disease among contacts of known cases	Size of contact population at risk	Varies: 10^n where $n = 2,3,4,5,6$
Point prevalence	No. current cases, new and old, of a specified disease at a given point in time	Estimated population at the same point in time	Varies: 10^n where $n = 2,3,4,5,6$

[*Source*: CDC, 1992.[2]]

contacts of primary cases during the study period divided by the total number of contacts. To calculate the total number of household contacts we normally subtract the number of primary cases from the total number of people residing in those households.

For example, 7 cases of hepatitis A occurred among 70 children attending a child care center. Each infected child came from a different family. The total number of persons in the seven affected families was 32, including the 7 infected children and 25 contacts. One generation period later, 5 family contacts also developed hepatitis A. The secondary attack rate then is: 5 infected contacts/ 25 contacts or 20%.[2]

Multiple cases in households or other living groups could also arise from food, water, or factors other than person-to-person transmission. Accordingly, you should determine that the timing between the cases in a household is compatible with secondary transmission. Also, you should always compare rates in these groups to the rates in the general population without the presumption that the cases are secondary.

Person–Time Incidence Rates

A person–time incidence rate directly incorporates time into the denominator. Typically, each person is observed from a set beginning point to an established end point (onset of disease, death, migration out of the group, or into the group). The numerator is still the number of new cases, but the denominator is a little different. The denominator is a sum of the time each person is observed, totaled for all persons. Therefore, the person–time rate equals the number of cases detected during the observation period divided by the time each person was observed, totaled for all persons.

For example, a person enrolled in a study who develops a disease of interest 5 years later contributes 5 person-years to the denominator. A person who is disease free is followed for 1 year, and, subsequently, is lost to follow-up and contributes 1 person-year plus one-half of the subsequent year (if the follow-up intervals are years) to the denominator.

Person–time rates are often used in cohort (follow-up) studies of diseases with long incubation or latency periods, such as some occupationally related diseases, AIDS, and chronic diseases. In addition, the person–time rates may be very useful in acute outbreaks or special surveillance systems where individuals may spend extremely variable periods of time in the general area of exposure (e.g., in nosocomial infection outbreaks where duration in the hospital may vary markedly between individuals).

Prevalence Rates

Prevalence rates reflect the proportion of the population that has an existing condition (prevalent cases). Point prevalence means that the measurement on each individual is made at one point in time. In the example (see Fig. 6–1), the 7 prevalent cases on April 1 were among 18 (living) individuals yielding a point prevalence rate of 7/18 = 39%.

Historically, prevalence has been less utilized than incidence in field epidemiology. However, more recently, a number of conditions measured by prevalence (e.g., blood lead levels, birth defects, and behavioral risk factors) have come under surveillance and, accordingly, been routinely scrutinized by field epidemiologists. In addition, the prevalence rates before, during, and after an outbreak may be compared to make estimations of incidence in situations when incidence cannot be measured directly.

Ratios and Alternative Denominators

In some situations the population at risk is unknown, costly to determine, or even inappropriate. In these situations you must consider using alternative denominators to estimate risk or compare risks among population groups. These resultant quotients are properly termed *ratios* rather than rates.

Commonly used ratios include an infant mortality rate, a maternal mortality ratio, and a case-to-death ratio (Table 6–3). To assess adverse effects from a vaccine or pharmaceutical you might use total doses distributed, since the actual numbers of individuals who received the product may be difficult to obtain. Similarly, in a food-borne outbreak you might use restaurant receipts or the number of portions of a suspect food served as a denominator rather than the actual number of persons visiting the restaurant or eating a food. Injuries from snowmobile usage have been calculated, both as ratios per registered vehicles and as per crash incident (Fig. 6–2).[3]

TIME, PLACE, AND PERSON

In the preceding overview we have referred to counts or rates in populations. In order to identify and depict epidemiologically relevant patterns, these counts and rates should be organized by time, place, and person.

Depicting Data by Time

Since all field studies take place over a certain time frame, the field epidemiologist will need to know how to organize and describe these time patterns in the effort to understand the health event being studied. Rates should be used whenever possible. However, for short time periods in stable populations, you may safely organize only numerator data to identify time patterns.

Health events may present with several important time characteristics. Most critical are the time of exposure to risk factors and the time of onset of health events. Other relevant events should also be placed in temporal sequence to help create an accurate chronologic framework for investigating the problem.

The accuracy of this information can vary considerably by situation or disease and may be greater for acute problems that have occurred recently than for those that are chronic in nature. For certain types of problems, the time of precipitating events must be carefully distinguished from the time of occurrence of the outcome (e.g., injury and death).

Events in time may be related to one another. If you know both time of onset and time of known or presumed exposure, you can estimate the incubation or latency period. When the agent is unknown, the time interval between presumed exposure and onset of symptoms is critical in hypothesizing the etiology. If an agent is suspected, then a similar comparison may help to either dispel or reinforce suspicions. For example, the consistent time interval between rotavirus vac-

Table 6–3. Frequently Used Measures of Mortality

MEASURE	NUMERATOR (x)	DENOMINATOR (y)	EXPRESSED PER NUMBER AT RISK (10^N)
Crude death rate	Total number of deaths reported during a given time interval	Estimated midinterval population	1000 or 100,000
Cause-specific death rate	No. deaths assigned to a specific cause during a given time interval	Estimated midinterval population	100,000
Proportional mortality	No. deaths assigned to a specific cause during a given time interval	Total number of deaths from all causes during the same interval	100 or 1000
Death-to-case ratio	No. deaths assigned to a specific disease during a given time interval	No. new cases of that disease reported during the same time interval	100
Neonatal mortality rate	No. deaths under 28 days of age during a given time interval	No. live births during the same time interval	1000
Postneonatal mortality rate	No. deaths from 28 days to, but not including, 1 year of age, during a given time interval	No. live births during the same time interval	1000
Infant mortality rate	No. deaths under 1 year of age during a given time interval	No. live births reported during the same time interval	1000
Maternal mortality rate	No. deaths assigned to pregnancy-related causes during a given time interval	No. live births during the same time interval	100,000

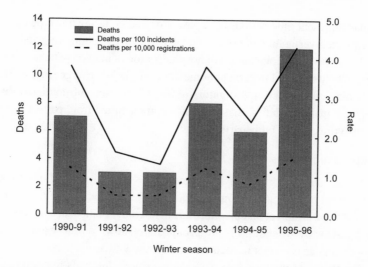

Figure 6–2. Number of deaths and death rates per snowmobile-related incident and per snowmobile registration—Maine, 1990–91 through 1995–96 winter seasons. [*Source*: CDC, 1997.[3]]

cination and onset of intussusception (see Table 6–1) helped build the hypothesis that the vaccine precipitated the disease. Similarly, when the incubation period is known, the time interval of exposure may be estimated and potential exposures during that interval may be identified.

Identification of special events or certain unusual circumstances temporally related to the problem may also help in the formulation of relevant hypotheses. These principles are illustrated in the depiction of the incidence of malaria in the United States as shown for the period 1930–1998, which compares incidence rates to important modifying events (see Fig. 3–1).[4]

Graphic display of time data provides a simple visual depiction of the relative magnitude, past and current trends, potential future course of the problem, and the impact of specified related events. Depending on the health event you are studying, the time period may include years, months, weeks, days, or even hours. For chronic diseases or other conditions, time is usually depicted as a secular trend—the annual rate plotted over many years or decades. For more acute conditions, incident cases or incidence rates are plotted. For acute disease the ideal point in time to plot is the onset of disease. However, in surveillance systems the date of report is often the only available time information.

Time line

For small numbers of cases the critical times may be graphed on a simple time line. Points on time lines can represent disease onset or point exposures, while bars may represent time periods of exposure or illness. Using this type of graphic device for an investigation of nosocomial malaria, investigators were able to demonstrate a time–space coincidence of hospitalization of malaria patients with other patients who developed malaria at home after hospital discharge (Fig. 6–3). This data display quickly led investigators to the hypothesis, substantiated through subsequent analytic studies, that malaria was transmitted from patient to patient through syringes used on heparin locks.[5]

Epidemic curves

As case numbers increase, a histogram gives a better view of onset times of a health event (see Figure A–1 in Appendix at end of book). If the time period of interest is the duration of an epidemic, this histogram is called an epidemic curve. Time intervals by which onsets are grouped are shown on the x axis while the corresponding case counts in each interval on the y axis.

The choice of the time interval used is critical. Intervals that are too short (like hours for diseases with long incubation periods) may overemphasize random noise in the underlying pattern and hinder interpretation. Intervals that are too long (like weeks for diseases with short incubation periods) will group many cases into a few intervals and obscure the real pattern. As a general rule, intervals between one-fourth to one-half an incubation/latency period work best at revealing the time pattern of an epidemic. As case numbers increase, shorter intervals will reveal more detail to the pattern (Fig. 6–4, A, B).[6]

A second point is where to begin and end the x axis. You should show when the epidemic started with a sufficient lead period to demonstrate the pre-epidemic background. Similarly, extend the time sufficiently after the last case to convinc-

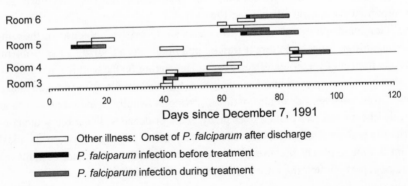

Figure 6–3. Duration of hospitalization in days and location by rooms of 7 *Plasmodium falciparum* patients and 14 other patients who developed *P. falciparum* infections after discharge from Riyadh Central Hospital, Pediatric ward 2, Riyadh, Saudi Arabia, December 1991–April 1992.

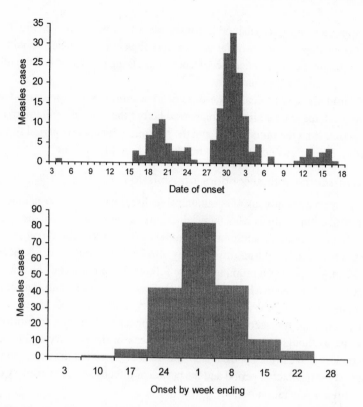

Figure 6–4. Measles cases by (A) day or (B) week of rash onset—Saint Louis County, Missouri, and Jersey County, Illinois, April 4–May 17, 1994. [*Source:* CDC, 1994.[6]]

ingly show the end of the epidemic. Usually two incubation periods before and after are necessary and in some situations more may be necessary. This will also reveal possible source cases, secondary transmission, and other outliers of interest.

Labels should be used to designate cases of special importance (e.g., those suspected of introducing the disease agent or playing an essential role in propagating the outbreak), time periods, or events related to the outbreak.

As mentioned in Chapter 2, there are a variety of ways diseases are transmitted. The epidemic curves you draw will often reveal these modes of transmission. The following are certain kinds of epidemic situations that can frequently be "diagnosed" by simple, appropriate plotting of cases on graph paper.

Point source

An epidemic curve that shows a tight clustering of cases in time (less than 1.5 times the range of the incubation period if the agent is known) with a sharp upslope and a trailing downslope is consistent with a point source (Fig. 6–5).[7] Variations in slopes (e.g., bimodal or a broader than expected peak) should suggest ideas about the appearance, persistence, and disappearance of and the differences in exposure to the source.

In point source outbreaks, the time of exposure may be approximated by counting back the average incubation period before the peak, the minimum incubation period from the initial cases, and the maximum incubation period from the last cases. These three points should bracket the time of exposure.

Point source with secondary transmission

A point source outbreak of communicable disease produces substantial numbers of infected individuals who, themselves, may serve as sources of the agent to infect others. Although such transmission may often be through direct personal contact, other vehicles of transmission may also lead to secondary cases. Secondary cases may appear as a prominent wave following a point source by one incubation period, as noted in a hepatitis E outbreak resulting from repairs on a broken water main (Fig. 6–6).[8] With diseases of shorter incubation and lower rates of secondary spread, the secondary wave may appear only as a more prolonged downslope. Although the period between the peak of the primary outbreak and the secondary wave often approximates the incubation period, it is really a combination of the incubation period and the period of infectivity of the primary cases and is called a generation period.[9,10]

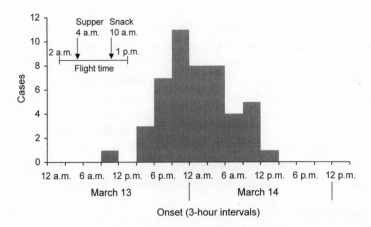

Figure 6–5. Cases of Salmonellosis in passengers on a flight from London to the United States, by time of onset, March 13–14, 1984. [*Source:* Tauxe et al., 1987.[7]]

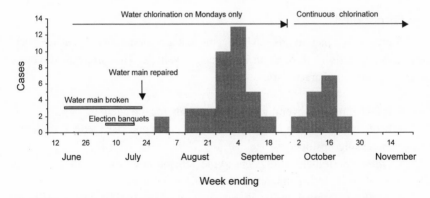

Figure 6–6. Cases of jaundice by week of onset, June–October 1999, Jaf'r, Ma'an Governorate, Jordan. [*Source*: Ministry of Health, Jordan, 1999.[8]]

Continuing common source

Outbreaks may arise from common sources that continue over time. The epidemic curve will rise sharply as with a point source. Rather than rise to a peak, this type of epidemic curve will find a plateau. The downslope may be precipitous if the common source is removed or gradual if it exhausts itself. All three of these features can be seen on an epidemic curve for a salmonellosis outbreak involving cheese distributed to multiple restaurants (Fig. 6–7).[11]

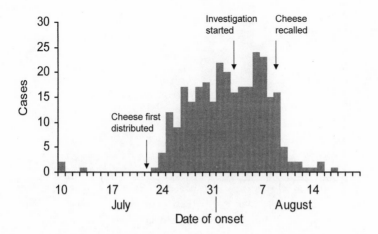

Figure 6–7. Cases of *Salmonella heidelberg* infection, by onset, Colorado, July 10–August 17, 1976. [*Source*: Fontaine et al., 1980.[11]]

Propagated

A propagated pattern arises with agents that are communicable between persons either directly or through an intermediate vehicle. This propagated pattern has four principal characteristics:

- It encompasses several generation periods for the agent.
- It often begins with a small number of cases and rises with a gradually increasing upslope.
- Often a periodicity equivalent to the generation period for the agent may be obvious during the initial stages of the outbreak.
- After the outbreak peaks, the exhaustion of susceptible hosts usually results in a rapid downslope.

An outbreak of rubella illustrates these features including an approximate 3 week periodicity (Fig. 6–8).[12] Certain behaviors such as drug addiction and mass sociogenic illness may propagate from person to person, but the epidemic curve will not necessarily reflect generation times. Propagation between individuals generally represents a circumscribed, localized occurrence. Epidemic curves for large areas such as states, large cities, or heavily populated counties may not reveal the periodicity or the characteristic rise and fall of a propagated outbreak. For these larger areas it is important to stratify the epidemic curves by smaller subunits.

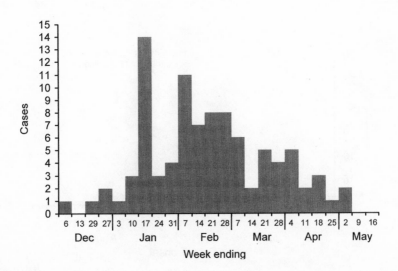

Figure 6–8. Confirmed cases of rubella, by week of rash onset—Westchester County, New York, December 1997–May 1998. [*Source*: CDC, 1999.[12]]

Environmental

Epidemic curves from environmentally spread diseases reflect complex inter-actions between the agent and the environment and the factors that lead to exposure of humans to the environmental source. Outbreaks that arise from environmental sources will usually encompass several generation or incubation periods for the agent. They differ from propagated outbreaks in that they normally do not show the peri-odicity that approximates the generation time of the agent. In addition, a gradually increasing upslope and a rapid downslope are normally seen only with zoonoses where the natural animal host itself is experiencing a propagated outbreak.

The epidemiologist should attempt to include on the epidemic curve a repre-sentation of the suspected environmental factor as is done in Figure 6–9 with rain-fall for an outbreak of leptospirosis.[13] In this example nearly every peak of rainfall precedes a peak in leptospirosis, supporting the hypothesis of the importance of water in transmission.

Zoonotic

The epidemic curve for a zoonotic disease in humans will generally repre-sent the variations in prevalence among the reservoir animal population as it is

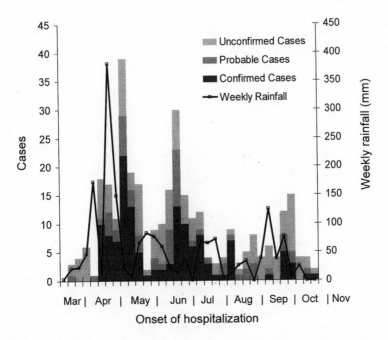

Figure 6–9. Cases of leptospirosis by week of hospitalization and rainfall in Sal-vador, Brazil, March 10–November 2, 1996. [*Source*: Ko et al., 1999.[13]]

modified by the variability of contact between humans and the reservoir animal. Since zoonoses often grow rapidly among reservoir hosts, the epidemic curve among humans may also appear as a rapid rise. This tendency can be appreciated in the West Nile virus outbreak in New York City (Fig. 6–10).[14]

Vector-borne

Vector-borne diseases (excluding mechanical transmission) propagate between an arthropod vector and a vertebrate host. Because two incubation periods (an extrinsic one in the vector and an intrinsic one in the human) are involved, the generation times tend to be longer than for person-to-person outbreaks. The early phase of these outbreaks tends to develop more slowly. Three additional biologic factors profoundly affect the shape of the epidemic curve.

- Arthropod vectors, once infected, characteristically remain so until they perish. This tends to prolong and stabilize vector-borne outbreaks and smear any underlying propagative periodicity.
- Environmental temperatures exert a marked effect on the development and multiplication of infectious agents in an arthropod.
- Arthropod populations may grow explosively and can "crash" even more rapidly.

These last two factors will lead to irregular peaks during the progression of the outbreak and precipitous decreases.

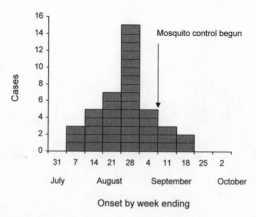

Figure 6–10. Number of seropositive cases of West Nile virus, by week of onset—New York City, 1999. [*Source*: CDC, 1999.[14]]

An outbreak of *Plasmodium falciparum* malaria under highly favorable environmental conditions in Saudi Arabia shows several of these features (Fig. 6–11).[15] The outbreak developed very slowly until after week 7. Although periodic peaks typical of a propagated outbreak are not apparent, a stepwise increase with a 3–4 week period is noticeable. Finally, the outbreak declines abruptly after control of adult vectors.

Many vector-borne diseases are zoonoses in which the agent propagates in a non-human host while humans are a dead-end host. The West Nile virus epidemic in New York in 1999 revealed a rapid rise and a fairly abrupt decrease, perhaps related to a sudden decline in the vector population or exhaustion of the susceptible zoonotic population in late August of that year (see Fig. 6–10).[14]

Multiple strata display

To assess whether critical epidemiologic times show distinctive internal patterns (e.g., by exposure, method of case detection, place, or personal characteristics) epidemic curves should be stratified. For example, in a continuing common source outbreak of typhoid fever, stratification revealed that confirmed cases both began and ended earlier among hospital staff than among the community or military base personnel (Fig. 6–12).[16] The reason for the time difference was related to the hospital's obtaining water from a commercial well while its own well was under repair. New cases among hospital staff ceased to occur 1 week after the hospital began using its own well again. The commercial well also sold water

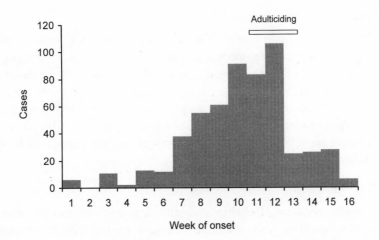

Figure 6–11. *Plasmodium falciparum* infections by week of onset of fever, Gelwa, Al-Baha Region, Saudi Arabia, January–April 1996. [*Source:* Ministry of Health, Saudi Arabia, 1996.[15]]

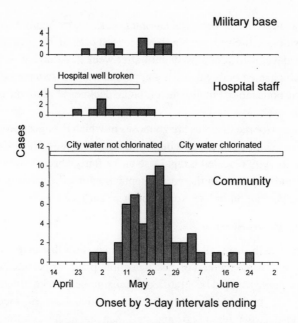

Figure 6–12. Cases of typhoid fever by date of onset, Tabuk, Saudi Arabia, April–June 1992. [*Source*: Al-Qawari et al., 1995.[16]]

through three outlets in the community, and cases decreased in both the community and a nearby military base about 1 to 2 weeks after chlorination was enforced.

Examining rates in time

Whereas case counts over time are usually graphed as a histogram, disease rates over time are usually graphed with a line graph or a frequency polygon (see Appendix 6–1). The x axis represents a period of time of interest: decades, years, months, or days of the week. The y axis represents the rate of the health event. For most conditions, when the rates vary over one or two orders of magnitude, an arithmetic scale is appropriate. For rates which vary more widely and/or when comparisons are to be made, a logarithmic scale for the y axis may be more appropriate.

Secular trend

For some conditions, including many chronic diseases, the time characteristic of interest is the secular trend—the rate of disease over many years. Review of these secular trends may suggest or indicate key events, improvements in control, sociologic phenomena, or other factors that have modified the epidemiology of the condition. Secular trends are most often shown on a line graph along with important modifying factors. The secular trend of malaria from 1930 to 1998 may thus be compared to important events that influenced malaria incidence (see Fig. 3–1).

Cyclical, seasonal, and other cycles

For many conditions, a description by season, month, day of the week, or even time of day may be revealing. For example, the incidence of varicella appears to be seasonal, since outbreaks tend to occur between March and May (Fig. 6–13).[17] Seasonal patterns may also be summarized in a seasonal or cyclical curve (see Appendix 6–1). These in turn may be stratified by place or person or other features to compare or contrast patterns. For instance, the pattern of seasonality shows distinct differences between villages and *Plasmodium* species in El Salvador (Fig. 6–14).[18]

Examining Data by Place

Place represents another dimension for organizing and identifying patterns of epidemiologic data. Indeed, careful localization of cases can provide clear insight into an epidemiologic process. As with time, rates are important, but not necessary in every situation.

Information on place may include residence, workplace, school, recreation site, other relevant locales, or even movement between these fixed geographic points. Always distinguish between place of onset, place of exposure, and place of case identification: they are often different and have distinct epidemiologic implications. Information on place may range in precision from the geographic

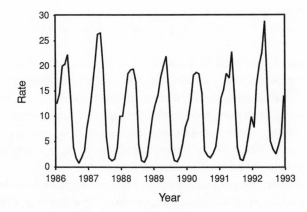

Figure 6–13. Rate (reported cases per 100,000 population) of Varicella (Chickenpox)—United States, 1986–1992. [*Source*: CDC, 1992.[17]]

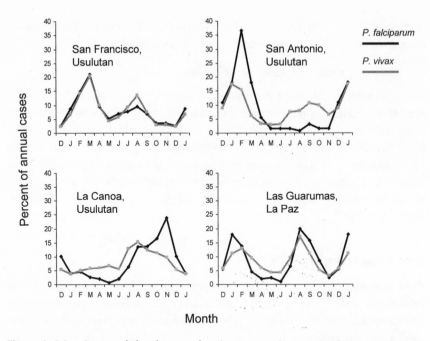

Figure 6–14.   Seasonal distribution of malaria cases by month of detection by voluntary collaborators in four villages, El Salvador, 1970–1977. [*Source*: Fontaine et al., 1984.[18]]

coordinates of a residence or bed in a hospital to simply the state of residence. Since population estimates or censuses are limited to standard geographic areas (e.g., city, census tract, county, state, or country), determination of rates is also restricted to these same areas.

Maps

Place data are best organized, displayed, and examined on maps. Maps give you the ability to compare rates of disease by place. Maps display a wealth of underlying detail to compare with disease distribution. And maps allow quick recognition and comparisons relative to tables or other data displays. A simple, comparative display of rates by place on a table or chart may appear to show only minor differences. However, on a map, a spatial trend or aggregation of higher rates in one area might be more evident.

Spot Maps: In outbreak investigations, cases can be plotted on a base map, a floor plan, or other spatially accurate diagram to create a spot map. Cases may be represented as dots, other symbols, or even case identification numbers for indexing with a line-listing. With the availability of hand-held geographic positioning units and satellite images of the earth's surface, cases may be plotted precisely over a detailed picture of the earth's surface.

A spot map of an airplane cabin (Fig. 6–15) shows where passengers (who later became ill) sat in relation to the source case.[19] Although a map scale or scale bar is normally a necessity on maps, in this example the distances between seats on a Boeing 747 are familiar. Spot maps that do not show spatial aggregation of cases may suggest a widespread environmental source, a distribution system (e.g., for food, water, or other product), or dispersal of individuals from a common area.

Instead of showing the location of individual cases within a town (or other small geographic unit), spots or symbols may represent affected houses, towns, or other population units. In this situation the spots may also represent rates or ratios, if sufficient cases are present in each unit and a denominator is known.

Spot maps that show only numerator data have a general weakness. The pattern of cases could represent a distinctive quality of the health event, variability in the underlying population distribution, or a combination of the two. Accordingly, the epidemiologist should only use case spot maps within areas of relatively uniform population density such as inside town boundaries. Even fairly uniform populations may encompass unpopulated areas (e.g., parks, vacant lots, abandoned warehouses). Inspect the base maps carefully before interpreting the case distributions.

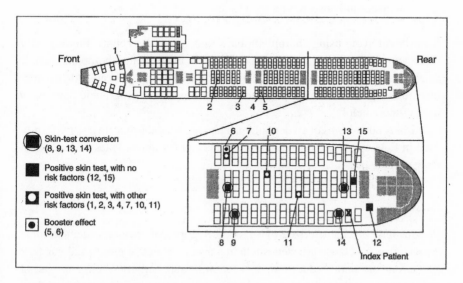

Figure 6–15. Diagram of the Boeing 747-100 with seat assignments of the passengers and flight crew on Flight 4 who had positive tuberculin skin tests. [*Source:* Kenyon et al., 1996.[19]]

Area Maps and Rates: Rates are normally shown by areas on a choropleth (from the Greek *choros* = place, and *plethos* = magnitude) map. The map is divided into population enumeration areas for which rates (or ratios) may be computed. The areas are then ranked according to their respective rates, and the ranking is broken up into intervals and shaded (see Appendix 6–1). Choropleth maps represent an essential tool in descriptive epidemiology, because they are very easy to construct and give good representations of spatial distributions of rates and ratios.

To reveal underlying patterns in the data, try to increase the data density on these maps by computing rates for the smallest area possible. For example, the county map of Lyme disease in the United States effectively displays several levels of risk for human infection (Fig. 6–16).[20]

Although choropleth maps are the epidemiologic standard for geographic displaying of rates and ratios, they have several disadvantages:

- They lack the detailed geographic localization provided by spot maps.
- They visually overemphasize large, sparsely populated areas.
- Areas with unstable rates (small numerators and denominators) may confuse the visual display.
- The areas are portrayed as if they were internally homogeneous, thus masking any internal variability within the geographic unit.
- Features from other map layers that might be used for epidemiologic comparisons are obscured by the shading.

You should avoid using choropleth maps to display case counts. Plotting only numerators loses the advantages of both the spot map and the choropleth map. If small numbers of cases must be shown over a wide geographic area, then a spot map showing the relationship of the cases to important geographic features is usually more helpful.

Many other forms of epidemiologic maps are available but are less frequently used in field epidemiology (e.g., cartograms and isarithmic maps). More detail on these may be found in other texts.[21–23]

Person

Persons may be characterized by several categories of attributes: demographic characteristics of those affected (including age, race, ethnic group, and gender); socioeconomic status; education; occupation; leisure activities; religion; marital status; contact with other persons or groups; and other personal variables (such as pregnancy, blood type, immunization status, underlying illnesses, or use of medi-

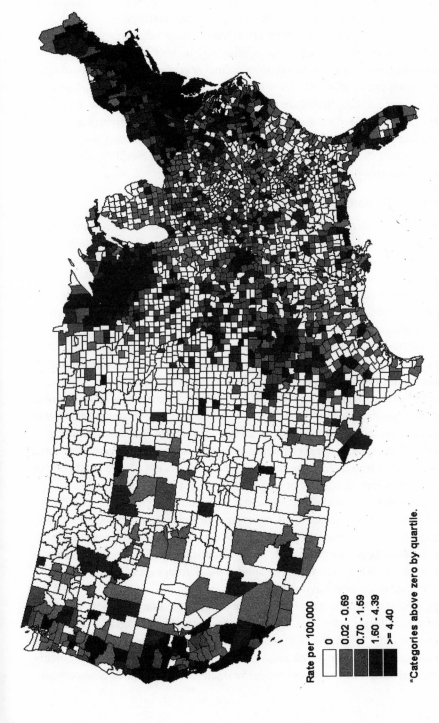

Rate per 100,000

☐ 0
▨ 0.02 - 0.69
▨ 0.70 - 1.59
▨ 1.60 - 4.39
■ >= 4.40

*Categories above zero by quartile.

Figure 6–16. Average annual rate of Lyme disease cases per 100,000 per year in the United States, 1992–1998.
[Source: CDC, 1999.[20]]

cations). The recognition of disease patterns, according to these personal attributes, constitutes the third essential step in descriptive epidemiology.

Information on person can be presented in either tabular or graphic form. Graphic displays of personal characteristics may be very illuminating when one or more personal characteristics is on an ordinal or continuous scale, for example, age or body mass index. Rates for nominative variables alone, such as gender, ethnicity, race, or other traits, are best presented in tabular format. Two important qualifications apply to the assessment of person data. First, determination of rates for person data is far more critical than for time and place. Second, age is one of the strongest independent determinants for many causes of morbidity and mortality and, accordingly, deserves primary consideration.

Personal contact and network groups

Humans characteristically form social groupings. These groups may be as well defined and compact as a family living together in a home or as diffuse as a group linked together only by common interests or behaviors. Description of diseases by family, other well-defined groups, or as diffuse social networks can often uncover patterns that may assist in developing hypotheses. Data concerning these personal linkages are often obtained during initial, exploratory interviews of reported cases.

The underlying epidemiologic process may produce distributions that range from strong aggregation to randomness or to uniformity in a family or household. Clustered distributions may suggest common exposures of household members, an agent that is transmissible from one family member to another, an environmental exposure from the living quarters themselves, localization of the houses near or within an environmental area of high risk, or even human–vector–human transmission in situations where the vector is not highly mobile. In contrast, random or even distributions among households suggest that the exposure lies outside the family unit or that it is uniformly distributed among all units (e.g., a town water supply).

Since census data provide household sizes and numbers of households, denominator data are available, if necessary, to make comparisons. However, assessment of risk among large numbers of small population groups (i.e., families) leads to highly unstable rates. Several statistical packages are available to assess aggregation by household or similar small groupings of people.

For diseases or behaviors spread through personal association or contact (e.g., measles, sexually transmitted diseases, tuberculosis, addiction, and mass sociogenic illness), data concerning linkages between affected individuals are often revealing. Diagrams of these networks showing closeness and quality of relationships, timing between onsets, and places of contact provide a quickly interpretable overview and may reveal key details, such as index cases or outliers (Fig. 6–17).[24]

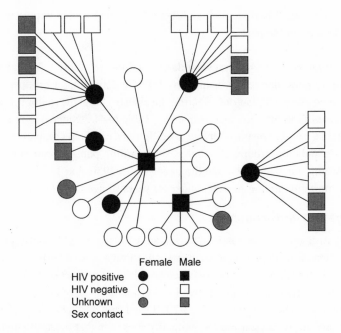

Figure 6–17. Sex network of seven persons with HIV infection—Mississippi, 1999. [*Source*: CDC, 2000.24]

Age

The epidemiologist will determine disease rates by age in virtually all field investigations. This may be as simple as finding that a health event is affecting only a limited age group or as complicated as comparing age-specific incidence rates among several groups of people. Remember that age actually represents three different categories of determinants of disease risk.

- The condition of the host and its susceptibility to disease: Individuals of different ages often differ in susceptibility or predisposition to disease. Clearly, age is one of the most important determinants in the expression of chronic diseases, many infectious diseases, and mortality.
- Differing intensities of exposure to causative agents: For example, infants and young children may be at far greater risk of exposure to organisms spread through the fecal–oral route than older individuals.
- The passage of time: Older individuals will simply have had greater overall time of exposure or may have been exposed at different periods of time when background exposures to certain agents were greater. A disease with

a long latent period, such as tuberculosis, may reflect exposures several decades in the past.

In an analysis of farm tractor–related fatalities in Georgia, age group–specific fatality rates, derived by using two different denominator groups, draws attention to potential risk factors affecting the elderly and to the major difference in risk between farm and nonfarm residence (Table 6–4).[25] Since age is a continuous variable, graphic displays of age-specific rates can help compare differences between population groups. A graph, using semilog paper, comparing age-specific mortality rates in the United States for 1910, 1950, and 1998 reveals reductions of mortality among persons under 60 years of age (Fig. 6–18).[26–28]

Age standardization

Because age is a pervasive determinant of disease and because population groups often differ in their age structures, adjustment or standardization by age is a useful tool for comparing rates between population groups. For example, a comparison of the crude death rates of two Florida counties—Dade and Pinellas counties—for 1960, shows a rate of 15.3/1000 for Dade and 8.9/1000 for Pinellas. Age-specific death rates, however, generally show a higher mortality rate in Dade County. This seemingly contradictory finding can be explained simply by unequal distributions of persons in the various age groups. To "adjust" for these differences you can create a "standard" population by pooling both these two population groups or by using an age distribution from another "representative" population. Finally, you would apply age-specific death rates from each county (or the "representative" population) to those pooled numbers and create new,

Table 6–4. Annual Fatality Rates per 100,000 Males in Accidents Associated with Farm Tractors, Georgia, 1971–1981

AGE GROUP (YEARS)	NUMBER OF DEATHS	FARM RESIDENTS		ALL RURAL RESIDENTS	
		RATE	STANDARD ERROR	RATE	STANDARD ERROR
<20	21	6.7	±1.5	0.5	±0.1
20–39	32	32.3	±4.0	1.1	±0.2
40–59	65	27.6	±3.4	3.1	±0.4
≥60	80	54.1	±6.1	6.4	±0.1
Total	198	23.6		1.9	

[*Source*: Goodman et al., 1992.[25]]

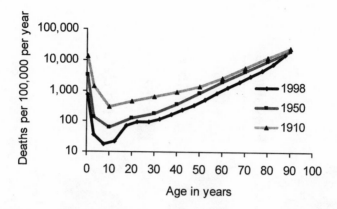

Figure 6-18. Age-specific mortality rates per 100,000 per year, United States, 1910, 1950, and 1998. [*Source:* NCHS, 2001.[26-28]]

supposed age-specific death rates for each county. If you do this, the crude death rates then become 10.9/1000 for Dade County and 10.4/1000 for Pinellas County.[29]

Age-adjusted rates may be used to compare rates among populations from different areas, from the same area at different times, and among any other characteristic such as ethnicity or socioeconomic status. Adjustment produces a summary rate for each population with the effect of age removed. However, at the same time, adjustment hides potentially illuminating patterns in age-specific incidence rates. Accordingly, it is highly advisable to examine age-specific rates in graphic or tabular form before embarking on age standardization.

Other personal attributes

The use of other personal attributes in descriptive epidemiology is limited only by the availability of denominators for computing rates. Most commonly these include gender, ethnicity, race, education, and socioeconomic level.

Combinations of Time, Place, and Person

Often comparisons in descriptive epidemiology will require evaluation of two or even all three of the principal epidemiologic variables. These comparisons are best visualized through a series of small, multiple figures. For instance, the progression of a disease in time across a geographic area may be best shown with a series of small maps (Fig. 6–19).[30] When the shape of the epidemic curve must be compared for different localities or different population groups, a series of small epidemic curves offers an efficient method of comparison (see Fig. 6–12). To reveal tempo-

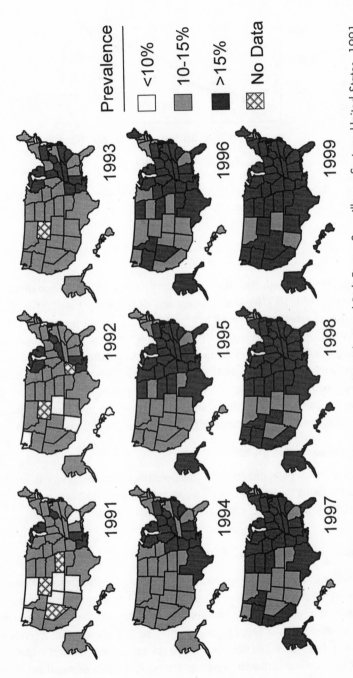

Figure 6-19. Prevalence of overweight among adults, Behavioral Risk Factor Surveillance System, United States, 1991–1999. [*Source: Mokdad et al., 1999.*[30]]

ral or spatial variation, a series of small line graphs may be created for comparison (see Fig. 6–14).

DATA QUALITY

Throughout this chapter we have described epidemiologic data as if they were free of mistakes or artifacts. This is not always true. Interpretation of patterns that arise from poor quality or haphazardly collected data leads to confusion, loss of valuable time and resources, and, most important of all, invalid assumptions. To assess the quality of descriptive data, you should first try to identify and understand the factors that might be leading you astray. These could include incomplete data; uneven reporting in time, place, or person; combining prevalent with incident cases; changes or nonuniform application of case definitions; using date of report to represent date of onset; and so forth. Where place is concerned, reports may come from reporting sites that do not correspond to residence or exposure. You should also recognize that some categories of data are inherently more accurate (age) than others (e.g., socioeconomic status). Review the data set, and look for problems such as terminal digit bias, onset dates that follow diagnosis dates, or age or gender that is incompatible with the disease, as examples.

Finally, descriptive epidemiology deals with population-level characteristics. Accordingly, be aware of two separate problems: aggregation bias that comes from loss of information when individuals are grouped; and specification bias that comes from the definition of the group itself.[31] Problems with the data may be diverse and are not always or fully under your control. It is important to be alert for them, recognize them when they occur, and correct them or take them into account in your interpretation.

SUMMARY

Descriptive epidemiology includes both numbers and rates to document how much of a health condition is present or occurring in a population. It also includes the three critical dimensions for describing health conditions: time, place, and person. Time refers to acute changes in disease occurrence, such as an epidemic, and changes over longer time periods, such as seasonal patterns and secular trends. Time data are usually displayed graphically. Place refers to geopolitical boundaries, topography, or locations of rooms, buildings, and other structures. Place data are best displayed with maps. Person refers to demographic and other personal characteristics of the populations under study. Person data are usually displayed in tables or graphs. When done well, descriptive epidemiology can characterize the health problem in the community; provide clues that can be turned into testable hypotheses; and promote effective communication with scientific, policy-making, and lay audiences alike.

APPENDIX 6–1. GRAPHS, MAPS, AND CHARTS IN DESCRIPTIVE EPIDEMIOLOGY

GENERAL PRINCIPLES

Graphs, charts, maps, diagrams, and tables should give the viewer a rapid, objective, and coherent grasp of the data. The simplest graphs are most effective. No more lines or symbols should be used in a single graph than the eye can easily follow or that the viewer can easily understand. To compare several strata use several miniaturized and identically scaled graphs arranged on the page to facilitate comparison. Avoid unnecessary decoration. Above all emphasize the data without distortion. The best graphs synthesize large amounts of data yet preserve the necessary detail in the data. For more comprehensive coverage of graphic techniques the reader is referred to a series of books by Tufte.[21,32,33]

Follow these guidelines:

- Every graph should be titled and labeled correctly so that no text is needed to orient the viewer.
- When more than one variable is shown on the graph, each should be clearly differentiated by means of legends or keys.
- Frequencies are usually represented on the vertical scale and method of classification on the horizontal scale.
- Adhere to basic mathematical principles in plotting data and scaling axes.
- On an arithmetic scale, equal numerical units must be represented by equal distances on the scale.
- Scale divisions should be clearly indicated, as well as the units into which the scale is divided.
- Emphasize the data while minimizing background. Frames, gridlines, axes, should be reduced to the absolute essentials.
- Use graphic designs that reveal the data from the broad overview to the fine detail.
- Lastly, ask yourself, "What do I want the viewer to walk away with? What is my take-home message?" There should be only one, two, or, perhaps, three clear, simple, and understandable messages from each figure, table, or chart.

GRAPHING TIME AND OTHER NUMERICALLY SCALED VARIABLES

Histograms (epidemic curves) and frequency polygons are best used for displaying counts in time. The basic options for displaying and assessing epidemiologic rates include arithmetic and semilogarithmic graphs.

Time or other numerically scaled variables (e.g., age) are best shown on the *x* axis either on a continuous scale or divided into intervals. Case counts, rates, or ratios are best shown on the *y* axis. A graph may indicate the timing of events thought to be related to the health problem, such as a period of exposure or the date of implementation of a control measure. Depending on the health event you are studying, the time period may include years, months, weeks, or may be limited to a period in which the observed number of cases exceeds the expected (e.g., an epidemic).

Arithmetic Scale Line Graph

In an arithmetic scale line graph, an equal distance on the *y* axis represents an equal quantity anywhere on a given *x* axis. The shape of the line will depend upon the scaling of the axes, and judgment should be used to avoid distorting the data or obscuring important features of the line. The scale should be defined in such a way as to make it easy to understand. When possible, a break in the scale should *not* be used with a scale line graph. If large differences in rates must be shown then consider using a box inset into the graph to show a portion of the line at a different scale.

Semilogarithmic Scale Line Graph

In a semilogarithmic scale line graph, one coordinate or axis (usually the *y* axis) is transformed to logarithms of units, whereas the other axis is scaled in arithmetic units. Consider this approach for examining the relative changes rather than the absolute change (i.e., actual amount of change). It is particularly helpful when comparing two or more variables whose rates differ by several orders of magnitude. The advantages of semilogarithmic graphing are that:

- A straight line indicates a constant rate of change,
- The slope of the line indicates the rate of change,
- Two or more lines following parallel paths show identical rates of change, and
- A wide range of values (three to four orders of magnitude) can be displayed effectively on a single graph.

DISPLAYS OF FREQUENCY DISTRIBUTIONS

Histograms

A histogram presents the frequency distribution of individual measurements. A measurement—normally a continuous variable, such as time, age, height, weight, blood pressure—is partitioned into intervals along the *x* axis. Counts of individuals or cases are then shown as vertical columns scaled against the *y* axis. The area under the curve represents the *frequency distribution*. Thus, adjacent columns are not separated by space, and scale breaks should not be used. Do not use unequal intervals. However, if unequal intervals are unavoidable (e.g., for a frequency distribution by age), the height of each column should be adjusted to maintain the ratio of area to frequency.

Histograms of incident cases by time intervals, constructed for outbreak investigation, are referred to as *epidemic curves*. In general, only lines representing the height of each column are drawn. With only a few cases, a common practice is to divide each column to show individual cases. At the other extreme a dot alone may be used to mark the top of each column with dense data such as emergency room visits per day.

Comparing more than one frequency distribution

Comparing the frequency distributions of two or more subgroups will often be necessary. For example, you may want to analyze an epidemic by looking at different districts in a city. To allow the eye to rapidly compare graphs of individual strata, avoid stacking all subgroups upon one another on the same baseline. This can hopelessly distort interpretation of the patterns. Consider using multiple histograms, simple graphical figures, that can be reduced in size and repeated for different strata without losing sight of the patterns shown in the graphic. Also strongly consider using *frequency polygons*. Frequency polygons are constructed from histograms. A line is drawn between the midpoints of the tops of each column. Several frequency polygons may then be plotted on the same axes as long as the individual lines do not become entangled and difficult to interpret.

Seasonal curves

For a single year either a simple histogram of case counts or a line graph of monthly rates may be constructed. Since the idea of the seasonal curve is to observe the relative difference from month to month, comparisons of seasonal curves in different places must be adjusted to depict relative rather than absolute differences. The epidemiologist may make semilogarithmic plots. This method has the advantage of conserving the comparison of rates but tends to suppress the visual perception of peaks and valleys in the distribution. A second method converts the data to percentage of total (see Fig. 6–14). This will put all localities on the same relative axis and accentuate the visual perception of seasonal peaks. However, localities with more extended seasonal increases will appear as if they had less intense incidence. Consider including a redundant beginning point and end point (see Fig. 6–14). This allows the viewer to see the trend between the last and first intervals of the cycle.

Tables

Tables are the best way to show exact numerical values. Tables are preferable for many small data sets. They also work well when data presentation requires many localized comparisons.[21] A well-structured table that is organized to focus on comparisons may prove to be a superior presentation than a graph or chart.

Charts

Charts are instruments for presenting statistical information symbolically using only one coordinate. Charts presented here include those based on length and proportion.

Bar charts

Bar charts allow rapid visualization and comprehension of differences in rates or counts among nominative categories. Alternatively, a table may show the same data with similar effectiveness. Avoid using bar charts for showing different categories of a numerically scaled variable. These are better presented as line graphs.

All categories in a bar chart have a uniform column width. The columns are separated by spaces. The bars may be arranged horizontally or vertically. Arrangement in either an ascending or descending order helps interpretation. Scale breaks should never be used in bar charts. However, the columns may be shaded, hatched, or colored to index the variable shown by each bar. Bars should be labeled at their base.

Simple bar chart

Counts, rates, percentages, ratios, or any other numerical derivative of several categories of a nominative variable may be compared using this basic format (Fig. 6–20).[34] Each column rises from a baseline. The length of the column is gauged against the other columns and the y axis or, if a horizontal chart, the x axis. The numerical scale may be arithmetic or logarithmic, ratio-scaled or by any other derivative of the basic data. The tabular equivalent of this chart is a two-variable table.

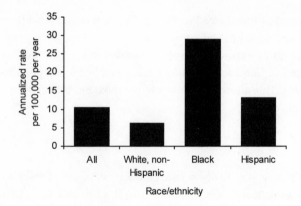

Figure 6–20. Annualized rates per 100,000 population for firearm-related injuries by race/ethnicity—United States, 1993–1998. [*Source*: CDC, 2001.[34]]

Two-category bar charts

Several designs allow simultaneous comparisons of a numerical variable among different categories and subcategories of a nominative value variable. For example, a major category, ethnic group, could be divided into a secondary nominative variable such as education attained. A legend is needed to index the subcategories. These charts correspond to three-variable tables.

Grouped (clustered) bar chart

A grouped bar chart can also be thought of as an aggregation of miniaturized, simple bar charts each one representing a different primary category (Fig. 6–21A).[34] Bars within each primary category are usually adjoining, whereas bar groupings are separated. Grouped bar charts may be shown as a series of charts along a single baseline or as miniaturized multiples arranged in columns and rows. Since all bars are on the same baseline, differences in bar length are more easily visualized than with a stacked or 100% bar chart. Grouped bar charts do not clearly show the differences in the totals among the major categories. Moreover, the display becomes confusing with more than a few subcategories.

Stacked bar chart

In a stacked bar chart, bar segments representing different subcategories of a primary category are stacked one atop another within a single bar (Fig. 6–21B).[33] The top of the bar represents a total for the primary category. However, subcategories (except for the bottom subcategories) rest on different baselines, making their comparisons less exact. The height of the top of each subcategory is not pro-

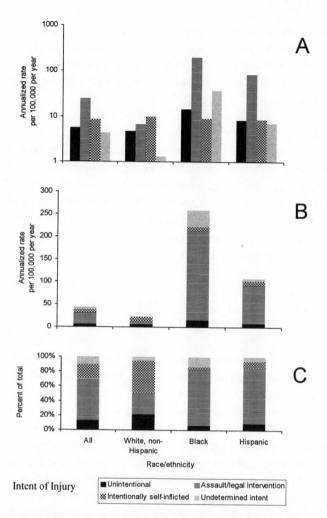

Figure 6–21. Annualized rates per 100,000 population for firearm-related injuries by race/ethnicity and intent of injury—United States, 1993–1998, as illustrated by the use of a grouped bar chart (A), a stacked bar chart (B), and a 100% bar chart (C). [*Source*: CDC, 2001.[34]]

portional to the actual value for that category. Accordingly, you must visually compare the relative size of the portion of the bar for each subcategory rather than the height of the top of the subcategory above the baseline.

100% bar chart

In the 100% bar chart, a variation of the stacked bar chart, proportional frequencies (percentage of total) are shown (Fig. 6–21C). The components or subcategories of each category are shown as a percentage of the total of the primary category. Unlike the normal stacked bar chart it is not useful in comparing the relative sizes of either the primary itself or the subcategories. Indeed, they suffer from all the potential distortions of any comparison of proportional frequencies in epidemiology.

Pie charts

Pie charts represent proportional frequencies with wedge-shaped portions of the circle. Pie charts are, in actuality, weak graphical instruments.[21] They present only a minimal amount of data relative to the amount of space used. The eye cannot quickly identify order to the categories. Finally, visual comparisons are easier on a linear arrangement. Always consider substituting a simple bar chart with a percentage scale or a two-variable table for a pie chart. A 100% bar chart always provides a visually superior data display than multiple pie charts.

SOME FINAL SUGGESTIONS FOR THE DESIGN AND USE OF TABLES, GRAPHS, AND CHARTS

- Choose the tool that is most effective for data and purpose. This means you should specify the point that must be communicated and then choose the method.
- Emphasize one idea at a time. Confine the presentation to one purpose or idea. Include only one kind of datum in each presentation.
- Use adequate and properly located labels. The title should include the "what, where, and when" that completely identify the data they introduce. All other labels should be equally clear, complete, and easy to understand. Like the title, they should be outside the frame of the data. Only keys and legends should appear within the field of a graph or chart. Keys and legends should be clearly distinguished from the data.
- The sources of the data should be provided. Verification or further analysis by the audience is difficult or impossible without full disclosure of sources.
- Recall that you may sometimes base your epidemiologic conclusions on more data than are actually displayed in your charts, tables, and graphs. Since these methods of presentation usually summarize data, some detail is necessarily lost. Thus, potential distortions should be compensated for both in design and in comment by using footnotes or other means to note important detail that has been obscured.
- Effective communication entails not only the ability to transfer facts to the viewer so that understanding is reached, but to do so in a believable and

persuasive way. So, remember who your audience is. Are they professional epidemiologists, other scientists, policy makers, administrators, news media, or the general public? Your presentations and language should fit with their level of understanding and intellect. However, no matter who the audience is, your challenge is to inform and simplify while showing an undistorted picture of the data as is possible.

REFERENCES

1. Centers for Disease Control and Prevention (1999). Intussusception among recipients of rotavirus vaccine—United States, 1998–1999. *Morb Mortal Wkly Rep* 48, 577–81.
2. Centers for Disease Control and Prevention. (1992). *Principles of Epidemiology. A Self-Study Course*, 2nd ed. Atlanta, GA.
3. Centers for Disease Control and Prevention (1997). Injuries and deaths associated with use of snowmobiles—Maine, 1991–1996. *Morb Mortal Wkly Rep* 46,1–4.
4. Centers for Disease Control and Prevention (1992). Summary of notifiable diseases, United States. *Morb Mortal Wkly Rep* 41, 38.
5. Abulrahi, H.A., Bohlega, E.A., Fontaine, R.E., et al. (1997). *Plasmodium falciparum* malaria transmitted in hospital through heparin locks. *Lancet* 349, 23–25.
6. Centers for Disease Control and Prevention (1994). Outbreak of measles among Christian Science students—Missouri and Illinois, 1994. *Morb Mortal Wkly Rep* 43, 463–65.
7. Tauxe, R.V., Tormey, M.P., Mascola, L., et al. (1987). Salmonellosis outbreak in transatlantic flights; Foodborne illness on aircraft: 1947–1984. *Am J Epidemiol* 125, 150–57.
8. Ministry of Health (1999). Field Epidemiology Training Program, Jordan. Unpublished data.
9. Mausner, J.S., Bahn, A.K. (1974). *Epidemiology: an introductory text*, W.B. Saunders, Philadelphia.
10. Anderson, R.M., May, R.M. (1992). *Infectious Diseases of Humans: dynamics and control*. Oxford University Press, Oxford.
11. Fontaine, R.E., Cohen, M.L., Martin, W.T., et al. (1980). Epidemic salmonellosis from cheddar cheese: surveillance and prevention. *Am J Epidemiol* 111, 247–53.
12. Centers for Disease Control and Prevention (1999). Rubella outbreak—Westchester County, New York, 1997–1998. *Morb Mortal Wkly Rep* 48, 560–63
13. Ko, A.I., Mitermayer, G.R., Ribero Dourado, C.M., et al. (1999). Urban epidemic of severe leptospirosis in Brazil. *Lancet* 354, 820–25.
14. Centers for Disease Control and Prevention (1999). Update: West Nile virus encephalitis—New York, 1999. *Morb Mortal Wkly Rep* 48, 944–55.
15. Ministry of Health (1996). Field Epidemiology Training Program, Saudi Arabia. Unpublished data.
16. Al-Qarawi, S.M., El Bushra, H.E., Fontaine, R.E., et al. (1995). Typhoid fever from water desalinized using reverse osmosis. *Epidemiol Infect* 114, 41–50.
17. Centers for Disease Control and Prevention (1992). Summary of notifiable diseases, United States. *Morb Mortal Wkly Rep* 41, 64.

18. Fontaine, R.E., van Severin, M., Houng, A. (1984). The stratification of malaria in El Salvador using available malaria surveillance data. Abstract 184, XIth International Congress for Tropical Medicine and Malaria, Calgary, Canada.16–22 September 1984.

19. Kenyon, T.A., Valway, S.E., Ihle, W.W., et al. (1996). Transmission of multidrug-resistant *Mycobacterium tuberculosis* during a long airplane flight. *N Engl J Med* 334, 933–38.

20. Centers for Disease Control and Prevention (1999). Unpublished data.

21. Tufte, E.R. (1987) *The Visual Display of Quantitative Information*. Graphics Press, Cheshire, CT.

22. Robinson, A.H., Sale, R.D., Morrison, J.L., et al. (1985). *Elements of Cartography*, 5th ed. John Wiley & Sons, New York.

23. Cliff, A.D., Haggett, P. (1988). *Atlas of Disease Distributions: analytic approaches to epidemiological data*. Blackwell Publishers, Cambridge, MA.

24. Centers for Disease Control and Prevention (2000). Cluster of HIV-infected adolescents and young adults—Mississippi, 1999. *Morb Mortal Wkly Rep* 49, 861–64.

25. Goodman, R.A., Smith, J.D., Sikes, R.K., et al. An epidemiologic study of fatalities associated with farm tractor injuries. *Public Health Rep* 100, 329–33.

26. National Center for Health Statistics (2001) http://www.cdc.gov/nchs/data/mx190039.pdf. April 2001.

27. National Center for Health Statistics (2001) http://www.cdc.gov/nchs/data/mx195059.pdf. April 2001.

28. National Center for Health Statistics (2001) http://www.cdc.gov/nchs/data/nvsr/nvsr48/nvsr48_11.pdf. April 2001.

29. Fleiss, J.C. (1981). *Statistical Methods for Rates and Proportions*. John Wiley & Sons, New York.

30. Mokdad, A.H., Serdula, M.K., Dietz, W.H., et al. (1999). The spread of the obesity epidemic in the United States, 1991–1998. *JAMA* 282, 1519–22.

31. Janes, G.R., Hutwagner, L., Cates, W., et al. (2000). Descriptive epidemiology: analyzing and interpreting surveillance data. In S.M. Teutsch, R.E. Churchill (Eds.) *Principles and Practices of Public Health Surveillance*, 2nd ed. Oxford University Press, New York.

32. Tufte, E.R. (1990). *Envisioning Information*. Graphics Press, Cheshire, CT.

33. Tufte, E.R. (1997). *Visual Explanations*. Graphics Press, Cheshire, CT.

34. Centers for Disease Control and Prevention (2001). Surveillance for fatal and non-fatal firearm-related injuries—United States, 1993–1998. *Morb Mortal Wkly Rep* CDC Surveillance Summaries, 50, 27–28.

7

DESIGNING STUDIES IN THE FIELD

Richard C. Dicker

For all but the most straightforward field investigations, you are likely to design and conduct an epidemiologic study of some sort. This is sometimes called an analytic study, to distinguish it from a descriptive study. The basic ingredients of epidemiologic studies consist of two groups: the observed group, such as a group of ill or exposed persons, and a comparison group, which provides baseline or "expected" data. Using these groups is an efficient way to evaluate hypotheses about causes of disease and risk factors that have been raised in earlier phases of the investigation. By comparing the observed data with the expected data from the comparison group, you can quantify the relationship between possible risk factors and disease, and can test the statistical significance of the various hypotheses that have been raised.

The gold standard for an epidemiologic study is an experimental study such as a therapeutic trial, in which study participants are enrolled, randomly assigned into intervention or nonintervention (placebo) exposure groups, and then monitored over time. In public health practice, however, epidemiologists rarely conduct such experiments, because they are seldom in a position to assign exposures—exposures have generally already occurred through genetics, circumstance, or choice. As a result, almost all studies conducted by field epidemiologists are observational studies, in which the epidemiologists document rather than determine exposures.

You will likely conduct two types of epidemiologic studies. In a *cohort* or *follow-up study*, enrollment of the study group is based on exposure characteristics or membership in a particular group. The occurrence of health-related outcomes (like diseases) is then determined and the frequency of those occurrences is compared among exposure groups. In a *case-control study*, enrollment is based on the presence ("case") or absence ("control") of disease, and the frequency of exposures is compared between the cases and controls. Each type of study has its strengths and limitations, but each has an important place in field investigations.

This chapter provides an overview of these two study designs, emphasizing methodologic considerations in the field. For more in-depth discussion of the theory and other features of study design, the reader is referred to other epidemiology texts.[1-3]

DEFINING EXPOSURE GROUPS

Since both cohort and case-control studies are used to quantify the relationship between exposure and disease, defining what is meant by "exposure" and "disease" is critical. In general, exposure is used quite broadly, meaning demographic characteristics, genetic or immunologic makeup, behaviors, environmental exposures, and other factors that might influence one's risk of disease.

Since precise exposure information is essential to accurate estimation of an exposure's effect on disease, exposure measures should be as objective and standard as possible. An exposure may be a relatively discrete event or characteristic, and developing a measure of exposure is conceptually straightforward, for example, whether a person ate the shrimp appetizer at Restaurant A or whether a person had received influenza vaccine this year. While these exposures may be straightforward in theory, they are subject to the whims of memory. Memory aids, such as Restaurant A's menu, and exposure documentation, such as a vaccination card or medical record, may help in these situations.

Some exposures can be subdivided by dose or duration (number of glasses of apple cider, number of years working in a coal mine). A pathogen may require a minimum (threshold) level of exposure to cause disease and may be more likely to cause disease with increasing exposures. The disease may require prolonged exposure or have a long latency or incubation period. These relationships may be missed by characterizing exposure simply as "yes" or "no." Similarly, the vehicle of infection, for example, may be a component or ingredient of other measured exposures. One could then create a composite measure, such as whether a person ate any item with mayonnaise as an ingredient.

Some exposures are subtle or difficult to quantify. Surrogate measures may be used (census track or level of education as a surrogate for socioeconomic status, which in turn may be a surrogate for access to health care, adequacy of housing, nutritional status, etc.), but should be interpreted with caution.

DEFINING OUTCOMES ("CASE DEFINITION")

A case definition is a set of standard criteria for deciding whether an individual should be classified as having the health condition of interest. A case definition consists of clinical criteria and, particularly in the setting of an outbreak investigation, certain restrictions on time, place, and person. The clinical criteria may include confirmatory laboratory tests, if available, or combinations of symptoms, signs, and other findings, but in general they should be kept simple and objective, for example, the presence of elevated antibody titers, three or more loose bowel movements per day, illness severe enough to require hospitalization, or primary hospital discharge diagnosis of ICD-9 code 480-486). The case definition may be restricted by time (e.g., to persons with onset of illness within the past 2 months), by place (e.g., to employees at a particular manufacturing plant or to residents of a town), and by person (e.g., to persons who had previously tested negative for chlamydia or to children at least 9 months old). Whatever the criteria, they must be applied consistently and without bias to all persons under investigation to ensure that persons with illness are characterized consistently over time, locale, and clinical practice.

A case definition can have degrees of certainty, for example, a suspect case (usually based on clinical and sometimes epidemiologic criteria) versus a confirmed case (based on laboratory confirmation). For example, during an outbreak of measles, a person with fever and rash may be categorized as having a suspect, probable, or confirmed case of measles, depending on the strength of the additional laboratory and epidemiologic evidence. Sometimes a case is temporarily classified as suspect or probable while awaiting laboratory results. Depending on the lab results, the case will be reclassified as either confirmed or "not a case." Sometimes a case is permanently classified as suspect or probable, because, in the midst of a large outbreak of a known agent, investigators need not use precious time and resources to identify the same agent from every person with consistent clinical findings and history of exposure.

The case definition may also vary depending on the purpose. For case finding in a local area, the case definition should be relatively sensitive to capture as many potential cases as possible, that is, throw the net wide. However, for enrolling persons into an epidemiologic study to identify risk factors, a relatively specific or narrow case definition will minimize misclassification and bias.

For an epidemiologic study, a definition for controls may be just as important as the definition for cases. That is, since misclassification and bias may result if some controls actually have the disease under study, you may wish to adopt a control definition to exclude persons with mild or asymptomatic cases of the disease. In a study of a cluster of thyrotoxicosis, a surprise finding was that 75% of asymptomatic family members of cases had elevated thyroid function tests.[4] Had these family members been enrolled as controls, the epidemiologic study would not have identified a difference in exposure between cases and controls, and the association with consumption of locally produced ground beef that inadvertently included bits of thyroid gland would have been missed.

COHORT STUDIES

In concept, a cohort study, like an experimental study, begins with a group of persons without the disease under study but with different exposure experiences, and follows them over time to find out if they develop disease or a health condition of interest. In a cohort study, though, each person's exposure status is merely recorded rather than assigned randomly by the investigator. Then, the occurrence of disease among persons with different exposures is compared to assess whether the exposures are associated with increased risk of disease.

A cohort study sometimes begins by enrolling everyone in a population regardless of exposure status, then characterizing each person's exposure status after enrollment. Alternatively, a sample rather than the whole population could be enrolled. The enrollees are then followed over time for occurrence of the disease(s) of interest. Examples of large cohort studies that span many years include the Framingham Study, a study of cardiovascular disease among residents of Framingham, Massachusetts,[5] and the Nurses' Health Study, a study of the effects of oral contraceptives, diet, and lifestyle risk factors among over 100,000 nurses.[6] Another example of this type of cohort study is one that enrolls all employees of a manufacturing plant before ascertaining each person's job type or exposure to a manufacturing process or chemical. A third example is a study that enrolls all persons who attended a banquet, then elicits food consumption histories to determine exposure. Note that in cohort studies that enroll all or a sample of a population without regard to exposure status, a wide variety of exposures as well as a wide variety of outcomes can be examined.

A cohort study can also begin with the enrollment of persons based on their exposure status. In this type of cohort study, two or more groups defined by their exposure status are enrolled. For example, an investigator may decide to enroll 100 persons exposed to some agent and 100 persons who were not exposed but are otherwise comparable. In this type of cohort study, while a wide variety of outcomes can be examined, assessment of exposure may be restricted to the one used to define the enrollment groups.

In a *prospective cohort study*, enrollment takes place before the occurrence of disease. In fact, any potential subject who is found to have the disease at enrollment will be excluded. Thus each subsequently identified case is an *incident* case. Incidence may be quantified as the number of cases over the sum of time that person was followed (*incidence rate*), or as the number of cases over the number of persons being followed (*attack rate* or *risk*). A major challenge for prospective studies is to maintain follow-up that is as complete as possible and comparable for each exposure group.

Note that, for a prospective study, disease should not have already occurred. Therefore, in field epidemiology, a prospective study is only likely to be conducted after a known exposure and a long incubation or latency period before illness. One example is the follow-up study of persons exposed to nuclear tests in Utah.[7] More commonly, cohort studies are conducted by field epidemiologists in response to a noted cluster or outbreak of disease in a well-defined population. A cohort study in which persons are enrolled after disease has already occurred is called a *retrospective cohort study*. In the typical "church picnic" outbreak where all or a representative sample of participants provide information on both their food exposures and whether they became ill, the investigator can calculate attack rates of disease in those who did or did not eat each food, and compare those attack rates to identify the food associated with the greatest increase in risk (see Appendix at end of book). This retrospective cohort type of study is the technique of choice for an acute outbreak in a well-defined population, particularly one for which a roster of names and contact information such as telephone numbers are available. Examples include not only the church picnic for which membership lists are available but also weddings and other gatherings, cruise ships, nursing homes, and schools. Retrospective cohort studies can also be used in a noninfectious disease context and are popular in occupational epidemiology. For example, a group of persons exposed to a worksite hazard years ago or over many years (e.g., workers exposed to vinyl chloride during the manufacturing process) and a comparable group not exposed (e.g., workers in a different part of the same plant) are constructed from available employment records, and the morbidity or mortality of the two groups is determined and compared[8] (see Chapter 17). However, when the population at risk is not known (e.g., as with nationwide epidemics), the only expedient and scientifically sound way to analyze the problem is to use the case-control method.

CASE-CONTROL STUDIES

Whereas a cohort study proceeds conceptually from exposure to disease, a case-control study begins conceptually with disease and looks backward at prior exposures. Specifically, in a case-control study, a group of people with the disease of interest (cases or case–patients) and an appropriate group of people without disease are enrolled, and their prior exposures are ascertained. Differences in exposure between the two groups indicate an association between the exposure and disease under study.

Selection of Subjects

The case-control study begins with the identification of cases and the selection of controls. The case group represents the "observed" exposure experience, while the control group is needed to provide the "expected" level of exposure.

The cases in a case-control study must meet the case definition, that is, they must have the disease in question. The case definition must be independent of the exposure(s) under study. Ideally, the cases will be limited to new or incident cases rather than prevalent cases, so that the study does not confuse factors associated with disease occurrence with those associated with survival. Because field investigations rarely find all the cases, because you often are under strong pressure to find an answer, and because having only 70% to 80% of all cases is usually enough to perform an adequate study, you will usually attempt to enroll all persons who are eligible and meet the case definition. Since one goal of an analytic study is to quantify the relationship between exposure and disease, you should use a relatively narrow or specific case definition to ensure that cases truly have the disease—minimizing one source of misclassification bias.

A comparable group of controls must be identified and enrolled. While this statement is simple, debates about the selection of controls can be among the most complex in epidemiology.[9] The controls should not have the disease in question and, like the cases, should be identified independently of exposure. As a general rule, the controls should be representative of the population from which the cases arose, so that if a control had developed the disease, he or she would have been included as a case in the study. Suppose the cases are persons with community-acquired pneumonia admitted to a single hospital. The controls should be persons who would be admitted to the same hospital if they had the disease. This condition helps ensure comparability between cases and controls, since persons admitted to a different hospital may reflect a different population with a variety of different host characteristics and other exposures that may affect risk of disease. Commonly, controls for hospital-based cases are selected from the group of patients admitted to the same hospital, but with diagnoses other than the case-defining illness. Similarly, cases diagnosed in the outpatient setting may be compared to controls from the same clinical practices. Cases scattered through a community are often compared with community-based controls.

Controls should be free of the disease under study. This underscores the importance of both the case definition and the control definition in distinguishing persons who have the disease from those who do not. In some studies, controls are required to have laboratory or other confirmation that they are disease free. In other studies, lack of symptoms and signs of illness are presumed to indicate absence of disease. However, the stricter the definition of the controls, the less opportunity for misclassification (enrolling someone with mild or asymptomatic disease as a control) and bias.

Consider the thyrotoxicosis outbreak mentioned earlier, with about 75% of asymptomatic family members with elevated thyroid function tests because they ate the same contaminated ground beef as the cases. Had the investigators not tested the family members, and had the family members thus been included in the control group, they would have had exposures similar to the cases, making the exposure-disease association harder to identify.

In general, controls should be at risk for the disease. While this can be challenged on academic grounds, the assertion has face validity and needs little justification. For example, in a case-control study of risk factors for uterine cancer, most epidemiologists would not include men in the control group. While men might adequately represent the distribution of A-B-O blood groups in the population, they surely would represent an inappropriate estimate of the "expected" levels of sexual activity, contraceptive choices, and the like.

Sometimes the choice of a control group is so vexing that investigators decide to use more than one type of control group. For example, in a study where the cases are persons hospitalized with West Nile encephalitis, you might want to select a hospital-based control group (since only a minority of persons with West Nile infection require hospitalization and are the cases most easily found) and a community-based control group. If the two control groups provide similar results and conclusions about risk factors for West Nile infection, then the credibility of the findings is increased. On the other hand, if the two control groups yield conflicting results, then you must struggle to develop plausible explanations.

Types of Controls

Controls come from a variety of sources, each with potential strengths and weaknesses. As noted previously, two of the guiding principles in selecting a control group are whether they represent the population from which the cases came, and whether they will provide a good estimate of the level of exposure one would expect in that population. Some common sources of controls include persons served by the same health-care institutions or providers as the cases; members of the same institution or organization; relatives, friends, or neighbors; or a random sample of the community from which the cases came.

For outbreaks in hospitals or nursing homes, the source of controls is usually other patients or residents of the facility. For example, in the investigation of postoperative surgical site infections the epidemiologist might select as controls persons who had similar surgery but who did not develop postoperative infections. The advantages of using such controls are that they come from the same catchment area as the cases, have similar access to medical care, have comparable medical records, have time on their hands, and are usually cooperative. The disadvantage is that they may have conditions that are associated either positively or negatively with the disease or risk factors of interest. For example, hospitalized patients are more likely to be current or former smokers than the general population. Depending on the disease and risk factors under study, the best strategy may be to select controls with only a limited number of diagnoses known to be independent of the exposures and disease, or, alternatively, to select controls with as broad a range of diagnoses as possible, so that no one diagnosis has undue influence.

In other settings with a well-defined or easily enumerated population, controls generally come from lists of persons in that population who did not become ill. For example, controls for an outbreak of nausea, lightheadedness, and fainting among seventh graders at a middle school might be seventh grade students at the same school who did not experience those symptoms. Similarly, on a cruise ship, controls might be selected as a random sample of well passengers or perhaps cabin mates of cases who ate together but remained well. These population-based controls have advantages similar to those listed for hospital-based controls, but without the disadvantage of having another disease.

When an outbreak occurs in a community at large, controls may be randomly selected from that community. However, the epidemiologist is not likely to have an available list of all persons from which to choose. Therefore, he or she must enlist controls either by telephoning a randomly or systematically selected set of telephone numbers, or by mailings to residents, or by conducting a door-to-door neighborhood survey. Each approach has its relative strengths and weaknesses, and associated potential biases. For example, both telephone dialing and door-to-door canvassing are labor intensive and are best done in the evenings when people are likely to be home. Even so, the public has become wary of telephone solicitations and even more so of strangers, however well intentioned, knocking on their doors. Mailings require far less labor but have notoriously low response rates, and those who respond may be a skewed rather than representative group (see Chapter 11).

When an investigation is not limited to a specific location but, for instance, involves the entire United States (e.g., toxic shock syndrome and tampon use or HIV infection and sexual practices), the selection of an appropriate control group is not as straightforward. In such circumstances epidemiologists have successfully used friends, relatives, or neighbors as controls. Typically, the investigator interviews a case, then asks for the names and telephone numbers of perhaps three friends to call as possible controls. One advantage is that the friends of an ill person are usually quite willing to participate, knowing that their cooperation may help solve the puzzle. On the other hand, they may be too similar to the cases, sharing personal habits and other exposures. The consequence of enrolling controls who are too similar to the cases—called "overmatching"—makes it harder to identify exposure-disease associations.

Sampling Methods for Selecting Controls

A variety of approaches can be used to select controls, depending on the hypotheses to be evaluated, the urgency of the investigation, the resources available, and the setting.

All persons at risk

Occasionally, an outbreak occurs in a well-defined, relatively small population. Examples include a food-borne outbreak among persons who attended a wedding, or a nosocomial outbreak among patients in the intensive care unit of a hospital. All persons with the disease under study could be called cases, and all persons who did not become ill could be called controls. However, since the entire population is available for study, you could and should analyze the data as a cohort study, computing and comparing rates of disease among exposed and unexposed groups, rather than analyzing the data in case-control fashion.

Random or systematic sampling

When an outbreak occurs in a population with a large number of potential controls, you can choose a random or systematic sample of the population. If a roster is available, you could choose a random sample by using a table or computer-generated list of random numbers to select individuals. For a systematic sample, you would select every tenth or thirtieth (or other appropriate interval) person on the list. When no roster is available you might resort to the technique called "random digit dialing," dialing random telephone numbers with the same area codes and exchanges as the cases. Whichever strategy is used, potential controls with symptoms and signs similar to the cases should either be excluded, or if they meet the definition for a case, be evaluated and included as cases, if appropriate.

Pair matching

Pair matching is the selection of one or more controls for each case, who have the same or similar specified characteristics as that case. For example, if the criteria for pair matching were same gender, school, and grade as the case, and the control-to-case ratio were one-to-one, then a female ninth grade case at Lincoln High School would need to be matched to a female Lincoln High School ninth grade control. Although the term *pair matching* implies one case and one control, the term may also refer to two, three, or even four controls matched to each case.

In field epidemiology, pair matching is used in two circumstances—to control for potential confounding, or for logistical ease. In the first circumstance, one or more factors may be suspected to confound the relationship between exposure and disease; that is, the factor may be linked to the exposure and, independently, be a risk factor for the disease. To help eliminate the intertwining of the effect of the confounder with the effect of the other exposures of interest, the epidemiologist may choose to match on the confounder. The result is that the cases and controls are the same in terms of the confounding factor, and, when analyzed properly, any apparent association between the exposure and the disease cannot be due to confounding by the matching factor. Note that matching in the design of the study, that is, choosing controls matched to the cases, requires the use of matched analysis methods (see Chapter 8).

A second reason for pair matching is simple expedience. As noted earlier, sometimes the quickest and most convenient method of selecting controls is to ask the cases for the names of friends, or to walk next door to a neighbor's home. This is pair matching because Jane's friend or neighbor in Seattle is not the friend or neighbor of Mary in Chicago. While such pair matching may be done for expedience, the net result is that cases and controls generally do wind up being matched for such difficult-to-measure factors such as socioeconomic status, cultural influence, exposure to local advertising, and the like.

Frequency matching

Frequency matching, also called category matching, is an alternative to pair matching. Frequency matching involves the selection of controls in proportion to the distribution of certain characteristics of the cases. For example, if 70% of the cases were ninth graders, 20% were eighth graders, and 10% were seventh graders, then the same proportion of controls would be selected from those grades. Frequency matching works best when all the cases have been identified before control selection begins.

Matching has several advantages. Matching is conceptually simple. It can save time and resources, as noted above with friend controls, and it can control for confounding by numerous social factors that are difficult to quantify and, hence, otherwise difficult to control for in an analysis. Finally, if the matching factor would have been a strong confounder, then matching improves the precision or power of the analysis.

However, matching has important disadvantages as well. First and foremost, if you match on a factor, you can no longer evaluate its effect on disease in your study, because you have made the controls and cases alike on that factor. For example, if infants with nosocomial infections in a neonatal intensive care unit were matched by birth weight to other newborns, then investigators would not be able to study birth weight itself as a risk factor for infection. Therefore, you should only match on factors that you do not need to evaluate. Second, if you use too many or too rigid matching criteria, it may be hard to find appropriate controls, and you may have to toss out cases if appropriately matched controls cannot be found. For example, one disadvantage of using sibling controls is that cases who are only children in a family have no eligible controls and cannot be included in the study. Finally, matching on factors that are not confounders tends to decrease a study's precision.

Size of Control Group

The size of the control group may be determined by circumstances, resources, or power considerations. Circumstance, for example, the number of eligible controls, sometimes is a limiting factor. At other times, time and resources may limit the number of controls that can be enrolled. However, when the size of the population from which the cases arose is large and resources are adequate, power calculations may be performed to determine the optimal number of controls needed to identify an important association. Most case-control studies use a control-to-case ratio of either 1:1, 2:1, or 3:1. In general, little power is gained with control-to-case ratios in excess of 3:1 or 4:1.

COMPARISONS OF COHORT AND CASE-CONTROL STUDIES

Some outbreaks occur in settings that are amenable to either a retrospective cohort or case-control study design. Others are better suited to one study type or the other. The advantages and disadvantages of these two approaches are listed in Table 7–1.

Risk Measurement

One of the most important advantages of the cohort design is that you can directly measure the disease risk (attack rate) of disease. This information is particularly important if the exposure is at the discretion of the individual. Only a cohort study can fill in the blank of "What is my risk of developing [name of disease] if I choose to [be exposed]?" The case-control study, with a set number of cases and an arbitrary number of controls, does not permit calculation of disease risk for a given exposure group.

Rare Exposure

Cohort studies are better suited than case-control studies for examining health effects following a relatively rare exposure. With a cohort approach, all persons

Table 7–1. Features of Case-Control and Retrospective Cohort Studies

FEATURE	CASE-CONTROL STUDY	RETROSPECTIVE COHORT STUDY
Sample size	Smaller	Larger
Costs	Less	More because of size
Study time	Short	Short
Rare disease	Efficient	Inefficient
Rare exposure	Inefficient	Efficient
Multiple exposures	Can examine	Often can examine
Multiple outcomes	Cannot examine	Can examine
Natural history	Cannot ascertain	Can ascertain
Disease risk	Cannot measure	Can measure
Recall bias	Potential problem	Potential problem
Loss to follow-up	Not an issue	Potential problem
Selection bias	Potential problem	Potential problem

with the exposure can be enrolled and monitored, as well as a sample of comparable persons who were not exposed. This rationale explains the popularity of retrospective cohort studies in occupational epidemiology, where a group of workers with an exposure common among that group but relatively rare in the community at large can be followed over time.

Rare Disease

Case-control studies are the design of choice for sporadic occurrences of an otherwise rare disease in a population. All cases and an appropriate number of controls can be enrolled and exposures evaluated for association with disease. In contrast, a cohort study would have to enroll an extremely large number of persons to have enough with the outcome of interest.

POTENTIAL PITFALLS IN THE DESIGN AND CONDUCT OF EPIDEMIOLOGIC STUDIES

Designing and conducting a good epidemiologic study in the field is not easy. In designing a study you must make many choices. Many of these choices have no right answer but involve trade-offs or compromises between theory and practical issues such as time constraints and resources. Other choices involve deciding between two less-than-perfect options, such as two different control groups each with potential flaws. Some of the pitfalls that result from less-than-ideal study design and conduct are described below.

Selection Bias

Selection bias is a systematic error in choosing the study groups to be enrolled (e.g., cases and controls in a case-control study, exposed and unexposed groups in a cohort study) or in the enrollment of study participants that results in a mistaken estimate of an exposure-disease association. Consider, for example, a disease with low pathogenicity, that is, one with many asymptomatic cases. If a case-control study were conducted but controls were not tested for evidence of asymptomatic infection, then at least some of the controls may have the infection under study. The exposures among these mislabeled controls will be the same as the cases, resulting in an underestimate of the exposure-disease relationship. Another source of selection bias is diagnostic bias, in which knowledge of the exposure-disease hypothesis may prompt a clinician to make a diagnosis. For example, a physician may be more likely to diagnose pulmonary embolism in a woman he knows to be taking oral contraceptives—any subsequent analyses will show an association between oral contraceptives and pulmonary embolism! A third source of selection bias is nonresponse bias, in which persons who choose to participate may differ in important ways from persons who choose not to participate or cannot be found. In occupational epidemiology a well-known source of selection bias is called the *healthy worker effect*, wherein workers who remain on the job are, in general, more healthy and fit than the population at large, and comparisons between workers and the general population may not be appropriate. The list of types of selection bias is lengthy, so investigators must be careful to use an objective and consistent case definition; select controls that represent the population from which the cases arose, using objective and consistent control criteria; and work hard to promote high response rates among all groups.

Information Bias

Information bias is a systematic error in the collection of exposure or outcome data about the study participants that results in a mistaken estimate of an exposure's effect on the risk of disease. One of the most common types of information bias is recall bias, in which one group is more likely than the other to remember and report an exposure. For example, persons who developed severe diarrhea are very likely to have thought about all the preceding meals and foods they had eaten, while healthy controls are not. Interviewer bias occurs when interviewers are more probing about exposures with the cases than with the controls. To minimize information bias, good studies use standard and pretested questionnaires or data collection forms, and interviewers or abstractors who are trained in the objective use of the forms. Memory aids, such as calendars, menus, or photographs of medications, can often aid participants' recall.

Confounding

Confounding is the distortion of an exposure-disease association by a third factor that is related to both exposure and disease. Consider, for example, a study of an investigational cancer drug versus "usual treatment." Suppose that most people who received the drug had early-stage disease, and most people who received usual treatment had later-stage disease. Then even if the investigational drug had no beneficial effect, it might look efficacious because its effect was intertwined with that of disease stage. For a factor to be a confounder it must be an independent risk factor for the disease, and it must be unequally distributed among the exposure groups. Since age is independently associated with almost every health condition imaginable, age automatically fulfills one of the two criteria for confounding, so it must always be considered a potential confounder.

In observational studies, confounding can be addressed through restriction, matching, stratified analysis, or modeling. Restriction means, simply, that the study population is limited to a narrowly defined population. In the investigational drug example above, if the study had been limited to persons with early-stage disease, the disease stage could not confound the results. Similarly, if age is a suspected confounder, the study could be limited to a narrow age range. Matching in the study design has been addressed previously in this chapter. Matching in the analysis, as well as stratified analysis and modeling, is addressed in Chapter 8.

Small Sample Size

Sample size and power calculations can provide estimates of the number of subjects needed to find an association that is statistically significant and that you consider important. In practice, the size of a study is sometimes limited by the number of cases, time, and resources available. While the two most popular measures of effect—risk ratio and odds ratio—are not influenced by the size of the study, their measures of precision—confidence intervals—and measures of statistical significance, such as chi-square tests and p values, are all affected by study size. Many an investigator has wished for a larger study after calculating a large and potentially important risk ratio or odds ratio that, alas, is not statistically significant and has a wide confidence interval. Would a larger study confirm the association statistically different from the null, or would it show that the apparent association was indeed just chance variation from the null? Often, the investigator will never know. Determination of an adequate sample size in advance could avoid this situation.

SUMMARY

Cohort and case-control studies are the two types of analytic studies used most commonly by field epidemiologists. They are effective mechanisms for evaluating—quantifying and testing—hypotheses suggested in earlier phases of the investigation. Cohort studies, which are oriented conceptually from exposure to disease, are appropriate in settings in which an entire population is well defined and available for enrollment, such as invited guests at a wedding reception. Cohort studies are also appropriate when you can define and enroll groups by exposure, such as employees working in different parts of a manufacturing plant. Case-control studies, on the other hand, are quite useful when the population is less clearly defined. Case-control studies, oriented from disease to exposure, identify persons with disease ("cases") through, say, surveillance, and a comparable group of persons without disease ("controls"), then the exposure experiences of the two groups are compared. While conceptually straightforward, the design of a good epidemiologic study requires many decisions including who make up an appropriate comparison group, whether or not to match, and how best to avoid potential biases.

REFERENCES

1. Rothman, K.J. (1986). *Modern Epidemiology*. Little, Brown, Boston.
2. Schlesselman, J.J. (1982). *Case-Control Studies*. Oxford University Press, New York.
3. Breslow, N.E., Day, N.E. (1997). *Statistical Methods in Cancer Research*, vol 2. *The design and analysis of cohort studies*. IARC Scientific Publications, Lyon, France.
4. Hedberg, C.W., Fishbein, D.B., Janssen, R.S., et al. (1987). An outbreak of thyrotoxicosis caused by the consumption of bovine thyroid gland in ground beef. *N Engl J Med* 316, 993–98.
5. Dawber, T.R., Kannel, W.B., Lyell, L.P. (1963). An approach to longitudinal studies in a community: the Framingham study. *Ann NY Acad Sci* 107, 539–56.
6. Colditz, G.A. (1995). The Nurses' Health Study: a cohort of US women followed since 1976. *J Am Med Womens Assoc* 50, 40–44, 63.
7. Caldwell, G.G., Kelley, D.B., Zack, M., et al. (1983). Mortality and cancer frequency among military nuclear test (smoky) participants, 1957–1979. *J Am Med Assoc* 250, 620–24.
8. Waxweiler, R.J., Stringer, W., Wagoner, J.K., et al. (1976). Neoplastic risk among workers exposed to vinyl chloride. *Ann NY Acad Sci* 271, 40–48.
9. Wacholder, S., McLaughlin, J.K., Silverman, D.T., et al. (1992). Selection of controls in case-control studies: I. Principles. *Am J Epidemiol* 135, 1019–28.
10. Morse, L.J., Bryan, J.A., Hurley, J.P., et al. (1972). The Holy Cross College football team hepatitis outbreak. *J Am Med Assoc* 219, 706–8.

8

ANALYZING AND INTERPRETING DATA

Richard C. Dicker

The purpose of many field investigations is to identify causes, risk factors, sources, vehicles, routes of transmission, or other factors that put some members of the population at greater risk than others of having an adverse health event. In some field investigations, identifying a "culprit" is sufficient; if the culprit can be eliminated, the problem is solved. In other field settings, the goal may be to quantify the relationship between exposure (or any population characteristic) and an adverse health event. Quantifying this relationship may lead not only to appropriate interventions but also to advances in knowledge about disease causation. Both types of field investigation require appropriate but not necessarily sophisticated analytic methods. This chapter describes the strategy for planning an analysis, methods for conducting the analysis, and guidelines for interpreting the results.

PREANALYSIS PLANNING

What to Analyze

The first step of a successful analysis is to lay out an analytic strategy in advance. A thoughtfully planned and carefully executed analysis is just as critical for a field investigation as it is for a protocol-based study. Planning is necessary to assure that the appropriate hypotheses will be considered and that the relevant data will be appropriately collected, recorded, managed, analyzed, and interpreted to evaluate those hypotheses. Therefore, the time to decide on what (and how) to analyze the data is before you design your questionnaire, *not* after you have collected the data. As illustrated in Figure 8–1, the hypotheses that you wish to evaluate drive the analysis. (These hypotheses are usually developed by considering the common causes and modes of transmission of the condition under investigation; talking with patients and with local medical and public health staff; observing the dominant patterns in the descriptive epidemiologic data; and scrutinizing the outliers in these data.) Depending on the health condition being investigated, the hypotheses should address the source of the agent, the mode (and vehicle or vector) of transmission, and the exposures that caused disease. They should obviously be testable, since the role of the analysis will be to evaluate them.

Once you have determined the hypotheses to be evaluated, you must decide which data to collect in order to test the hypotheses. (You will also need to determine the best study design to use, as described in the previous chapter.) There is a saying in clinical medicine that "If you don't take a temperature, you can't find a fever".[1] Similarly, in field epidemiology, if you neglect to ask about a potentially important risk factor in the questionnaire, you cannot evaluate its role in the outbreak. Since the hypotheses to be tested dictate the data you need to collect, the time to plan the analysis is before you design the questionnaire.

Questionnaires and other data collection instruments are not limited to risk factors, however. They should also include identifying information, clinical information, and descriptive factors. Identifying information (or ID codes linked to identifying information stored elsewhere) allows you to recontact the respondent to ask additional questions or provide follow-up information. Sufficient clinical information should be collected to determine whether a patient truly meets the case definition. Clinical data on spectrum and severity of illness, hospitalization, and sequelae may also be useful. Descriptive factors related to time, place, and person should be collected to adequately characterize the population, assess comparability between groups (cases and controls in a case-control study; exposed and unexposed groups in a cohort study), and help you generate hypotheses about causal relationships.

Data Editing

Usually, data for an analytic study are collected on paper questionnaires. These data are then entered into a computer. Increasingly, data are entered directly into a computer as they are obtained. In either situation, good data management practices will facilitate the analysis. These practices include, at the very least,

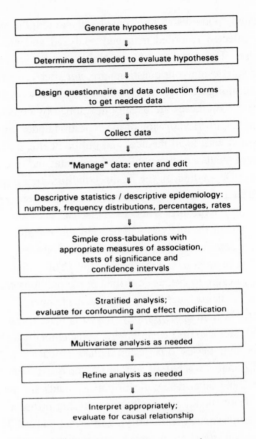

Figure 8–1. Steps in an analysis.

- Ensuring that you have the right number of records, with no duplicates
- Performing quality-control checks on each data field

Check that the number of records in the computerized database matches the number of questionnaires. Then check for duplicate records. It is not uncommon for questionnaires to be skipped or entered twice, particularly if they are not all entered at one sitting.

Two types of quality-control checks should be performed before beginning the analysis: range checks and logic (or consistency) checks. A range check identifies values for each variable that are "out of range" (i.e., not allowed, or at least highly suspicious). If, for the variable "gender," "male" is coded as 1 and "female" as 2, the range check should flag all records with any value other than 1 or 2. If 3's, F's, or blanks are found, review the original questionnaire, recontact the respondent, or recode those values to "known missing." For the variable "weight (in pounds)," an allowable range for adults might be 90 to 250. It is quite possible that some respondents will weigh more or less than this range, but it is also possible that values outside that range represent coding errors. Again, you must decide whether to attempt to verify the information or leave it as entered. The effort needed to confirm and complete the information should be weighed against the effect of lost data in the analysis—for a small study, you can ill afford missing data for the key variables but can tolerate it for less important variables. Under no circumstances should you change a value just because "it doesn't seem right."

A logic check compares responses to two different questions and flags those that are inconsistent. For example, a record in which "gender" is coded as "male" and "hysterectomy" is coded as "yes" should probably be flagged! Dates can also be compared—date of onset of illness should usually precede date of hospitalization (except in outbreaks of nosocomial infection, when date of hospitalization *precedes* date of onset), and date of onset should precede date of report. Again you must decide how to handle inconsistencies.

Two additional principles should guide data management. First, document everything, particularly your decisions. Take a blank copy of the questionnaire and write the name of each variable next to the corresponding question on the questionnaire. If, for the variable "gender," you decide to recode F's as 2's and recode 3's and blanks as 9's for "known missing," write those decisions down as well, so that you and others will know how to recode unacceptable values for gender in the future.

Note that you cannot create logic checks in advance for every possible contingency. Many inconsistencies in a database come to light during the analysis. Treat these inconsistencies the same way—decide how best to resolve the inconsistency (short of making up better data!) and then document your decision.

The second principle is, "Never let an error age." Deal with the problem as soon as you find it. Under the pressures of a field investigation, it is all too common to forget about a data error, analyze the data as they are, and then be embarrassed during a presentation when calculations or values in a table do not seem to make sense.

Developing the Analysis Strategy

After the data have been edited, they are ready to be analyzed. But before you sit down to analyze the data, first develop an analysis strategy (Table 8–1). The analysis strategy is comparable to the outline you would develop before sitting down to write a term paper. It lays out the key components of the analysis in a logical sequence and provides a guide to follow during the actual analysis. An analytic strategy that is well planned in advance will expedite the analysis once the data are collected.

Table 8–1. Sequence of an Epidemiologic Analysis Strategy

---

1. Establish how the data were collected and plan to analyze accordingly.
2. Identify and list the most important variables in light of what you know about the subject matter, biologically plausible hypotheses, and the manner in which the study will be (or was) conducted:
   Exposures of interest
   Outcomes of interest
   Potential confounders
   Variables for subgroup analysis
3. To become familiar with the data, plan to perform frequency distributions and descriptive statistics on the variables identified in step 2.
4. To characterize the study population, create tables of clinical features and descriptive epidemiology (table shells should be created in advance).
5. To assess exposure-disease associations, create two-way tables based on study design, prior knowledge, and hypotheses (table shells should be created in advance).
6. Create additional two-way tables based on interesting findings in the data.
7. Create three-way tables, refinements (e.g., dose-response; sensitivity analysis) and subgroup analysis based on design, prior knowledge, hypotheses, or interesting findings in the data.

The first step in developing the analysis strategy is recognizing how the data were collected. For example, if you have data from a cohort study, think in terms of exposure groups and plan to calculate rates. If you have data from a case-control study, think in terms of cases and controls. If the cases and controls were matched, plan to do a matched analysis. If you have survey data, review the sampling scheme—you may need to account for the survey's design effect in your analysis.

The next step is deciding which variables are most important. Include the exposures and outcomes of interest, other known risk factors, study design factors such as variables you matched on, any other variables you think may have an impact on the analysis, and variables you are simply interested in. In a small questionnaire, perhaps all variables will be deemed important. Plan to review the frequency of responses and descriptive statistics for each variable. This is the best way to become familiar with the data. What are the minimum, maximum, and average values for each variable? Are there any variables that have many missing responses? If you hope to do a stratified or subgroup analysis by, say, race, is there a sufficient number of responses in each race category?

The next step in the analysis strategy is sketching out table shells. A table shell (sometimes called a "dummy table") is a table such as a frequency distribution or two-way table that is titled and fully labeled but contains no data. The numbers will be filled in as the analysis progresses.

You should sketch out the series of table shells as a guide for the analysis. The table shells should proceed in a logical order from simple (e.g., descriptive epidemiology) to complex (e.g., analytic epidemiology). The table shells should also indicate which measures (e.g., odds ratio) and statistics (e.g., chi-square) you will calculate for each table. Measures and statistics are described later in this chapter.

One way to think about the types and sequence of table shells is to consider what tables you would want to show in a report. One common sequence is as follows:

Table 1: Clinical features (e.g., signs and symptoms, percent lab-confirmed, percent hospitalized, percent died, etc.)

Table 2: Descriptive epidemiology

Time: usually graphed as line graph (for secular trends) or epidemic curve

Place: county of residence or occurrence, spot or shaded map

Person: "Who is in the study?" (age, race, gender, etc.)

For analytic studies,

Table 3: Primary tables of association (i.e., risk factors by outcome status)

Table 4: Stratification of Table 3 to separate effects and to assess confounding and effect modification

Table 5: Refinements of Table 3 (e.g., dose-response, latency, use of more sensitive or more specific case definition, etc.)

Table 6: Specific subgroup analyses

The following sequence of table shells (A through I) was designed before conducting a case-control study of Kawasaki syndrome (a pediatric disease of unknown cause that occasionally occurs in clusters). Since there is no definitive diagnostic test for this syndrome, the case definition requires that the patient have fever plus at least four of five other clinical findings listed in Table Shell A. Three hypotheses to be tested by the case-control study were the syndrome's purported association with antecedent viral illness, recent exposure to carpet shampoo, and increasing household income.

Since descriptive epidemiology has been covered in Chapter 5, the remainder of this chapter addresses the analytic techniques most commonly used in field investigations.

Figure 8–2 depicts a screen from *Epi Info*'s Analysis module (see Chapter 12). It shows the output from the "Tables" command for data from a typical field investigation. Note the four elements of the output: (*1*) a two-by-two table; (*2*) measures of association; (*3*) tests of statistical significance; and (*4*) confidence intervals. Each of these elements is discussed below.

Table Shell A. Diagnostic Criteria for Kawasaki Syndrome Cases
with Onset October–December

CRITERION	NUMBER	PERCENT
1. Fever ≥5 days	—	(%)
2. Bilateral conjunctival injection	—	(%)
3. Oral changes	—	(%)
Injected lips	—	(%)
Injected pharynx	—	(%)
Dry, fissured lips	—	(%)
Strawberry tongue	—	(%)
4. Peripheral extremity changes	—	(%)
Edema	—	(%)
Erythema	—	(%)
Periungual desquamation	—	(%)
5. Rash	—	(%)
6. Cervical lymphadenopathy > 1.5 cm	—	(%)

Table Shell B. Days of Hospitalization, Kawasaki Syndrome Cases
with Onset October–December

DAYS OF HOSPITALIZATION	FREQUENCY
0	—
1	—
2	—
3	—
4	—
5	—
6	—
7	—
8	—
9	—
and so on to maximum	—
Unknown	—
Range:	—
Mean:	—
Median:	—

Table Shell C. Frequency Distribution of Serious Complications among
Kawasaki Syndrome Cases with Onset October–December

CRITERION	NUMBER	PERCENT
Arthritis	__	(%)
Coronary artery aneurysm	__	(%)
Other complications (list:)	__	(%)
Death	__	(%)

Table Shell D. Demographic Characteristics of Kawasaki Syndrome Cases
with Onset October–December

DEMOGRAPHIC CHARACTERISTIC		NUMBER	PERCENT
Age	< 1 yr	__	(%)
	1 yr	__	(%)
	2 yr	__	(%)
	3 yr	__	(%)
	4 yr	__	(%)
	5 yr	__	(%)
	≥ 6 yr	__	(%)
Gender	Male	__	(%)
	Female	__	(%)
Race	White	__	(%)
	Black	__	(%)
	Asian	__	(%)
	Other	__	(%)

Table Shell E. Frequency Distribution by County of Residence,
Kawasaki Syndrome Cases, October–December

COUNTY	NUMBER	PERCENT	POPULATION	ATTACK RATE
County A	__	(%)	__	__
County B	__	(%)	__	__
County C	__	(%)	__	__
County D	__	(%)	__	__
County E	__	(%)	__	__
County F	__	(%)	__	__

Table Shell F. Frequency Distribution by Household Income, Kawasaki Syndrome Cases, October–December

ANNUAL HOUSEHOLD INCOME[a]	NUMBER	PERCENT
< $15,000	—	(%)
$15,000–$29,999	—	(%)
$30,000–$44,999	—	(%)
≥ $45,000	—	(%)

[a]May need to revise categories of household income to portray range.

Table Shell G. Kawasaki Syndrome and Antecedent Illness, Case-Control Study

		CASES	CONTROLS	TOTAL	
	YES	—	—	—	Odds ratio = ___
					95% CI = (,)
ANTECEDENT ILLNESS	NO	—	—	—	$x^2 = $ _____,
					P value = _____
	TOTAL	—	—	—	

Table Shell H. Kawasaki Syndrome and Carpet Shampoo, Case-Control Study

		CASES	CONTROLS	TOTAL	
	YES	—	—	—	Odds ratio = ___
					95% CI = (,)
CARPET SHAMPOO	NO	—	—	—	$x^2 = $ _____,
					P value = _____
	TOTAL	—	—	—	

Table Shell I. Kawasaki Syndrome and Carpet Shampoo, Case-Control Study

		CASES	CONTROLS	TOTAL	
HOUSEHOLD	<15	—	—	—	
INCOME	15–30	—	—	—	$x^2 = $ _____,
(IN THOUSANDS	30–45	—	—	—	P value = _____
OF DOLLARS)	45+	—	—	—	
	TOTAL	—	—	—	

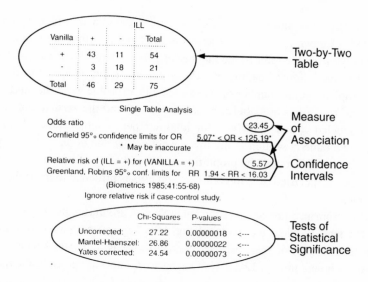

Figure 8–2. Typical *Epi Info* output from the analysis module, using the tables command. [*Source:* Dean, A.G. et al., 1994.[2]]

The Two-by-Two Table

"Every epidemiologic study can be summarized in a two-by-two table."

—H. Ory

In many epidemiologic studies, exposure and the health event being studied can be characterized as binary variables (e.g., "yes" or "no"). The relationship between exposure and disease can then be cross-tabulated in a *two-by-two table*, so named because both the exposure and disease have just two categories (Table 8–2). One can put disease status (e.g., ill vs. well) along the top and exposure status along the side. (*Epi Info*, a microcomputer program written for field use, also follows this convention, although some epidemiologic textbooks do not [see

Table 8–2. Data Layout and Notation for Standard Two-by-Two Table

	ILL	WELL	TOTAL	ATTACK RATE
EXPOSED	a	b	h_1	a/h_1
UNEXPOSED	c	d	h_0	c/h_0
TOTAL	v_1	v_0	t	v_1/t

Chapter 12].) The intersection of a row and a column in which a count is recorded is known as a *cell*. The letters a, b, c, and d within the four cells of the two-by-two table refer to the number of persons with the disease status indicated in the column heading and the exposure status indicated to the left. For example, c is the number of unexposed ill/case subjects in the study. The *horizontal* row totals are labeled h_1 and h_0 (or h_2), and the *vertical* column totals are labeled v_1 and v_0 (or v_2). The total number of subjects included in the two-by-two table is written in the lower right corner and is represented by the letter t or n. Attack rates (the proportion of a group of people who develop disease during a specified time interval) are sometimes provided to the right of the row totals.

Data from an outbreak investigation in South Carolina are presented in Table 8–3. The table provides a cross-tabulation of turkey consumption (exposure) by presence or absence of *Salmonella* gastroenteritis (outcome). Attack rates (56.4% for those who ate turkey; 12.2% for those who did not) are given to the right of the table.

MEASURES OF ASSOCIATION

A measure of association quantifies the strength or magnitude of the statistical association between the exposure and the health problem of interest. Measures of association are sometimes called measures of effect because—if the exposure is causally related to the disease—the measures quantify the effect of having the exposure on the incidence of disease. In cohort studies, the measure of association most commonly used is the relative risk. In case-control studies, the odds ratio is the most commonly used measure of association. In cross-sectional studies, either a prevalence ratio or a prevalence odds ratio may be calculated.

Table 8–3. Turkey Consumption and Gastrointestinal Illness,
Salmonella Outbreak, South Carolina, 1990

		ILL	WELL	TOTAL	ATTACK RATE
ATE	YES	115	89	204	56.4%
TURKEY?	NO	5	36	41	12.2%
	TOTAL	120	125	245	49.0%

[*Source*: Luby et al., 1993.[3]]

Relative Risk (Risk Ratio)

The relative risk is the risk in the exposed group divided by the risk in the unexposed group:

$$\text{Relative risk (RR)} = \text{risk}_{\text{exposed}} / \text{risk}_{\text{unexposed}} = (a/h_1) / (c/h_0)$$

The relative risk reflects the excess risk in the exposed group compared with the unexposed (background, expected) group. The excess is expressed as a ratio. In acute outbreak settings, risk is represented by the attack rate. The data presented in Table 8–3 show that the relative risk of illness, given turkey consumption, was 0.564/0.122 = 4.6. That is, persons who ate turkey were 4.6 times more likely to become ill than those who did not eat turkey. Note that the relative risk will be greater than 1.0 when the risk is greater in the exposed group than in the unexposed group. The relative risk will be less than 1.0 when the risk in the exposed group is less than the risk in the unexposed group, as is usually the case when the exposure under study is vaccination.

Odds Ratio (Cross-Product Ratio, Relative Odds)

In most case-control studies, because you do not know the true size of the exposed and unexposed groups, you do not have a denominator with which to calculate an attack rate or risk. However, using case-control data, the relative risk can be approximated by an odds ratio. The odds ratio is calculated as

$$\text{Odds ratio (OR)} = ad/bc$$

In an outbreak of group A *Streptococcus* (GAS) surgical wound infections in a community hospital, 10 cases had occurred during a 17 month period. Investigators used a table of random numbers to select controls from the 2600 surgical procedures performed during the epidemic period. Since many clusters of GAS surgical wound infections can be traced to a GAS carrier among operating room

Table 8–4. Surgical Wound Infection and Exposure to Nurse A, Hospital M, Michigan, 1980

		CASE	CONTROL	TOTAL
EXPOSED TO NURSE A?	YES	8	5	13
	NO	2	49	51
	TOTAL	10	54	64

[*Source*: Berkelman et al., 1982.[4]]

personnel, investigators studied all hospital staff associated with each patient. They drew a two-by-two table for exposure to each staff member and calculated odds ratios. The two-by-two table for exposure to nurse A is shown in Table 8–4. The odds ratio is calculated as $8 \times 49/2 \times 5 = 39.2$. Strictly speaking, this means that the *odds* of being exposed to nurse A were 39 times higher among cases than among controls. It is also reasonable to say that the odds of developing a GAS surgical wound infection were 39 times higher among those exposed to nurse A than among those not exposed. For a rare disease (say, less than 5%), the odds ratio approximates the relative risk. So in this setting, with only 10 cases out of 2600 procedures, the odds ratio could be interpreted as indicating that the *risk* of developing a GAS surgical wound infection was 39 times higher among those exposed to nurse A than among those not exposed.

The odds ratio is a very useful measure of association in epidemiology for a variety of reasons. As noted above, when the disease is rare, a case-control study can yield an odds ratio that closely approximates the relative risk from a cohort study. From a theoretical statistical perspective (beyond the scope of this book), the odds ratio also has some desirable statistical properties and is easily derived from multivariate modeling techniques.

Prevalence Ratio and Prevalence Odds Ratio

Cross-sectional studies or surveys generally measure the prevalence (existing cases) of a health condition in a population rather than the incidence (new cases). Prevalence is a function of both incidence (risk) and duration of illness, so measures of association based on prevalent cases reflect both the exposure's effect on incidence and its effect on duration or survival.

The prevalence measures of association analogous to the relative risk and the odds ratio are the *prevalence ratio* and the *prevalence odds* ratio, respectively.

In the two-by-two table (Table 8–5), the prevalence ratio = $0.20/0.05 = 4.0$. That is, exposed subjects are four times as likely as are unexposed subjects to have the condition. In the example above, the prevalence odds ratio = (20) (380) / (80) (20) = 4.75. The *odds* of having disease is 4.75 times higher for the exposed than the unexposed group. Note that when the prevalence is low, the values of the prevalence ratio and the prevalence odds ratio will be similar.

MEASURES OF PUBLIC HEALTH IMPACT

A measure of public health impact places the exposure-disease association in a public health perspective. It reflects the apparent contribution of an exposure to the frequency of disease in a particular population. For example, for an exposure associ-

Table 8–5. Data from a Hypothetical Cross-Sectional Survey

		HAVE CONDITION?			
		YES	NO	TOTAL	PREVALENCE
EXPOSED?	YES	20	80	100	0.20
	NO	20	380	400	0.05
	TOTAL	40	460	500	

ated with an increased risk of disease (e.g., smoking and lung cancer), the attributable risk percentage represents the expected reduction in disease load if the exposure could be removed (or never existed). The population attributable risk percentage represents the proportion of disease in a population attributable to an exposure. For an exposure associated with a decreased risk of disease (e.g., vaccination), a prevented fraction could be calculated that represents the actual reduction in disease load attributable to the current level of exposure in the population.

Attributable Risk Percent (Attributable Fraction [or Proportion] among the Exposed, Etiologic Fraction)

The attributable risk percent is the proportion of cases in the exposed group presumably attributable to the exposure. This measure assumes that the level of risk in the unexposed group (assumed to be the baseline or background risk of disease) also applies to the exposed group, so that only the *excess* risk should be attributed to the exposure. The attributable risk percent can be calculated with either of the following formulas (which are algebraically equivalent):

$$\text{Attributable risk percent} = (\text{risk}_{\text{exposed}} - \text{risk}_{\text{unexposed}}) / \text{risk}_{\text{exposed}}$$
$$= (RR - 1) / RR$$

The attributable risk percent can be reported as a fraction or can be multiplied by 100 and reported as a percent. Using the turkey consumption data in Table 8–3, the attributable risk percent is $(0.564 - 0.122) / 0.564 = 78.4\%$. Therefore, over three-fourths of the gastroenteritis that occurred among persons who ate turkey may be attributable to turkey consumption. The other 21.6% is attributed to the baseline occurrence of gastroenteritis in that population.

In a case-control study, if the odds ratio is thought to be a reasonable approximation of the relative risk, you can calculate the attributable risk percent as

$$\text{Attributable risk percent} = (OR - 1) / OR$$

Population Attributable Risk Percent (Population Attributable Fraction)

The population attributable risk percent is the proportion of cases in the entire population (both exposed and unexposed groups) presumably attributable to the exposure. Algebraically equivalent formulas include

$$\text{Population attributable risk percent} = (\text{risk}_{overall} - \text{risk}_{unexposed}) / \text{risk}_{overall}$$
$$= P(RR - 1) / [P(RR - 1) + 1]$$

where P = proportion of population exposed = h_1/t

Applying the first formula to the turkey consumption data, the population attributable risk percent is $(0.490 - 0.122) / 0.490 = 75.1\%$. In situations in which most of the cases are exposed, the attributable risk percent and population attributable risk percent will be close. For diseases with multiple causes (e.g., many chronic diseases) and uncommon exposures, the population attributable risk percent may be considerably less than the attributable risk percent.

The population attributable risk percent can be estimated from a population-based case-control study by using the OR to approximate the RR and by using the proportion of controls exposed to approximate P; that is, $P = b/v_0$ (assuming that the controls are representative of the entire population).

Prevented Fraction in the Exposed Group (Vaccine Efficacy)

If the risk ratio is less than 1.0, you can calculate the prevented fraction, which is the proportion of potential new cases that would have occurred in the absence of the exposure. In other words, the prevented fraction is the proportion of potential cases prevented by some beneficial exposure, such as vaccination. The prevented fraction in the exposed group is calculated as

$$\text{Prevented fraction among the exposed} = (\text{risk}_{unexposed} - \text{risk}_{exposed}) / \text{risk}_{unexposed}$$
$$= 1 - RR$$

Table 8–6 presents data from a 1970 measles outbreak along the Texas-Arkansas border. Because some cases had occurred among children vaccinated against measles, the public questioned the effectiveness of the measles vaccine. As shown in Table 8–6, the risk of measles among vaccinated children was about 4% of the risk among unvaccinated children. Vaccine efficacy was calculated to be 96%, indicating that vaccination prevented 96% of the cases that might have otherwise occurred among vaccinated children had they not been vaccinated.

Table 8–6. Vaccination Status and Occurrence of Measles, Texarkana, 1970

	MEASLES	NO MEASLES	TOTAL	RISK PER 1,000
VACCINATED	27	6,323	6,350	4.2
NOT VACCINATED	512	4,323	4,835	105.9
TOTAL	539	10,646	11,185	48.2

Relative risk = 4.2 / 105.9 = 0.04

Vaccine efficacy = (105.9 – 4.2) / 105.9 = 0.96

[*Source*: Landrigan, 1972.[5]]

Note that the terms "attributable" and "prevented" convey much more than statistical association. They imply a cause-and-effect relationship between the exposure and disease. Therefore, these measures should not be presented routinely but only after thoughtful inference of causality.

TESTS OF STATISTICAL SIGNIFICANCE

Tests of statistical significance are used to determine how likely it is that the observed results could have occurred by chance alone, if exposure was not actually related to disease. In the paragraphs that follow, we describe the key features of the tests most commonly used with two-by-two tables. For discussion of theory, derivations, and other topics beyond the scope of this book, we suggest that you consult one of the many biostatistics textbooks, which cover these subjects well.

In statistical testing, you assume that the study population is a sample from some large "source population." Then assume that, in the source population, incidence of disease is the same for exposed and unexposed groups. In other words, assume that, in the source population, exposure is not related to disease. This assumption is known as the *null hypothesis*. (The *alternative hypothesis*, which may be adopted if the null hypothesis proves to be implausible, is that exposure *is* associated with disease.) Next, compute a measure of association, such as a relative risk or odds ratio. Then, calculate the test of statistical significance such as a chi-square (described below). This test tells you the probability of finding an association as strong as (or stronger than) the one you have observed if the null hypothesis were really true. This probability is called the *P value*. A very small *P* value means that you would be very unlikely to observe such an association if the null hypothesis were true. In other words, a small *P* value indicates that the null hypothesis is implausible, given the data at hand. If this *P* value is smaller than some predetermined cutoff (usually 0.05 or 5%), you can discard ("reject") the null hypothesis in favor of the alternative hypothesis. The association is then said to be "statistically significant."

In reaching a decision about the null hypothesis, be alert to two types of error. In a *type I error* (also called *alpha error*), the null hypothesis is rejected when in fact it is true. In a *type II error* (also called *beta error*), the null hypothesis is not rejected when in fact it is false.

Both the null hypothesis and the alternative hypothesis should be specified in advance. When little is known about the association being tested, you should specify a null hypothesis that the exposure is not related to disease (e.g., RR = 1 or OR = 1). The corresponding alternative hypothesis states that exposure and disease are associated (e.g., RR ≠ 1 or OR ≠ 1). Note that this alternative hypothesis includes the possibilities that exposure may either increase or decrease the risk of disease.

When you know more about the association between a given exposure and disease, you may specify a narrower ("directional") hypothesis. For example, if it is well established that an exposure increases the risk of developing a particular health problem (e.g., smoking and lung cancer), you can specify a null hypothesis that the exposure does not increase risk of that condition (e.g., RR ≤ 1 or OR ≤ 1) and an alternative hypothesis that exposure does increase the risk (e.g., RR > 1 or OR > 1). Similarly, if you were studying a well-established protective relationship [measles-mumps-rubella (MMR) vaccine and measles], you could specify a null hypothesis that RR ≥ 1 and an alternative hypothesis that RR < 1.

A nondirectional hypothesis is tested by a "two-tailed" test. A directional hypothesis is tested with a "one-tailed" test. In general, the cutoff for a one-tailed test is twice the cutoff of a two-tailed test (i.e., 0.10 rather than 0.05). Since raising the cutoff for rejecting the null hypothesis increases the likelihood of making a type I error, epidemiologists in field situations generally use a two-tailed test.

Two different tests, each with some variations, are used for testing data in a two-by-two table. These two tests, described below, are the Fisher exact test and the chi-square test. These tests are not specific to any particular measure of association. The same test can be used regardless of whether you are interested in risk ratio, odds ratio, or attributable risk.

Fisher Exact Test

The Fisher exact test is considered the "gold standard" for a two-by-two table and is the test of choice when the numbers in a two-by-two table are small. Assume that the null hypothesis is true in the source population and that the values in the four cells but not the row and column totals of the two-by-two table could change. The Fisher exact test involves computing the probability of observing an association in a sample equal to or greater than the one observed. The technique for deriving this probability is outlined in Appendix 8–1.

As a rule of thumb, the Fisher exact test is the test of choice when the *expected* value in any cell of the two-by-two table is less than 5. The expected value is calculated by multiplying the row total by the column total and dividing by the table total. However, calculating the Fisher exact test, which is tedious at best for small numbers, becomes virtually impossible when the numbers get large. Fortunately, with large numbers, the chi-square test provides a reasonable approximation to the Fisher exact test.

Chi-Square Test

When you have at least 30 subjects and the expected value in each cell of the two-by-two table is at least 5, the chi-square test provides a reasonable approximation to the Fisher exact test. Plugging the appropriate numbers into the chi-square formula, you get a value for the chi-square. Then look up its corresponding two-tailed P value in a chi-square table (see Appendix 8–2). A two-by-two table has one degree of freedom,* and a chi-square larger than 3.84 corresponds to a two-tailed P value smaller than 0.05.

At least three different formulas of the chi-square for a two-by-two table are in common use; *Epi Info* presents all three.

$$\text{Pearson uncorrected } \chi^2 = \frac{t\ (ad-bc)^2}{(v_1)\ (v_0)\ (h_1)\ (h_0)}$$

$$\text{Yates corrected } \chi^2 = \frac{t\ \left(|ad-bc| - \left(\frac{t}{2}\right)\right)^2}{(v_1)\ (v_0)\ (h_1)\ (h_0)}$$

$$\text{Mantel-Haenszel } \chi^2 = \frac{(t-1)\ (ad-bc)^2}{(v_1)\ (v_0)\ (h_1)\ (h_0)}$$

For a given set of data in a two-by-two table, the Pearson chi-square formula gives the largest chi-square value and hence the smallest P value. This P value is often somewhat smaller than the "gold standard" P value calculated by the Fisher exact method. So the Pearson chi-square is more apt to lead to a type I error (concluding that there is an association when there is not). The Yates corrected chi-square gives the largest P value of the three formulas, sometimes even larger than the corresponding Fisher exact P value. The Yates correction is preferred by those epidemiologists who want to minimize their likelihood of making a type I error, but it increases the likelihood of making a type II error. The Mantel-Haenszel formula, popular in stratified analysis,

---

*Degrees of freedom equals the number of rows in the table minus 1 times the number of columns in the table minus 1. So for a two-by-two table, degrees of freedom = $(2 - 1) \times (2 - 1) = 1$.

yields a P value which is slightly larger than that from the Pearson chi-square but often smaller than the P value from the Yates corrected chi-square and Fisher exact P value. Table 8–7 shows the data for macaroni consumption and risk of gastroenteritis from the South Carolina *Salmonella* outbreak. For these data, the Pearson and Mantel-Haenszel chi-square formulas yield P values smaller than 0.05 (the usual cutoff for rejecting the null hypothesis). In contrast, the corrected chi-square formula yields a P value closer to but slightly larger than the Fisher exact P value (the "gold standard"). Both P values are larger than 0.05, indicating that the null hypothesis should *not* be rejected. Fortunately, for most analyses the three chi-square formulas provide similar enough P values to make the same decision regarding the null hypothesis based on all three.

Which Test to Use?

The Fisher exact test should be used if the expected value in any cell is less than 5. Remember that the expected value for any cell can be determined by multiplying the row total by the column total and dividing by the table total.

Table 8–7. Macaroni Consumption and Gastroenteritis, *Salmonella* Outbreak, South Carolina, 1990

	ILL	WELL	TOTAL	RISK	
EXPOSED	76	63	139	54.7%	Relative risk = 1.3
UNEXPOSED	44	62	106	41.5%	Odds ratio = 1.7
TOTAL	120	125	245		

$$\text{Uncorrected } \chi^2 = \frac{(245)\,(76 \times 62 - 63 \times 44)^2}{(120)\,(125)\,(139)\,(106)} = 4.17$$

$$\text{Mantel-Haenszel } \chi^2 = \frac{(245 - 1)\,(76 \times 62 - 63 \times 44)^2}{(120)\,(125)\,(139)\,(106)} = 4.16$$

$$\text{Corrected } \chi^2 = \frac{(245)\,[|76 \times 62 - 63 \times 44| - \left(\frac{245}{2}\right)]^2}{(120)\,(125)\,(139)\,(106)} = 3.66$$

The corresponding two-tailed P values are as follows:
Uncorrected $\chi^2 = 4.17$, P value = 0.041
Mantel-Haenszel $\chi^2 = 4.16$, P value = 0.042
Corrected $\chi^2 = 3.66$, P value = 0.056

Fisher exact P value (two-tail) = 0.053

[*Source*: Luby et al., 1993.[3]]

If all expected values in the two-by-two table are 5 or greater, then you can choose among the chi-square tests. Each of the three formulas shown above has its advocates among epidemiologists, and *Epi Info* provides all three. Many field epidemiologists prefer the Yates corrected formula because they are least likely to make type I error (but most likely to make a type II error). Epidemiologists who frequently perform stratified analyses are accustomed to using the Mantel-Haenszel formula, so they tend to use this formula even for simple two-by-two tables.

Measure of Association versus Test of Significance

The measures of association, such as relative risk and odds ratio, reflect the strength of the relationship between an exposure and a disease. These measures are generally independent of the size of the study and may be thought of as the "best guess" of the true degree of association in the source population. However, the measure gives no indication of its reliability (i.e., how much faith to put in it).

In contrast, a test of significance provides an indication of how likely it is that the observed association may be due to chance. Although the chi-square test statistic is influenced both by the magnitude of the association and the study size, it does not distinguish the contribution of each one. Thus the measure of association and the test of significance (or a confidence interval, see below) provide complementary information.

Interpreting Statistical Test Results

"Not significant" does not necessarily mean "no association." The measure of association (relative risk, odds ratio) indicates the direction and strength of the association. The statistical test indicates how likely it is that the observed association may have occurred by chance alone. Nonsignificance may reflect no association in the source population but may also reflect a study size too small to detect a true association in the source population.

Statistical significance does not by itself indicate a cause-effect relationship. An observed association may indeed represent a causal relationship, but it may also be due to chance, selection bias, information bias, confounding, and other sources of error in the design, execution, and analysis of the study. Statistical testing relates only to the role of chance in explaining an observed association, and statistical significance indicates only that chance is an unlikely (though not impossible) explanation of the association. You must rely on your epidemiologic judgment in considering these factors as well as consistency of the findings with those from other studies, the temporal relationship between exposure and disease, biological plausibility, and other criteria for inferring causation. These issues are discussed at greater length in the last section of this chapter.

Finally, statistical significance does not necessarily mean public health significance. With a large study, a weak association with little public health (or clinical) relevance many nonetheless be "statistically significant." More commonly, relationships of public health and/or clinical importance fail to be "statistically significant" because the studies are too small.

CONFIDENCE INTERVALS FOR MEASURES OF ASSOCIATION

We have just described the use of a statistical test to determine how likely the difference between an observed association and the null state is consistent with chance variation. Another index of the statistical variability of the association is the *confidence interval*. Statisticians define a 95% confidence interval as the interval that, given repeated sampling of the source population, will include or "cover" the true association value 95% of the time. The confidence interval from a single study may be roughly interpreted as the range of values that, given the data at hand and in the absence of bias, has a 95% chance of including the "true" value. Even more loosely, the confidence interval may be thought of as the range in which the "true" value of an association is likely to be found, or the range of values that is consistent with the data in your study.

The chi-square test and the confidence interval are closely related. The chi-square test uses the observed data to determine the probability (*P* value) under the null hypothesis, and you "reject" the null hypothesis if the probability is less than some preselected value, called alpha, such as 5%. The confidence interval uses a preselected probability value, alpha, to determine the limits of the interval, and you can reject the null hypothesis if the interval does not include the null association value. Both indicate the precision of the observed association; both are influenced by the magnitude of the association and the size of the study group. While both measure precision, neither addresses validity (lack of bias).

You must select a probability level (alpha) to determine limiting values of the confidence interval. As with the chi-square test, epidemiologists traditionally choose an alpha level of 0.05 or 0.01. The "confidence" is then $100 \times (1 - \text{alpha})\%$ (e.g., 95% or 99%).

Unlike the calculation of a chi-square, the calculation of a confidence interval is a function of the particular measure of association. That is, each association measure has its own formula for calculating confidence intervals. In fact, each measure has several formulas. There are "exact" confidence intervals and a variety of approximations.

Interpreting the Confidence Interval

As noted above, a confidence interval is sometimes loosely regarded as the range of values consistent with the data in a study. Suppose that you conducted a study in your area in which the relative risk for smoking and disease X was 4.0, and the 95% confidence interval was 3.0 to 5.3. Your single best guess of the association in the general population is 4.0, but your data are consistent with values anywhere from 3.0 to 5.3. Note that your data are *not* consistent with a relative risk of 1.0; that is, your data are *not* consistent with the null hypothesis. Thus, the values that are included in the confidence interval and values that are excluded both provide important information.

The width of a confidence interval (i.e., the values included) reflects the precision with which a study can pinpoint an association such as a relative risk. A wide confidence interval reflects a large amount of variability or imprecision. A narrow confidence interval reflects little variability and high precision. Usually, the larger the number of subjects or observations in a study, the greater the precision and the narrower the confidence interval.

As stated earlier, the measure of association provides the "best guess" of our estimate of the true association. If we were in a casino, that "best guess" would be the number to bet on. The confidence interval provides a measure of the confidence we should have in that "best guess," that is, it tells us how much to bet! A wide confidence interval indicates a fair amount of imprecision in our best guess, so we should not bet too much on that one number. A narrow confidence interval indicates a more precise estimate, so we might want to bet more on that number.

Since a confidence interval reflects the range of values consistent with the data in a study, one can use the confidence interval to determine whether the data are consistent with the null hypothesis. Since the null hypothesis specifies that the relative risk (or odds ratio) equals 1.0, a confidence interval that includes 1.0 is consistent with the null hypothesis. This is equivalent to deciding that the null hypothesis cannot be rejected. On the other hand, a confidence interval that does not include 1.0 indicates that the null hypothesis should be rejected, since it is inconsistent with the study results. Thus the confidence interval can be used as a test of statistical significance.

SUMMARY EXPOSURE TABLES

If the goal of the field investigation is to identify one or more vehicles or risk factors for disease, it may be helpful to summarize the exposures of interest in a single table, such as Table 8–8. For a food-borne outbreak, the table typically includes

Table 8–8. Food-Specific Attack Rates for Persons Who Ate Sunday Lunch, *Salmonella* Outbreak, South Carolina, 1990*

| | ATE | | | DID NOT EAT | | | | | |
FOOD	NO. CASES	TOTAL	AR %	NO. CASES	TOTAL	AR %	RR	(95% CI)	P VALUE
Turkey	115	204	56	5	41	12	4.6	(2.0, 10.6)	<0.001
Ham	65	121	54	54	122	44	1.2	(0.9, 1.6)	0.178
Dressing	99	186	53	21	59	36	1.5	(1.0, 2.2)	0.027
Gravy	85	159	53	35	85	41	1.3	(1.0, 1.7)	0.090
Macaroni	76	139	55	44	106	42	1.3	(1.0, 1.7)	0.056
Beans	96	183	52	23	61	38	1.4	(1.0, 2.0)	0.065
Corn	80	153	52	40	92	43	1.2	(0.9, 1.6)	0.229
Rolls	78	158	49	41	84	49	1.0	(0.8, 1.3)	0.958
Butter	47	88	53	73	157	46	1.2	(0.9, 1.5)	0.365
Tea	102	203	50	18	42	43	1.2	(0.8, 1.7)	0.482
Coffee	9	28	32	111	217	51	0.6	(0.4, 1.1)	0.090
Cranberries	42	74	57	78	171	46	1.2	(1.0, 1.6)	0.144

*AR = attack rate; RR = relative risk; and CI = confidence interval.
[*Source*: Luby et al., 1993.[3]]

each food item served, numbers of ill and well persons by food consumption history, food-specific attack rates (if a cohort study was done), relative risk (or odds ratio), chi-square and/or *P* value, and, sometimes, a confidence interval. To identify a culprit, you should look for a food item with two features:

1. An elevated relative risk, odds ratio, or chi-square (small *P* value), reflecting a substantial difference in attack rates among those exposed to the item and those not exposed.
2. Most of the ill persons had been exposed, so that the exposure could "explain" most if not all of the cases.

In Table 8–8, turkey has the highest relative risk (and smallest *P* value) and can account for 115 of the 120 cases.

STRATIFIED ANALYSIS

Although it has been said that every epidemiologic study can be summarized in a two-by-two table, many such studies require more sophisticated analyses than those described so far in this chapter. For example, two different exposures may appear to be associated with disease. How do you analyze both at the same time? Even when you are only interested in the association of one particular exposure and one particular outcome, a third factor may complicate the association. The two principal types of complications are *confounding* and *effect modification*. Stratified analysis, which involves examining the exposure-disease association within different categories of a third factor, is one method for dealing with these complications.

Stratified analysis is an effective method for looking at the effects of two different exposures on the disease. Consider a hypothetical outbreak of hepatitis A among junior high school students. The investigators, not knowing the vehicle, administered a food consumption questionnaire to 50 students with hepatitis A and to 50 well controls. Two exposures had elevated odds ratios and statistically significant *P* values: milk and donuts (Table 8–9). Donuts were often consumed with milk, so many people were exposed to both or neither. How do you tease apart the effect of each item?

Stratification is one way to tease apart the effects of the two foods. First, decide which food will be the exposure of interest and which will be the stratification variable. Since donuts has the larger odds ratio, you might choose donuts as the primary exposure and milk as the stratification variable. The results are shown in Table 8–10. The odds ratio for donuts is 6.0, whether milk was consumed or not. Now, what if you had decided to look at the milk-illness association, stratified by donuts? Those results are shown in Table 8–11. Clearly, from Table 8–10, consumption of donuts remains strongly associated with disease, regardless of milk consumption. On the other hand, from Table 8–11, milk consumption is not independently associated with disease, with an odds ratio of 1.0 among those who did and did not eat donuts. Milk only *appeared* to be associated with illness because so many milk drinkers also ate donuts.

Table 8–9. Hepatitis A and Consumption of Milk and Donuts

MILK	CASES	CONTROLS	TOTAL	
EXPOSED	37	21	58	Odds ratio = 3.9
UNEXPOSED	13	29	42	Yates-corrected χ^2 = 9.24
TOTAL	50	50	100	*P* value = 0.0002

DONUTS	CASES	CONTROLS	TOTAL	
EXPOSED	40	20	60	Odds ratio = 6.0
UNEXPOSED	10	30	40	Yates-corrected χ^2 = 15.04
	50	50	100	*P* value = 0.0001

Table 8–10. Hepatitis A and Donut Consumption, Stratified by Milk

		DRANK MILK					DID NOT DRINK MILK	
		CASES	CONTROLS				CASES	CONTROLS
ATE	YES	36	18		ATE	YES	4	2
DONUT?	NO	1	3		DONUT?	NO	9	27
		Odds ratio = 6.0					Odds ratio = 6.0	

Table 8–11. Hepatitis A and Milk Consumption, Stratified by Donuts

		ATE DONUT					DID NOT EAT DONUT	
		CASES	CONTROLS				CASES	CONTROLS
DRANK	YES	36	18		DRANK	YES	1	3
MILK?	NO	4	2		MILK?	NO	9	27
		Odds ratio = 1.0					Odds ratio = 1.0	

An alternative method for analyzing two exposures is with a two-by-four table, as shown in Table 8–12. In that table, exposure 1 is labeled "EXP 1"; exposure 2 is labeled "EXP 2." To calculate the risk ratio for each row, divide the attack rate ("risk") for that row by the attack rate for the group not exposed to either exposure (bottom row in Table 8–12). To calculate the odds ratio for each row, use that row's values for a and b in the usual formula, ad/bc.

With this presentation, it is easy to see the effect of exposure 1 alone (row 3) compared with the unexposed group (row 4), exposure 2 alone (row 2) compared with the unexposed group (row 4), and exposure 1 and 2 together (row 1) com-

Table 8–12. Data Layout for Two-by-Four Table, Analyzing Two Exposures at Once

EXP 1	EXP 2	ILL	WELL	TOTAL	RISK	RISK RATIO	ODDS RATIO
Yes	Yes	a_{YY}	b_{YY}	h_{YY}	a_{YY}/h_{YY}	$Risk_{YY}/Risk_{NN}$	$a_{YY}d/b_{YY}c$
No	Yes	a_{NY}	b_{NY}	h_{NY}	a_{NY}/h_{NY}	$Risk_{NY}/Risk_{NN}$	$a_{NY}d/b_{NY}c$
Yes	No	a_{YN}	b_{YN}	h_{YN}	a_{YN}/h_{YN}	$Risk_{YN}/Risk_{NN}$	$a_{YN}d/b_{YN}c$
No	No	c	d	h_{NN}	c/h_{NN}	1.0 (Ref)	1.0 (Ref)

pared with the unexposed group (row 4). Thus the separate and joint effects can be assessed.

From Table 8–13, you can see that donuts alone had an odds ratio of 6.0, whereas milk alone had an odds ratio of 1.0. Together, donuts and milk had an odds ratio of 6.0, the same as donuts alone. In other words, donuts, but not milk, were associated with illness. The two-by-four table summarizes the stratified tables in one and eliminates the need to designate one of the foods as the primary exposure and the other as the stratification variable.

Confounding

Stratification also helps in the identification and handling of confounding. *Confounding is the distortion of an exposure-disease association by the effect of some third factor (a "confounder").* A third factor may be a confounder and distort the exposure-disease association if it is

- Associated with the outcome independent of the exposure—that is, even in the nonexposed group. (In other words, it must be an independent "risk factor.")
- Associated with the exposure but not a consequence of it.

To separate out the effect of the exposure from the effect of the confounder, stratify by the confounder.

Consider the mortality rates in Alaska versus Arizona. In 1988, the crude mortality rate in Arizona was 7.9 deaths per 1000 population, over twice as high as the crude mortality rate in Alaska (3.9 deaths per 1000 population). Is living in Arizona more hazardous to one's health? The answer is no. In fact, for most age groups, the mortality rate in Arizona is about equal to or slightly lower than the mortality rate in Alaska. The population of Arizona is older than the population

Table 8–13. Hepatitis A and Consumption of Milk and Donuts,
in Two-by-Four Table Layout

DONUT	MILK	CASE	CONTROL	ODDS RATIO
Yes	Yes	36	18	6.0
No	Yes	1	3	1.0
Yes	No	4	2	6.0
No	No	9	27	1.0 (Ref)

of Alaska, and death rates rise with age. Age is a confounder that wholly accounts for Arizona's apparently elevated death rate—the age-adjusted mortality rates for Arizona and Alaska are 7.5/1000 and 8.4/1000, respectively. Note that age satisfies the two criteria described above: increasing age is associated with increased mortality, regardless of where one lives; and age is associated with state of residence (Arizona's population is older than Alaska's).

Return to the sequence in which an analysis should be conducted (see Fig. 8–1). After you have assessed the basic exposure-disease relationships using two-by-two tables, you should stratify the data by "third variables"—variables that are cofactors, potential confounders, or effect modifiers (described below). If your simple two-by-two table analysis has identified two or more possible risk factors, each should be stratified by the other or others. In addition, you should develop a list of other variables to be assessed. The list should include the known risk factors for the disease (one of the two criteria for a confounder) and matching variables. Then stratify or separate the data by categories of relevant third variables. For each stratum, compute a stratum-specific measure of association. Age is so often a real confounder that it is reasonable to consider it a potential confounder in almost any data set. Using age as an example, you could separate the data by 10 year age groups (strata), create a separate two-by-two table of exposure and outcome for each stratum, and calculate a measure of association for each stratum.

The result of this type of analysis is that, within each stratum, "like is compared with like." If the stratification variable is gender, then in one stratum the exposure-disease relationship can be assessed for women and in the other the same relationship can be assessed for men. Gender can no longer be a confounder in these strata, since women are compared with women and men are compared with men.

To look for confounding, first look at the smallest and largest values of the stratum-specific measures of association and compare them with the crude value. If the crude value does not fall within the range between the smallest and largest stratum-specific values, confounding is surely present.

Often, confounding is not quite that obvious. So the next step is to calculate a summary "adjusted" measure of association as a weighted average of the stratum-specific values. The most common method of controlling for confounding is by stratifying the data and then computing measures that represent weighted averages of the stratum-specific data. One popular technique was developed by Mantel and Haenszel. This and other methods are described in Reference 6. After calculating a summary value, compare the summary value to the crude value to see if the two are "appreciably different." Unfortunately, there are no hard-and-fast rules or statistical tests to determine what constitutes "appreciably different." In practice, we assume that the summary adjusted value is more accurate. The question then becomes, "Does the crude value adequately approximate the adjusted value, or would the crude value be misleading to a reader?" If the crude and adjusted values are close, you can use the crude because it is not misleading and it is easier to explain. If the two values are appreciably different (10%? 20%?), use the adjusted value.

After deciding whether the crude or adjusted or stratum-specific measures of association are appropriate, you can then perform hypothesis testing and calculate confidence intervals for the chosen measures.

Effect Modification

The third use of stratification is in assessing effect modification. *Effect modification* means, simply, that the degree of association between an exposure and an outcome differs in different subgroups of the population. For example, a measles vaccine (exposure) may be highly effective (strong association) in preventing disease (outcome) if given after a child is 15 months of age (stratification variable = age at vaccination, stratum 1 = ≥15 months), but less effective (weaker association) if given before 15 months (age stratum 2 = <15 months). As a second example, tetracycline (exposure) may cause (strong association) tooth mottling (outcome) among children (stratifier = age, stratum 1 = children), but tetracycline does not cause tooth mottling among adults. In both examples, the association or effect is a function of, or is modified by, some third variable. Effect modification is enlightening because it raises questions for further research. Why does the effect vary? In what way is one group different from the other? Studying these and related questions can lead to insights into pathophysiology, natural history of disease, and genetic or acquired host characteristics that influence risk.

Basically, evaluation for effect modification involves determining whether the stratum-specific measures of association differ from one another. Identification of effect modification is really a two-part process involving these questions:

1. Is the range of associations wide enough to be of public health or scientific importance? (A credo of field epidemiology is that "a difference, to be a difference, has to make a difference.")
2. Is the range of associations likely to represent normal sampling variation? Evaluation can be done either qualitatively ("eyeballing the results") or quantitatively (done with multivariate analysis such as logistic regression or with statistical tests of heterogeneity).

Another difference is important to note: confounding is extremely common because it is just an artifact of the data. True effect modification, on the other hand, usually represents a biological phenomenon and hence is much less common.

ADDITIONAL ANALYSES

Two additional areas are worth mentioning, although technical discussions are beyond the scope of this book. These two areas are the assessment of dose-response relationships and modeling.

Dose Response

In epidemiology, *dose-response* means increased risk of disease with increasing (or, for a protective exposure, decreasing) amount of exposure. Amount of exposure may reflect intensity of exposure (e.g., milligrams of L-tryptophan or number of cigarettes per day) or duration of exposure (e.g., number of months or years of exposure) or both.

If an association between an exposure and a health problem has been established, epidemiologists often take the next step to look for a dose-response effect. Indeed, the presence of a dose-response effect is one of the well-recognized criteria for inferring causation. Statistical techniques are available for assessing such relationships, even when confounders must be taken into account.

The first step, as always, is organizing your data. One convenient format is a 2-by-H table, where H represents the categories or doses of exposure.

As shown in Table 8–14, an odds ratio (or a risk ratio for a cohort study) can be calculated for each dose relative to the lowest dose or the unexposed group. You can calculate confidence intervals for each dose as well.

Merely eyeballing the data in this format can give you a sense of whether a dose-response relationship is present. If the odds ratios increase or decrease monotonically, a statistically significant dose-response relationship may be present. The Mantel extension test is one method of assessing the statistical significance of a dose-response effect. The mechanics of this test are described in Reference 7. The test yields a chi-square statistic with one degree of freedom.

Modeling

There comes a time in the life of many epidemiologists when neither simple nor stratified analysis can do justice to the data. At such times, epidemiologists may turn to modeling. Modeling is a technique of fitting the data to particular statistical equations. One group of models are regression models, where the outcome is a function of exposure variables, confounders, and interaction terms (effect modifiers). The types of data usually dictate the type of regression model that is most appropriate. For example, logistic regression is the model most epi-

Table 8–14. Data Layout and Notation for Dose-Response Table

	ILL	WELL		Odds ratio
Dose 5	a_5	b_5	h_5	$a_5 d/b_5 c$
Dose 4	a_4	b_4	h_4	$a_4 d/b_4 c$
Dose 3	a_3	b_3	h_3	$a_3 d/b_3 c$
Dose 2	a_2	b_2	h_2	$a_2 d/b_2 c$
Dose 1	a_1	b_1	h_1	$a_1 d/b_1 c$
Dose 0	c	d	h_0	1.0 (reference)
	v_1	v_0	t	

demiologists choose for binary outcome variables (ill/well, case/control, alive/dead, etc.).

In logistic regression, a binary outcome (dependent) variable is modeled as a function of a series of independent variables. The independent variables should include the exposure or exposures of primary interest and may include confounders and more complex interaction terms. Software packages provide beta coefficients for each independent term. If the model includes only the outcome variable and the primary exposure variable coded as (0,1), then e^β should equal the odds ratio you could calculate from the two-by-two table. If other terms are included in the model, then e^β equals the odds ratio adjusted for all the other terms. Logistic regression can also be used to assess dose-response relationships, effect modification, and more complex relationships. A variant of logistic regression called conditional logistic regression is particularly appropriate for pair-matched data.

Other types of models used in epidemiology include Cox proportional hazards models for life-table analysis, binomial regression for risk ratio analysis, and Poisson regression for analysis of rare-event data.

Keep in mind that *sophisticated analytic techniques cannot atone for sloppy data*. Analytic techniques such as those described in this chapter are only as good as the data to which they are applied. Analytic techniques, whether they be simple, stratified, or multivariate, use the information at hand. They do not ask or assess whether the proper comparison group was selected, whether the response rate was adequate, whether exposure and disease were properly defined, or whether the data coding and entry were free of errors. Analytic techniques are merely tools; as the analyst, you are responsible for knowing the quality of the data and interpreting the results appropriately.

MATCHING IN CASE-CONTROL STUDIES

Early in this chapter we noted that different study designs require different analytic methods. Matching is one design that requires methods different from those described so far. Because matching is so common in field studies, this section addresses this important topic.

Matching generally refers to a case-control study design in which controls are intentionally selected to be similar to case-subjects on one or more specified characteristics (other than the exposure or exposures of interest). The goal of matching, like that of stratified analysis, is to "compare like with like." The characteristics most appropriately specified for matching are those that are potential confounders of the exposure-disease associations of interest. By matching cases and controls on factors such as age, gender, or geographic area, the distribution of those factors among cases and controls will be identical. In other words, the matching variable will not be associated with case-control status in the study. As a result, if the analysis is properly done, the matching variable will not confound the association of primary interest.

Two types of matching schemes are commonly used in epidemiology. One type is *pair matching*, where each control is selected according to its similarity to a *particular* case. This method is most appropriate when each case is unique in terms of the matching factor, for example, 50 cases widely scattered geographically. Each case could be matched to a friend or neighborhood control. That control is suitably matched to that particular case-subject, but not to any other case-subject in the study. The matching by design into these unique pairs must be maintained in the analysis.

The term "pair matching" is sometimes generalized to include not only matched pairs (case and one control), but matched triplets (case and two controls), quadruplets, and so on. The term also refers to studies in which the number of matched controls per case varies, so long as the controls are matched to a specific case.

The other type of matching is *category matching*, also called *frequency matching*. Category matching is a form of stratified sampling of controls, wherein controls are selected in proportion to the number of cases in each category of a matching variable. For example, in a study of 70 male and 30 female case-subjects, if 100 controls were also desired, you would select 70 male controls at random from the pool of all non-ill males and 30 female controls from the female pool. The pairs are not unique; any male control is a suitable match to any male case-subject. Data collected by category matching in the study design must be analyzed using stratified analysis.

Matching has several advantages. Matching on factors such as neighborhood, friendship, or sibship may control for confounding by numerous social factors that would be otherwise impossible to measure and control. Matching may be cost-

and time-efficient, facilitating enrollment of controls. For example, matched friend controls may be identified while interviewing each case-subject, and these friends are more likely to cooperate than controls randomly selected from the general population. And finally, matching on a confounder increases the statistical efficiency of an analysis and thus provides narrower confidence intervals.

Matching has disadvantages, too. The primary disadvantage is that matching on a factor prevents you from examining its association with disease. If the age and gender distribution of case-subjects and controls are identical because you matched on those two factors, you cannot use your data to evaluate age and gender as risk factors themselves. Matching may be both cost- and time-inefficient, if considerable work must be performed to identify appropriately matched controls. The more variables to be matched on, the more difficult it will be to find suitably matched controls. In addition, matching on a factor that is not a confounder or having to discard cases because suitable controls could not be found decreases statistical efficiency and results in wider confidence intervals. Finally, matching complicates the analysis, particularly if other confounders are present.

In summary, matching is desirable and beneficial when you know beforehand that (1) you do not wish to examine the relationship between the matching factor and disease; (2) the factor is related to risk of disease so it is a potential confounder; and (3) matching is convenient or at least worth the potential extra costs to you. When in doubt, do not match, or match only on a strong risk factor that is likely to be distributed differently between exposed and unexposed groups and that is not a risk factor you are interested in assessing.

Matched Pairs

The basic data layout for a matched-pair analysis appears at first glance to resemble the simple unmatched two-by-two tables presented earlier in this chapter, but in reality the two are quite different. In the matched-pair two-by-two table, each cell represents the number of matched pairs who meet the row and column criteria. In the unmatched two-by-two table, each cell represents the number of individuals who meet the criteria.

In Table 8–15, E+ denotes "exposed" and E– denotes "unexposed." Cell f thus represents the number of pairs made up of an exposed case and an unexposed control. Cells e and h are called *concordant pairs* because the case and control are in the same exposure category. Cells f and g are called *discordant pairs*.

In a matched-pair analysis, only the discordant pairs are informative. The odds ratio is computed as

$$\text{Odds ratio} = f / g$$

Table 8–15. Data Layout and Notation for Matched-Pair
Two-by-Two Table

		CONTROLS		
		E+	E–	Total
CASES	E+	e	f	e + f
	E–	g	h	g + h
	TOTAL	e + g	f + h	e + f + g + h

The test of significance for a matched pair analysis is the McNemar chi-square test. Both uncorrected and corrected formulas are commonly used.

$$\text{Uncorrected McNemar test} = \frac{(f - g)^2}{(f + g)}$$

$$\text{Corrected McNemar test} = \frac{(|f - g| - 1)^2}{(f + g)}$$

Table 8–16 presents the data from a pair-matched case-control study conducted in 1980 to assess the association between tampon use and toxic shock syndrome.[8]

Table 8–16. Continual Tampon Use during
Index Menstrual Period in Case-Control Pairs,
Toxic Shock Syndrome Study, 1980

		CONTROLS		
		YES	NO	TOTAL
CASES	YES	33	9	42
	NO	1	1	2
	TOTAL	34	10	44 pairs

Odds ratio = 9 / 1 = 9.0

McNemar uncorrected chi-square test = $(9 - 1)^2 / (9 + 1) = 6.40$ ($P = 0.01$)

McNemar corrected chi-square test = $(|9 - 1| - 1)^2 / (9 + 1) = 4.90$ ($P = 0.03$)

[*Source*: Shands et al., 1980.][8]

Matched Triplets

The data layout for a study in which two controls are matched to each case is shown in Table 8–17. Each cell is named f_{ij}, where i is the number of exposed cases (1 if the case is exposed, 0 if the case is unexposed), and j is the number of exposed controls in the triplet. Thus cell f_{02} contains the number of triplets in which the case is unexposed but both controls are exposed.

A formula for calculating an odds ratio with *any* number of controls per case is

$$OR = \frac{\text{Number of unexposed controls matched with exposed cases}}{\text{Number of exposed controls matched with unexposed cases}}$$

For matched triplets, this formula reduces to

$$\text{Odds ratio} = \frac{2f_{10} + f_{11}}{2f_{02} + f_{01}}$$

Table 8–17 shows data from a case-control study of Kawasaki syndrome in Washington State.[9] For each of 16 case-subjects, two age- and neighborhood-matched controls were identified. Although the study found no association with carpet cleaning, it did find the usual association with high household income (Table 8–18).

Larger Matched Sets and Variable Matching

Analogous analytic methods are available for matched sets of any fixed size and for sets with variable numbers of controls per case.[10] Such data are best analyzed with appropriate computer software, such as *Epi Info*.

Table 8–17. Data Layout and Notation for a
Matched Case Control Study with Two Controls per Case

| | | PERCENT EXPOSED CONTROLS | | |
		2 of 2	1 of 2	0 of 2
CASES	E+	f_{12}	f_{11}	f_{10}
	E–	f_{02}	f_{01}	f_{00}

Table 8–18. Kawasaki Syndrome and Annual Household
Income > $40,000, Washington State, 1986

		NUMBER OF EXPOSED CONTROLS		
		2 of 2	1 of 2	0 of 2
CASES	E+	0	1	7
	E–	0	4	4

Odds ratio = $(2 \times 7 + 1) / (2 \times 0 + 4) = 3.8$

[*Source*: Dicker, 1986.][9]

Does a Matched Design Require a Matched Analysis?

Does a matched design require a matched analysis? Usually, yes. In a pair-matched study, if the pairs are unique (siblings, friends, etc.), then pair-matched analysis is needed. If the pairs were based on a nonunique characteristic such as gender or race, stratified analysis is preferred. In a frequency matched study, stratified analysis is necessary.

In practice, some epidemiologists perform the appropriate matched analysis, then "break the match" and perform an unmatched analysis on the same data. If the results are similar, they may opt to present the data in unmatched fashion. In most instances, the unmatched odds ratio will be closer to 1.0 than the matched odds ratio ("bias toward the null"). Less frequently, the "broken" or unmatched odds ratio will be further from the null. These differences, which are related to confounding, may be trivial or substantial. The chi-square test result from unmatched data may be particularly misleading, usually being larger than the McNemar test result from the matched data. The decision to use a matched analysis or unmatched analysis is analogous to the decision to present crude or adjusted results. You must use your epidemiologic judgment in deciding whether the unmatched results are misleading to your audience or, worse, to yourself!

INTERPRETING FIELD DATA

"Skepticism is the chastity of the intellect. . . .
Don't give it away to the first attractive hypothesis that comes along."
                                                            M. B. Gregg,
                                                    after George Santayana

Does an elevated relative risk or odds ratio or a statistically significant chi-square test mean that the exposure is a true cause of disease? Certainly not. Although the association may indeed be causal, flaws in study design, execution, and analysis can result in apparent associations that are actually artifacts. Chance, selection bias, information bias, confounding, and investigator error should all be evaluated as possible explanations for an observed association.

One possible explanation for an observed association is chance. Under the null hypothesis, you assume that your study population is a sample from some source population and that incidence of disease is not associated with exposure in the source population. The role of chance is assessed through the use of tests of statistical significance. (As noted above, confidence intervals can be used as well.) A very small P value indicates that the null hypothesis is an *unlikely* explanation of the result you found. Keep in mind that chance can never be ruled out entirely— even if the P value is small, say 0.01. Yours may be the one sample in a hundred in which the null hypothesis is true and chance *is* the explanation! Note that tests of significance evaluate only the role of chance. They do not say anything about the roles of selection bias, information bias, confounding, or investigator error, discussed below.

Another explanation for the observed explanation is selection bias. *Selection bias* is a systematic error in the study groups or in the enrollment of study participants that results in a mistaken estimate of an exposure's effect on the risk of disease. In more simplistic terms, selection bias may be thought of as a problem arising from who gets into the study. Selection bias may arise either in the design or in the execution of the study. Selection bias may arise from the faulty design of a case-control study if, for example, too loose a case definition is used (so some persons in the case group do not actually have the disease being studied), asymptomatic cases go undetected among the controls, or an inappropriate control group is used. In the execution phase, selection bias may result if eligible subjects with certain exposure and disease characteristics choose not to participate or cannot be located. For example, if ill persons with the exposure of interest know the hypothesis of the study and are more willing to participate than other ill persons, then cell a in the two-by-two table will be artificially inflated compared to cell c, and the odds ratio will also be inflated. So to evaluate the possible role of selection bias, you must look at how cases and controls were specified and how they were enrolled.

Another possible explanation of an observed association is information bias. *Information bias* is a systematic error in the collection of exposure or outcome data about the study participants that results in a mistaken estimate of an exposure's effect on the risk of disease. Again, in more simplistic terms, information bias is a problem with the information you collect from the people in the study. Information bias may arise in a number of ways, including poor wording or understanding of a question on a questionnaire, poor recall (what did YOU have for lunch a week ago Tuesday?), or inconsistent interviewing technique. Information bias may also arise if a subject knowingly provides false information, either to hide the truth or, as is common in some cultures, in an attempt to please the interviewer.

As discussed earlier in this chapter, confounding can also distort an association. To evaluate the role of confounding, ensure that a list of potential confounders has been drawn up, that they have been evaluated for confounding, and that they have been controlled for as necessary.

Finally, investigator error has been known to be the explanation for some apparent associations. A missed button on a calculator, an erroneous transcription of a value, or use of the wrong formula can all yield artifactual associations! Check your work, or have someone else try to replicate it.

So before considering whether an association may be causal, consider whether the association may be explained by chance, selection bias, information bias, confounding, or investigator error. Now suppose that an elevated risk ratio or odds ratio has a small *P* value and narrow confidence interval, so chance is an unlikely explanation. Specification of cases and controls is reasonable and participation was good, so selection bias is an unlikely explanation. Information was collected using a standard questionnaire by an experienced and well-trained interviewer. Confounding by other risk factors was assessed and found not to be present or to have been controlled for. Data entry and calculations were verified. But before you conclude that the association is causal, you should consider the strength of the association, its biological plausibility, consistency with results from other studies, temporal sequence, and dose-response relationship, if any.

Strength of the Association

In general, the stronger the association, the more likely one is to believe it is real. Thus we are generally more willing to believe that a relative risk of 9.0 may be causal than a relative risk of 1.5. This is not to say that a relative risk of 1.5 cannot reflect a causal relationship; it can. It is just that a subtle selection bias, information bias, or confounding could easily account for a relative risk of 1.5. The bias would have to be quite dramatic to account for a relative risk of 9.0!

Biological Plausibility

Does the association make sense? Is it consistent with what is known of the pathophysiology, the known vehicles, the natural history of disease, animal models, or other relevant biological factors? For an implicated food vehicle in an infectious disease outbreak, can the agent be identified in the food, or will the agent survive (or even thrive) in the food? While some outbreaks are caused by new or previously unrecognized vehicles or risk factors, most are caused by those that we already know.

Consistency with Other Studies

Are the results consistent with those from other studies? A finding is more plausible if it can be replicated by different investigators, using different methods in different populations.

Exposure Precedes Disease

This criterion seems obvious, but in a retrospective study it may be difficult to document that exposure precedes disease. Suppose, for example, that persons with a particular type of leukemia are more likely to have antibodies to a particular virus. It might be tempting to conclude that the virus causes the leukemia, but from the serologic evidence at hand you could not be certain that exposure to the virus preceded the onset of leukemic changes.

Dose-Response Effect

Evidence of a dose-response effect adds weight to the evidence for causation. A dose-response effect is not a *necessary* feature for a relationship to be causal; some causal relationships may exhibit a threshold effect, for example. In addition, a dose-response effect does not rule out the possibility of confounding. Nevertheless, it is usually thought to add credibility to the association.

In many field investigations, a likely culprit may not meet all the criteria listed above. Perhaps the response rate was less than ideal, or the etiologic agent could not be isolated from the implicated food, or the dose-response analysis was inconclusive. Nevertheless, if the public's health is at risk, failure to meet every criterion should not be used as an excuse for inaction. As stated by George Comstock, "The art of epidemiologic reasoning is to draw sensible conclusions from imperfect data."[11] After all, field epidemiology is a tool for public health action to promote and protect the public's health based on science (sound epidemiologic methods), causal reasoning, and a healthy dose of practical common sense.

> All scientific work is incomplete—whether it be observational or experimental. All scientific work is liable to be upset or modified by advancing knowledge. That does not confer upon us a freedom to ignore the knowledge we already have, or to postpone the action it appears to demand at a given time.[12]
>
> Sir Austin Bradford Hill

APPENDIX 8–1. FISHER EXACT TEST

The probability that the value in cell "a" is equal to the observed value, under the null hypothesis, is

$$\Pr{(a)} = \frac{(v_1)\,!\,(v_0)\,!\,(h_1)\,!\,(h_0)\,!}{t!\,a!\,b!\,c!\,d!}$$

where k! ("k factorial") = $1 \times 2 \times \ldots \times k$,
(e.g., 5! = $1 \times 2 \times 3 \times 4 \times 5 = 120$)

The easiest way to compute a two-tailed Fisher exact test is compute a one-tailed test and multiply by 2. Computing the one-tailed test is the hard part!

To compute the one-tailed Fisher exact test, first calculate the exact probability that cell a equals the observed value, using the formula shown above. Next, keeping all of the row and column totals the same, add or subtract 1 to the observed value in cell a to get a value even more extreme than the value observed. Modify the values in the other cells as necessary (add or subtract 1 to get the right row and column totals), and use the formula shown above to compute this new value's exact probability. Continue adding or subtracting 1 and computing probabilities until no more extreme values are possible without changing the marginal totals. Finally, sum these individual probabilities to get the one-tailed P value. For a two-tailed P value, add any smaller probabilities from the other tail.

Example:

	ILL	WELL	TOTAL	
EXPOSED	4	17	21	Odds ratio = undefined
UNEXPOSED	0	19	19	(cannot divide by zero)
TOTAL	4	36	40	

Based on the margins of this two-by-two table, cell a can take on values from 0 to 4, but none more extreme than 4. The probabilities for each value from 0 to 4 are

a	b	c	d	Probability	
4	17	0	19	4!36!21!19! / 40!4!17!0!19!	= 0.07
3	18	1	18	4!36!21!19! / 40!3!18!1!18!	= 0.28
2	19	2	17	4!36!21!19! / 40!2!19!2!17!	= 0.39
1	20	3	16	4!36!21!19! / 40!1!20!3!16!	= 0.22
0	21	4	15	4!36!21!19! / 40!0!21!4!15!	= 0.04.

Since there are no possible values of cell a more extreme than 4, the one-tailed P value is simply 0.07. The two-tailed P value is 0.07 + 0.04 = 0.11. Given a cutoff of 0.05, we could not reject the null hypothesis.

APPENDIX 8–2.

Chi-Square Table

DEGREE OF FREEDOM	PROBABILITY						
	0.50	0.20	0.10	0.05	0.02	0.01	0.001
1	0.455	1.642	2.706	3.841	5.412	6.635	10.827
2	1.386	3.219	4.605	5.991	7.824	9.210	13.815
3	2.366	4.642	6.251	7.815	9.837	11.345	16.268
4	3.357	5.989	7.779	9.488	11.668	13.277	18.465
5	4.351	7.289	9.236	11.070	13.388	15.086	20.517
10	9.342	13.442	15.987	18.307	21.161	23.209	29.588
15	14.339	19.311	22.307	24.996	28.259	30.578	37.697
20	19.337	25.038	28.412	31.410	35.020	37.566	43.315
25	24.337	30.675	34.382	37.652	41.566	44.314	52.620
30	29.336	36.250	40.256	43.773	47.962	50.892	59.703

Note: The Pearson chi-square test and the Yates corrected chi-square test from a two-by-two table have one degree of freedom. The Mantel-Haenszel chi-square also has one degree of freedom, whether from a single two-by-two table or from stratified analysis.

REFERENCES

1. Shem, S. (1978). The House of God. Richard Marek Publishers, New York.
2. Dean A.G., Dean J.A., Coulombier D., et al. (1994). Epi Info, Version 6: A word processing, database, and statistics program for epidemiology or microcomputers. Centers for Disease Control and Prevention, Atlanta, Georgia.
3. Luby, S.P., Jones, J.L., Horan, J.M. (1993). A large salmonellosis outbreak catered by a frequently penalized restaurant. *Epidemiol and Infect* 110, 31–39.
4. Berkelman, R.L., Martin, D., Graham, D.R., et al. (1982). Streptococcal wound infections caused by a vaginal carrier. *J American Med Assoc* 247, 2680–82.
5. Landrigan, P.J. (1972). Epidemic measles in a divided city. *J American Med Assoc* 221, 567–70.
6. Kleinbaum, D.G., Kupper, L.L., Morgenstern, H. (1982). *Epidemiologic Research: Principles and Quantitative Methods*. Lifetime Learning Publications, Belmont, California.
7. Schlesselman, J.J. (1982). *Case-control studies: Design, conduct, analysis*. Oxford University Press, New York.
8. Shands, K.N., Schmid, G.P., Dan, B.B., et al. (1980). Toxic-shock syndrome in menstruating women: Association with tampon use and *Staphylococcus aureus* and clinical features in 52 cases. *N Eng Med*, 303, 1436–42.
9. Dicker, R.C. (1986). Kawasaki syndrome. *Washington Morbid Rep*,(Oct);1–4.

10. Robins, J., Greenland, S., Breslow, N.E. (1986). A general estimator for the variance of the Mantel-Haenszel odds ratio. *Am J Epidemiol*, 124, 719–23.
11. Comstock, G.W. (1990). Vaccine evaluation by case-control or prospective studies. *Am J Epidemiol*, 131, 205–7.
12. Hill, A.B. (1965). The environment and disease: association or causation? *Proc R Soc Med* 58, 295–300.

9

DEVELOPING INTERVENTIONS

Richard A. Goodman
James W. Buehler
Jeffrey P. Koplan
Duc J. Vugia

Epidemiologic field investigations are often done in response to acute public health problems. When outbreaks of disease occur, there is usually an urgent need to identify the source and/or cause of the problem as a basis for initiating control measures or other interventions. Alternatively, the identification of environmental or occupational hazards frequently demands evaluation of exposed persons and an assessment of the risks of disease. Regardless of the nature of such problems, however, there will be an immediate need to investigate, to recommend control and preventive measures, and to convince the affected community to accept public health recommendations.

When circumstances require an immediate response, you must sometimes take and/or recommend specific public health actions without incontrovertible epidemiologic "proof," such as the determination of a causal relation. Under such circumstances, the key issue for the field epidemiologist and the decision makers revolves around the following question: To what extent must an acute health problem be epidemiologically defined and understood before action should be initiated? This chapter outlines factors that influence the conduct of field investigations and the decisions relating to interventions.

This chapter was adapted with permission of editors from: Goodman, R.A., Buehler, J.W., Koplan, J.P. (1990) The epidemiologic field investigation: science and judgment in public health practice. *Am J Epidemiol* 132, 91–96.

REASONS FOR INITIATING FIELD INVESTIGATIONS

In addition to the need to develop and implement control measures to end threats to the public's health, other reasons for field investigations include: (*1*) statutory and program considerations; (*2*) public and political concerns; (*3*) legal obligations; (*4*) opportunities for research; and (*5*) training.

Statutory and Program Considerations

Certain disease control programs at national, state, and local levels have specific and extensive requirements for epidemiologic investigation. For example, as part of the measles elimination effort in the United States, a measles outbreak is considered to exist in a community whenever one case of measles is confirmed.[1] Accordingly, every case of measles is investigated in order to identify and immunize susceptible persons and to evaluate such other control strategies as the exclusion from school of those children who cannot provide proof of immunity. A potentially detrimental effect of such policies is that costly investigations may yield limited public health benefit—as illustrated by the investigation of a single case of cholera in Texas in 1972.[2]

Because they can be costly in personnel time and resources, field investigations may detract from other activities. Thus, the capacity to do fieldwork may be limited by competing demands of other programs within an agency, whether at national, state, or local levels. Under these circumstances, failure to investigate a specific problem could result in a public health problem of greater magnitude, which, if controlled earlier, would have caused less human and economic loss. More specifically, emerging infections, such as the Hanta virus epidemic in the southwestern United States, and the anthrax bioterrorism attacks have forced local and state health departments to devote more time and energy to such realities.[3-6] Single cases of unusual or rare diseases now require greater scrutiny and more careful investigation than before—work that demands more staff and more money.

Public and Political Concern

Although the public's perceptions of hazards may differ from those of epidemiologists, these perceptions, more than ever before, drive the political process that mandates investigations or actions. In rare instances, a citizens' alert can lead to recognition of a major public health problem, such as with Lyme disease in Lyme, Connecticut, in 1976.[7] In some cases, however, public concerns mandate investigations that are premature or unlikely to be fruitful from a scientific perspective but are critical in terms of community relations. Small clusters of disease (e.g., leukemia or adverse fetal outcomes) are an example of problems that frequently generate great public concern. Small cluster outbreaks often occur by chance alone and only occasionally yield new research information when investigated.[8] However, because community members may perceive a health threat and because certain clusters do represent specific preventable risks, some public health agencies have developed standard procedures for investigating such clusters even though the likelihood of identifying a remediable cause is low.

On a much larger scale, for example, was an investigation of an encephalitis epidemic purported to have occurred in Lee County, Florida, in 1978. A private physician reported 300 to 400 cases of encephalitis over a 12 month period, monumentally more than any other physician in the county. The possibility of a mosquito-borne epidemic of encephalitis in southern Florida became real and frightening, so extensive investigations were done by the local and state health departments. No supportive evidence was found for the epidemic, but some citizens demanded further study. CDC was called, sent two epidemiologists, investigated, and found no epidemic. Further local agitation forced a reexamination, this time requiring four epidemiologists from CDC to spend more than 2 weeks, reviewing over 3500 medical records. They still found no epidemic, yet two of them were called to Washington, D.C., to report their findings to a U.S. senator from Florida (M.B. Gregg, personal communication, and CDC, unpublished data).

At the other extreme, attempts at more thorough epidemiologic investigations can be misinterpreted as community experimentation or bureaucratic delay. In a large E. coli enteric disease outbreak at Crater Lake National Park in 1975, a one-day delay in implementing control measures to obtain more epidemiologic data resulted in a congressional hearing and charges of a "cover up."[9]

Research Opportunities

Because almost all outbreaks are "natural experiments," they also present opportunities to address questions of importance to both the basic scientist and those in the applied science of public health practice. Even when there is a clear policy for control of a specific problem, investigation may still provide opportunities to identify new agents and risk factors for infection or disease, define the clinical spectrum of disease, measure the impact of control measures or clinical interventions, or assess the usefulness of microbiologic or other biologic markers.

Some outbreaks that initially appear to be "routine" may lead to important epidemiologic discoveries. For example, in 1983 investigators pursued a cluster of diarrhea cases, an extremely common problem, to extraordinary lengths.[10] As a result, the investigators were able to trace the chain of transmission of a unique strain of multiply-antibiotic resistant Salmonella back from the affected persons to hamburger they consumed, to the meat supplier, and ultimately to the specific animal herd source. This investigation played a key role in clarifying the linkage between antibiotic use by the cattle industry and subsequent antibiotic-resistant infection in humans.

Moreover, on a broader scale, over the past 30 to 40 years, field epidemiologists have established the applied scientific basis for virtually all immunization recommendations in the United States. A few examples of field studies that have shaped the evolving changes in immunization practices include the scores of field studies of mumps, measles, and rubella outbreaks; vaccine trials of viral hepatitis and influenza; and case investigations of vaccine-associated poliomyelitis.

Legal Obligations

Field investigations frequently require access to patients' private records, identification of private enterprises putatively responsible for illness, review of these companies' proprietary information, or even the reporting of errors of health care providers. Each task is clearly necessary to complete an objective, defensible field investigation, but each is also fraught with considerable ethical and legal overtones (see Chapter 14).

Some investigations are likely to be used as testimony in civil or criminal trials. In these situations, investigations may be carried further than would otherwise be done. For example, in an investigation of a cluster of cardiac arrests in an intensive care unit in Maryland in 1986, the investigation went to the unusual length of attempting to determine the contents of charts that could not be located.[11,12]

Training

By analogy to clerkships in medical school and postgraduate residencies, outbreak investigations provide opportunities for training in basic epidemiologic skills. Just as clinical training often is accomplished at the same time as patient care is provided, training in field epidemiology often simultaneously assists in developing skills in disease control and prevention.[13] For the local epidemiologist, public health nurse, sanitarian, or environmental health specialist there is no substitute for hands-on experience.

DETERMINANTS FOR INTERVENTIONS

The severity of a specific problem is a key determinant of the urgency and course of a field investigation. Severity is indicated by correlates such as the degree and nature of complications (e.g., mortality), duration of illness, need for treatment and hospitalization, and economic impact. For example, virtually all cases of rabies occurring in humans in the United States trigger extensive epidemiologic investigations because of the vital need to prevent deaths by quickly identifying other exposures and the animal source. Similarly, nosocomial infection clusters—especially those in postsurgical or immunocompromised patients—are often investigated because of the potential for serious complications and greatly prolonged hospitalization and the possibility of iatrogenic illness—with its own special urgency as an unnecessary medical event.

In addition to the severity of a problem, a spectrum of other factors influences the aggressiveness, extent, and scientific rigor of an epidemiologic field investigation. In the prototypic investigation, control measures are formulated only after a series of other steps have been carried out (see Chapter 5). In practice, however, decisions about control measures may be appropriate or warranted at any step in the sequence. For most outbreaks of acute disease, the scope of an investigation is dictated by the levels of certainty about (1) the etiology of the problem (e.g., the specific pathogen or toxic agent); and (2) the source and/or mode of spread (e.g., water-borne or airborne). When the problem initially is identified, the levels of certainty regarding the etiology, source, and mode of spread may range from known to unknown (Fig. 9–1). These basic dichotomies are illustrated in the figure by four examples that probably represent the extremes. In many situations control measures can be implemented empirically, while in others interventions are appropriate only after exhaustive epidemiologic investigation.

Source/transmission mode

		Known	Unknown
Etiology	**Known**	Investigation + Control +++ Example: Hepatitis A in a day care	Investigation +++ Control + Example: Salmonella in marijuana
	Unknown	Investigation +++ Control +++ Example: Parathion poisoning	Investigation +++ Control + Example: Legionnaires' disease

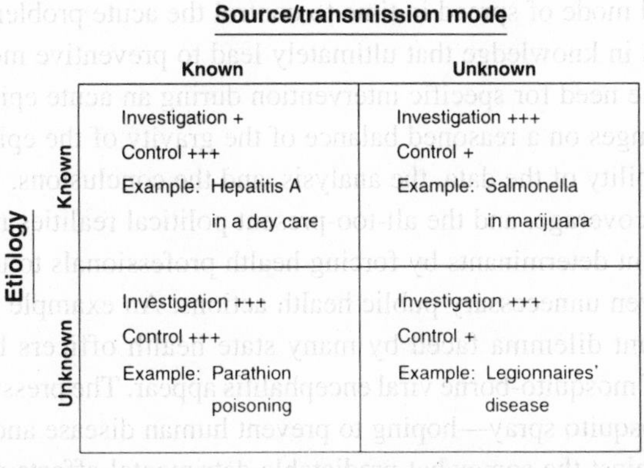

Figure 9–1. Relative emphasis of investigative and control efforts (response options) in disease outbreaks as influenced by levels of certainty about etiology and source/mode of transmission. *Investigation* means extent of the investigation; *control* means the basis for rapid implementation of control measures. Pluses show the level of response indicated (+ = low; +++ = high). [*Source:* Goodman et al., 1990.]

Preliminary control measures often can be started based on limited, initial information, and then can be modified as investigations proceed. For example, the occurrence of a single case of hepatitis A in a day care center may lead to the administration of immune globulin prophylaxis to an entire cohort of exposed children and staff.[14] In this instance, the response is predicated on routine policy and guidelines that have been developed by experts based on studies, previous outbreak experience, and virtual certainty about both the etiology of the problem and its mode of spread.

More commonly, there is some degree of uncertainty about the etiology or about sources and the mode of spread (Fig. 9–1). In most outbreaks of gastrointestinal disease, the control measures selected will depend on knowing whether transmission has resulted from person-to-person spread or from a common source exposure and, if the latter, identifying the source. For example, an outbreak of *Salmonella muenchen* in several states in 1981 required an extensive epidemiologic field investigation, including an analytic (case-control) study, before the mode of spread was found to be personal use or household exposure to marijuana.[15] The converse situation (i.e., in which the source is presumed, but the etiology is unknown) is illustrated by the nationwide outbreak of eosinophilia–myalgia syndrome (EMS) in the United States in 1989.[16] In that outbreak, L-tryptophan, a dietary supplement, was initially implicated as the source of the exposure and provided material for subsequent laboratory analysis to define the actual agent; in the interim, epidemiologists were able to make recommendations for preventing further exposures and cases. Finally, as illustrated by the legionnaires' disease outbreak in 1976, an extensive field investigation can fail to identify the cause, the source, and mode of spread in time to control the acute problem, but still enables advances in knowledge that ultimately lead to preventive measures.[17]

Indeed, the need for specific intervention during an acute epidemic investigation often hinges on a reasoned balance of the gravity of the epidemic and the scientific reliability of the data, the analysis, and the conclusions. Yet public demands, media coverage, and the all-too-present political realities may also serve as equally potent determinants by forcing health professionals to undertake controversial or even unnecessary public health actions. An example of such forces and the resultant dilemma faced by many state health officers happens when human cases of mosquito-borne viral encephalitis appear. The pressure of the public to apply mosquito spray—hoping to prevent human disease and death—must be weighed against the somewhat predictable detrimental effects of widespread, environmental chemical exposure. And in a situation involving meningococcal disease in New England, public and medical concern combined with social and political pressure resulted in a statewide vaccination campaign targeting all residents aged 2–22 years, although the situation did not meet criteria for an outbreak as defined by the Advisory Committee on Immunization Practices.[18]

Epidemiology and, particularly, field epidemiology are relatively young scientific disciplines in the medical world, acquiring academic and later public acceptance only slowly over the past four to five decades. Even slower acceptance of epidemiologic methods has been typical of many in the legal profession, private enterprise, and even certain regulatory agencies. And to some extent, rightly so—for, in the strictest sense, epidemiologic evidence establishes only associations, not hard proof. For example, several years elapsed after field studies had clearly linked aspirin use and Reye syndrome before industry and the Food and Drug Administration (FDA) accepted the association and issued warnings to that effect. The toxic shock syndrome story, so succinctly told in Chapter 18, further illustrates the reluctance of industry to accept epidemiologic evidence in the face of a nationwide epidemic.

As a related example, in 1996 and again in 1997, large outbreaks of *Cyclospora*, an emerging food-borne parasite, occurred in the United States and Canada.[19] Only epidemiologic evidence linked the outbreaks to fresh raspberries imported from Guatemala. In 1998, based primarily on that evidence, the FDA stopped importation of that product from Guatemala into the United States; Canada allowed continued importation, and a *Cyclospora* outbreak associated with these raspberries occurred in Ontario in May 1998.[20] Thus, acceptance of the relatively straightforward scientific thought process of epidemiology can significantly determine the course and outcome of interventions in the field.

CAUSATION AND THE FIELD INVESTIGATION

The need to determine whether a statistical association also supports a causal relation is as essential to an epidemiologic field investigation as it is to a planned prospective study. Thus, the criteria to assess causal associations are integral to the scientific framework of field investigations.[21,22] The challenge is to balance the need to assess causality through the process of scientific inquiry with the potentially conflicting need to intervene quickly to protect the public's health. Few epidemiologic field investigations appear to address the criteria of causality explicitly; however, when the criteria are applied to such investigations, they may be only partially attained.

The usefulness of individual criteria (e.g., temporality, strength of association, biologic gradient, consistency, plausibility) varies.[22] In any outbreak, multiple groups of persons may be exposed, affected, or involved in some respect. Because of differences in knowledge, beliefs, and perceived impact of the outbreak, each group may draw different conclusions about causality from the same information. For example, in a restaurant-associated food-borne outbreak, restaurant patrons, management, media, attorneys, and local health officials are each likely to have a different threshold for judging the food from the restaurant to be the source of disease. In this situation, your concerns might focus on strength of association and biologic gradient between exposure to a certain food item and illness, while a restaurant patron's primary concern may simply be plausibility. Attorneys, on the other hand, defending a restaurant epidemiologically associated with a food-borne epidemic, will often review each patient one by one. Their hope is to show that with each case there can be reasonable doubt that illness truly resulted from eating at the restaurant in question. By such tactics they hope to show there was no epidemic or no liability for the epidemic.

CONCLUSION AND FUTURE DIRECTIONS

Epidemiologic field investigations are usually initiated in response to epidemics or the occurrence of other acute disease, injury, or environmental health problems. Under such circumstances, the primary objective of the field investigation will be to employ the scientific principles of epidemiology to determine a rational and appropriate response for ending or controlling the problem. Key factors that influence decisions about the timing and choice of public health intervention(s) include a carefully crafted balance of the severity of the problem, the levels of scientific certainty of the findings, the extent to which causal criteria have been established, and, now, more than ever before, the public and political perceptions of what is the best course of action.

An important trend characterizing the nature of interventions to terminate outbreaks and control disease and injury occurrence is the increasing role of community involvement. For example, over the past decade, public health agencies have had to become innovative and to modify their responses to problems such as outbreaks of tuberculosis, clusters of cases of human immunodeficiency virus infection, and resurgent sexually transmitted diseases.[23,24] For some of these problems, traditional methods for investigation and contact evaluation have been supplanted by newer "social network" approaches—interventions that require increased involvement of community representatives. In such settings, community support is essential to the success of the investigation and longer-term prevention and control measures; conversely, failure to obtain community trust and support actually can disable an investigation. This may be especially true when problems disproportionately affect groups who are marginalized and who otherwise may be initially reluctant to work with public health officials. The increasing role of community involvement in and support for public health interventions applies not only to infectious diseases but also to the prevention and control of environmental hazards, injuries, and other noninfectious disease problems.

REFERENCES

1. Centers for Disease Control and Prevention (1998). Measles, mumps, and rubella—vaccine use and strategies for elimination of measles, rubella, and congenital rubella syndrome and control of mumps: recommendations of the Advisory Committee on Immunization Practices (ACIP). *MMWR* 47 (No. RR-8), 38–39.

2. Weissman, J.B., DeWitt, W.E., Thompson, J., et al. (1975). A case of cholera in Texas, 1973. *Am J Epidemiol* 100, 487–98.

3. Institute of Medicine (1992). *Emerging Infections: microbial threats to health in the United States.* National Academy Press, Washington, D.C.

4. Centers for Disease Control and Prevention (1994). *Addressing emerging infectious disease threats: a prevention strategy for the United States.* Atlanta.

5. Cieslak, T.J., Eitzen, E.M., Jr. (2000). Bioterrorism: agents of concern. *J Public Health Manag Pract* 6, 19–29.

6. Gallo, R.J., Campbell, D. (2000). Bioterrorism: challenges and opportunities for local health departments. *J Public Health Manag Pract* 6, 57–62.

7. Steere, A.C., Malawista, S.E., Snydman, D.R., et al. (1977). Lyme arthritis: an epidemic of oligoarticular arthritis in children and adults in three Connecticut communities. *Arthritis Rheum* 20, 7–17.

8. Schulte, P.A., Ehrenberg, R.L., Singal, M. (1987). Investigation of occupational cancer clusters: theory and practice. *Am J Public Health* 77, 52–56.

9. Rosenberg, M.L., Koplan, J.P., Wachsmith, I.K., et al. (1977). Epidemic diarrhea at Crater Lake from enterotoxigenic. Escherichia coli: a large waterborne outbreak. *Ann Intern Med* 86, 714–18.

10. Holmberg, S.D., Osterholm, M.T., Senger, K.A., et al. (1984). Drug-resistant Salmonella from animals fed antimicrobials. *N Engl J Med* 311, 617–22.

11. Sacks, J.J., Stroup, D.F., Will, M.L., et al (1988). A nurse-associated epidemic of cardiac arrests in an intensive care unit. *JAMA* 259, 689–95.

12. Sacks, J.J., Aung, H.K., Sniezek, J.S. (1988). The epidemiology of missing records (letter). *JAMA* 259, 685.

13. Thacker, S.B., Goodman, R.A., Dicker, R.C. (1990). Training and service in public health practice, 1951–90—CDC's Epidemic Intelligence Service. *Public Health Rep* 105, 599–604.

14. Centers for Disease Control and Prevention (1996). Prevention of hepatitis A through active or passive immunization: recommendations of the Advisory Committee on Immunization Practices (ACIP). *MMWR* 45 (No. RR-15), 24.

15. Taylor, D.N., Wachsmuth, K., Yung-Hui, S., et al. (1982). Salmonellosis associated with marijuana: a multistate outbreak traced by plasmic fingerprinting. *N Engl J Med* 306, 1249–53.

16. Kilbourne, E.M. (1992). Eosinophilia-myalgia syndrome: coming to grips with a new illness. *Epidemiol Rev* 14, 16–36.

17. Fraser, D.W., Tsai, T.R., Orenstein, W., et al. (1977). Legionnaires' disease: description of an epidemic of pneumonia. *N Engl J Med* 297, 1189–97.

18. Centers for Disease Control and Prevention (1999). Meningococcal disease—New England, 1993–1998. *MMWR* 48, 629–33.

19. Herwaldt, B.L., Beach, M.J., the Cyclospora Working Group (1999). The return of *Cyclospora* in 1997: another outbreak of cyclosporiasis in North America associated with imported raspberries. *Ann Intern Med* 130, 210–20.

20. Centers for Disease Control and Prevention (1998). Outbreak of cyclosporiasis—Ontario, Canada, May 1998. *MMWR* 47, 806–9.
21. Hill, A.B. (1965). Environment and diseases: association or causation? *Proc R Soc Med* 58, 295–300.
22. Rothman, K.J. (1986). *Modern Epidemiology*, pp. 16–20. Little, Brown, Boston.
23. Centers for Disease Control and Prevention (2001). Outbreak of syphilis among men who have sex with men—Southern California, 2000. *MMWR* 50, 117–20.
24. Centers for Disease Control and Prevention (2000). HIV-related tuberculosis in a transgender network—Baltimore, Maryland, and New York City area, 1998–2000. *MMWR* 49, 317–20.

10

COMMUNICATING EPIDEMIOLOGIC FINDINGS

Michael B. Gregg

Among the skills of a field epidemiologist is knowing how to communicate effectively. This chapter deals with some of the elements of both written and oral communication skills.

The single most important lesson to take home on this subject is that the data you collect are no more useful to fellow scientists and the public than your ability to communicate these findings convincingly.[1] Meaningful transfer of facts and their implications shapes medical and public health practice and drives the need to acquire new data. Therefore, communication stands as a prime function of the field epidemiologist.

A key word here is "convince." Supreme Court Justice Oliver Wendell Holmes once said, "a page of history is worth a volume of logic." What he meant was that if you want to move people to act, real-life illustrations, present-day success stories, and past experiences are much more persuasive than spelling out a series of logical analyses, which tend to be cold, academic, and unrelated to reality.

Another quotation from a famous American epidemiologist may also bring to light some of the more fundamental aspects of communicating epidemiologic findings. In defining epidemiology, Wade Hampton Frost, considered by many the "father" of American epidemiology, wrote, "Epidemiology is something more than the total of its established facts. It includes the orderly arrangement of facts into chains of inference that extend more or less beyond the bounds of direct observation." This tells us at least two things: first, that good epidemiology includes putting information into sensible order and, second, that the whole may be greater than the sum of the parts. Thus, once you assemble all the components, you may be able to draw more inferences from the aggregate than would appear to be possible when each fact is interpreted separately.

WRITING AN EPIDEMIOLOGIC PAPER

Basic Structure

Although varying somewhat from journal to journal, most formats of scientific papers include an introduction, a materials and methods section, and sections for results, discussion (or comment), and conclusions. Some articles have a summary, and most have an abstract of the article at the very beginning. Sometimes, particularly in epidemiologic papers, there is a background section. Over the past few years some medical journals changed their abstract to include subheadings such as: objective, design, setting, participants, interventions, main outcome measures, results, and conclusions. Because these divisions can be helpful to you in the overall organization of your epidemiologic paper,[2] let us look at each of the major sections briefly to get some ideas of their function.

Introduction

The introduction of virtually all scientific papers gives a very brief historical perspective. Epidemiologic papers are no exception. You should usually give some indication of why the investigation was done (i.e., because of an outbreak of illness or an apparent need to explain or explore why health events happened). You should also indicate the overall purpose of the paper and give some indication of the specific area to be covered. If the topic is cancer or an outbreak of salmonella infection, say what particular facet will be emphasized. Look at published papers in the target journal to get the acceptable format.

The introduction is not a literature review. You should pick out only the pertinent material and try to guide the reader's thinking into your own thought processes—where you are going and what will be covered.

Materials and Methods

Tell the readers what tools and methods you used, what was the design of the study, what rules and definitions were used, how they were applied, and what operations you actually did.

In an epidemiologic paper, a case definition is an absolute necessity because, if the readers do not know your definition, they do not know exactly what you are counting. Describe the case-finding techniques—contacting physicians, visiting all relevant clinics, doing a survey, analyzing an existing database, or various other methods of case finding. Outline the laboratory methods, but probably not in great detail in an epidemiologic paper. Describe surveys or other sampling techniques you used, statistical tests applied, and any allied areas such as animal, vector, and environmental studies.

Also, a statement concerning background or setting may fit appropriately here. Describe the area under investigation, the size of the community, or the hospital. Give the reader a denominator: "The community hospital served a population of 24,000 people"; "There were 200 discharges per month"; or "The community has a maximum population of 15,000 people, most of whom are migrant workers who come in during the peak harvesting season." Some detail about geographic, climatic, or physical features of where the investigation took place may be necessary. What was there when the investigation started and who was there? Key people may need to be identified (usually by title rather than by name). Such a section can also appear as part of the introduction or even be included in the results. After the first drafts of the paper are prepared, you will almost certainly have a better feeling of where a background statement best belongs.

Results

For a field investigation, the results section very often, but not always, starts with how the problem or epidemic was recognized and a very short description of the pertinent time, place, and person findings. Such a short paragraph prepares the reader and gives a feeling of time moving and a sense of the whole picture— important components of good communication.

Now comes the first major area of the results: *descriptive epidemiology*. Start with the clinical and laboratory aspects first. Usually, there will be a range of signs and symptoms from mild to very serious and even death. So describe the clinical findings in some detail. They will give the more clinically oriented reader an idea of the spectrum of disease and will often help justify the case definition. State what laboratory tests were done and their results. Avoid the tendency to defend the methods or to interpret the results at this point; that follows later in the discussion.

Next, in whatever detail is necessary, orient the reader to the time, the place, and the person of the investigation. This may involve considerable discussion about the timing and distribution of cases. It is the logical place to show an epidemic curve, if appropriate. Describe the figure and analyze it for the reader. Then describe the findings according to where the persons became ill or where they were placed at risk. Present the pertinent characteristics of the cases (age, gender, race, occupation, etc.) This section is still descriptive, but it should be as detailed as needed to help build the best possible foundation for developing a hypothesis and subsequent analysis. Include, if possible, pertinent negative findings. Such data are often as important as "positive" data and can materially help you lead the readers' minds in the direction you want them to go. You are not doing any real analysis yet, but you are setting the scene to do so.

Next comes the *transition of thought* between descriptive and analytic epidemiology. This often can be a difficult task, particularly for the beginner. Essentially, you are now taking the readers by the hand and leading them through an objective interpretation of the clinical, laboratory, and epidemiologic descriptive data. You should guide them down plausible avenues of inference that can be considered and discarded or considered and established as the most reasonable and defensible explanation for what was found. Present the pertinent information in an orderly way, blending the findings and existing knowledge in a persuasive path of logic. A possible order of considerations might be the following:

- What health problem (disease) do the clinical and laboratory data confirm or support?
- What do the facts of time, place, and person suggest? And, almost simultaneously:
- How well does the existing knowledge of this disease's pathogenesis and epidemiology fit with the investigative findings? Can these facts help one understand or suggest what happened?
- What possible exposures occurred and how can one postulate a chain of events happening that would explain the health problem?
- What hypotheses come to mind?

Here is an example, in somewhat truncated form:

Descriptive facts: In August 1980, a community hospital in Michigan recognized 7 cases of streptococcal wound infection in postoperative patients spanning the previous 4 months. Since this number represented more cases than usual, an investigation was begun.[3] A total of 10 cases of streptococcal infection, all of the same serotype, was ultimately found over the previous 4 months, all of whom were inpatients on several surgical wards. *Transition*: The temporal and geographic clustering of cases, the fact that all infections developed within 1 to 2 days after surgery, and the fact that all infections were of the same serotype strongly suggested a common exposure—presumably in the operating rooms. Since most streptococcal infections in the hospital setting are transmitted by humans, the field team hypothesized that contact with or exposure to a member of the hospital staff posed the unique risk to the infected patients.

This example shows how the descriptive data plus a knowledge of the epidemiology of the infectious agent were combined to lead the reader to the same logical hypothesis as the investigators.

Now comes *analytic epidemiology*, that is, comparisons of cases and controls or those exposed and not exposed (see Chapter 7). If there were no apparent associations between exposure and illness, you would probably not be writing the paper. If there were associations, what are the probabilities of them occurring? Here you will logically select risks and/or exposures that you compared and present them to the reader. Consider starting with those comparisons that showed no statistically significant differences, then lead on to those where differences were noted and focus on them.

To continue with the above example: The field team then compared infected patients to comparable noninfected postsurgical patients with respect to contact with 38 surgeons, anesthesiologists, and nursing staff. Rates of exposure to various hospital staff were not statistically different between cases and controls, except for one nurse. The nurse was then found to be a carrier of the epidemic strain of streptococcus. When she was removed from the surgical wards, no more cases of streptococcal infection occurred.

Sometimes the first analyses reveal nothing, requiring another level of analysis and/or collection of new data. This is particularly characteristic of nosocomial infections where numbers of cases are often small, such as in the outbreak above. In any event take your reader, logically, step by step through your analyses.

If control and/or prevention measures were taken, this is the place to include them in the paper.

Discussion

A good discussion highlights the significant findings without reviewing everything all over again. The most salient points can be restated for emphasis. You can now express your own judgment as to what the results mean and show how your findings relate to the current state of knowledge. You should weigh the possible inferences of all of your data as you go along, and then you should give your judgment in terms of a conclusion.

The discussion section is also a good place to integrate your findings with what is known about the subject. Moreover, consider how your investigation might serve as a stimulus for further research in the area of concern.

Be sure to review critically the definitions, the measurements, and the analytic tools that you used, for example, case definitions, survey instruments, levels of sensitivity and specificity, and statistical tests. How good were they? Were they the most appropriate instruments for the study? Weigh them fairly for the readers so they know how you view them. What were the weaknesses or difficulties you had in collecting important information? Did lack of relevant data have significant impact with regard to confounding or effect modification? Be a critic of your methods, yet defend them objectively and honestly. You will be much more believable if you do so. Exactly where in the discussion you include these remarks will depend a great deal upon their importance in verifying your findings. In fact, you may want to discuss the pros and cons of your methods as you interpret the findings. That is quite acceptable. However, in general, evaluations of methods will fall after the major points of the discussion.

Conclusions

Summarize the results and inferences of the work in one short paragraph. You may also want to include in a sentence or two what further work or research is needed to clarify or expand the findings of your study.

Order of Writing

Let us next talk about the sequence you might consider in starting to write an article. You have done the investigation, and you know the component parts; how do you write the article? The temptation is to start at the beginning, namely, the introduction, and go to the end. Consider avoiding this temptation and describe the facts first. It is a much more comfortable process. Some fledgling authors spend a great deal of time and effort spinning their wheels trying to write an introduction, not knowing how much of the literature to review, not yet knowing what their major points are going to be, not knowing how they want to orient the reader. So forget about the introduction, sit down and write about what you did and what you found—that is, what you know as nobody else knows.

Consider writing the body of the study—the background, the material and methods, and the results—first. The discussion and the introduction will still be there waiting and may appear in a better perspective if you first write about what you did and what you found out. Also, you will have exercised your descriptive and analytic mind so that by the time the discussion, the introduction, and the conclusion are ready to be written, you will see the major and minor findings quite clearly. In truth, you may not really be aware of some of the key issues, the new facts, and their ramifications and interplay until the facts are laid out in logical order in the descriptive and analytic narrative. Putting things on paper gives a perspective of what you know compared to what you thought you knew almost better than anything else you can do.

Lastly, after the first or second draft has been written, wait 10 days to 2 weeks before looking at your paper again. You will then often see your writing more objectively and critically. The evidence, the inferences, the logic, the "flow" of your paper may appear in a very different light and may need more changes.

Guidelines

Here are several guidelines that may help in presenting the results and in the discussion. Remember you are trying to convince and to persuade people to believe you.

1. Develop your findings logically. Write from the general to the specific; do not start with the minutiae and then try to encompass the whole world afterward. In the results section, try to grasp and explain the full extent of the findings at the beginning. Then focus on the individual elements one by one. In the discussion, start with the big picture to provide an overall context or consideration, and then fix attention upon the more specific aspects of your study. If the subject is influenza in the United States or about cancer of a particular type, write several sentences about influenza or cancer in general that orient the reader, so that all the subsequent facts and findings will fit into a more understandable context. In other words, concentrate on the unfolding of facts and transition in thought.

2. Consider "friendly persuasion" in the discussion. Do not hit your reader over the head with the hardest material to understand or even the best evidence at the beginning. Start with simple, understandable, and accepted statements. Present the weakest supporting evidence at the beginning, then slowly build to the strongest and most plausible explanation at the end. Let your sentences grow in complexity, all the while recognizing other possible explanations as you slowly present your case. Leave the really controversial aspects to the end of the discussion—you do not want to divert the readers' attention away from the conclusions you want them to accept.

3. Develop your thesis with an overall pathogenesis in mind. That is, when you elaborate on the factors that putatively contributed to the disease or health problem, consider the attributes of the inciting agent, the development of symptoms and signs, and the full-blown clinical presentations. How do they square with, support, and advance your presentation of the epidemiologic findings?

4. Make your style as simple as possible. Use short words (which are usually Anglo-Saxon in derivation), short sentences, and straightforward constructions. Use the active voice when possible. It is easier to understand and more forceful. Select words that denote rather than connote: you are an epidemiologist not a poet.

5. Use plenty of transition devices. Transitions are extremely important in any kind of writing. They prepare or cue the reader for further elaboration, a change in thinking, an exception, or an unusual observation. Additionally, transitions can create a time frame that helps move the action in a desired direction. Ideally, your exposition will have transitions in thought, but if it does not, at least transitional words will help. Subheadings also cue the reader to what is to come, including the size and complexity of the subject's component parts.

Problems

Here are a few problem areas to avoid:

1. Being wrong. One of the easiest ways to "turn readers off" is to be wrong. If you state the wrong percentage or the wrong bibliographic reference or your

numbers do not add up correctly, the reader may discount everything else you say. You have then lost the battle of communicating, of convincing.

2. "Talking down" to the reader. Declarative, unmodified statements, such as "all malaria is caused by mosquitoes," often invite error and make most readers angry. The use of long and highly technical words may seemingly command power and persuade, but seldom do these expressions, per se, convince scientifically experienced and critical audiences. More often, such words confuse rather than clarify, and their frequent use suggests a kind of professional insecurity.

3. Mixing opinion with fact. One may frequently see a statement or even a phrase stating a conclusion before all the evidence is presented. This most often happens when the author states the incubation period before the exposure has been established. Those inferences and opinions belong in the discussion after all the facts have been presented.

PRESENTING A SCIENTIFIC PAPER

Advance Preparation

The audience

Before preparing a scientific paper, you should know something about your audience. For the lay public, students, or scientists, you will necessarily select a special format of presentation, a vocabulary, appropriate audiovisuals, and perhaps even a demeanor or style of presentation. This means that you need to think carefully of how to communicate best—how to serve the needs and desires of that audience.

The facilities

How large is the auditorium? How is it lighted? How many does it seat? How many will be there? Who controls the lights and the projector? What kind of microphone will be used? Is there a lectern, a chalkboard, a flipchart? Do you have choices for any of those facilities? How far will you be from the first row of the audience, and how good are the acoustics? Sometimes the acoustics with a microphone are so bad that you are best understood by raising your voice unaided by the electronic media. Try to get answers to these questions as soon as possible. At scientific meetings at least try to attend several sessions in the same room a few hours in advance.

Slides, transparencies, or presentation software

The first rule of thumb is do not use more than one kind of projection method for your talk. To do so is confusing, wastes time, and is subject to easy error by you or the projectionist.

Slides and computer projections usually require a dark room. They are generally quicker to change. One can show the "real thing," that is, pictures of patients, places, and things. But slides are sometimes hard to make quickly and at the last minute. Equipment failures are not uncommon and can be absolutely devastating at an important scientific meeting or formal presentation. Parenthetically, it would be very smart to be sure, before you give your talk, that there are extra bulbs available for immediate replacement. With both slides and computer projections you frequently lose significant eye contact with your audience.

Transparencies are very easy to make at the last minute. They tend to promote good eye contact with the audience, particularly if you point at the transparency (not the screen) as you speak. However, they are often awkward to use because they collect static electricity, make noise, and there often is no logical place to put them when you are through. Moreover, unless you look at and check each transparency, one by one, as you show them, you can easily not center them correctly on the screen. For some, using transparencies gives the impression of teaching rather than lecturing or giving a scientific presentation. On the other hand, one can use transparencies for that delicate mixture of teaching and presenting material, because you can write on a transparency as you progress through your talk, underline, or circle, and emphasize certain points.

In some situations handouts can be very useful. They are particularly good for teaching and leaving your audience with the most important points you want to make, giving, in truth, a "take-home" lesson. They are ideal to use when, at the end of a field investigation, you are summarizing your findings to the local health officers. They are clearly very useful when you are concerned about electrical supply or the real possibility of equipment failure. Unfortunately, handouts have to be reproduced, they are noisy, the audience attention is not on you, but on the paper, and you lose control over them. Last, they really are not that frequently used at major scientific meetings.

The use of slides, presentation software, transparencies, or handouts is a personal choice. Knowing the setting and the formality of your talk, the nature of your audience, and the ultimate purpose of your presentation will be the best guides for deciding what audiovisual devices to use.[4]

To read or not to read

Another serious consideration is whether to read or not to read your presentation. Ideally, you will probably communicate best if you do not have to read your paper or talk. However, it usually requires years of practice, innate ability to extemporize, and a great deal of self-confidence to communicate scientific material effectively without reading it.

Again, the circumstances surrounding your talk will often dictate whether reading is essential, important, or inconsequential. Formal, major scientific presentations or guest lectureships will more likely than not necessitate reading a substantial part of your paper. This is particularly true if you are new at the game and not experienced in presenting scientific material. It is also true if there is a major time constraint (and there usually is). At most scientific meetings, one is given 10, maybe 15 minutes at most for presentations, and it is absolutely critical not to exceed your allotted time. This can best be accomplished by writing out the presentation and rehearsing it so that you are within 10 to 20 seconds of your allotted time. And, indeed, practice your talk—perhaps to a few of your colleagues or even your spouse. Get their reaction and input; it is well worth the time.

The size of the audience sometimes can help you decide whether to read or extemporize. Small audiences of 30 persons usually permit an informal atmosphere where your presentation can be done ad lib. When the audience is 50 or more, again depending upon a variety of circumstances, you may still be able to ad lib your presentation and refer frequently to notes to jog your memory. Scientific presentations to 75 persons or more probably dictate a formal, airtight presentation that is best read, unless you are a real professional. It is the rare professional who can present a paper ad lib at a scientific meeting in exactly 10 minutes in first-rate, smooth, and clear fashion. The vast majority of presenters read their papers; and with enthusiasm, knowledge of the subject, good projection of words, and modest eye contact, they can communicate extremely well to the audience.

The rule of thumb: when in doubt, read it out loud. If you rehearse and are enthusiastic, articulate, knowledgeable, and coherent, you should have little difficulty in communicating by informing and convincing.

The Actual Presentation

Be aware that you, almost as much as the substance of your talk, are under the close scrutiny of your audience. So try to eliminate any possible barriers that might arise between yourself and the audience such as: unfamiliar or odd clothing, unusual or inappropriate body language, or visible distractions. Suitable language and recognition of cultural norms go a long way to good communication as well. And do not endanger your credibility as an epidemiologist by self-deprecation or apologies.

When called upon to make your talk, walk briskly to the lectern. There is nothing more disappointing than seeing a lecturer or presenter saunter casually up to the stage. It gives the impression of not caring, of not being prepared. Get comfortable before you start talking. Make sure the microphone is exactly where you want it. Get your visuals, your notes, your glass of water, your position behind the lectern exactly the way you want them before you start. Frequently you may need to acknowledge the person who introduced you with thanks or perhaps a joke. More often, at a true scientific meeting, there will be no introduction, but it is usually good manners to acknowledge the moderator. Listen to a few talks before your own so you will know what manners are expected and appropriate. Position yourself close to the images on the screen so you do not have to walk halfway across the stage to point out something or find it yourself. Usually this is no problem. Minimize walking around on the stage unless you are really in a teaching mode or you are going to create a dialogue with your audience. Make eye contact with your audience as frequently as possible, not contact with the microphone, the screen, or the papers you are reading from. Look about the audience, not at one place or one person. This brings them in to you as you are talking. If there is a pointer, or electric arrow, keep it as still as possible and turn it off when you are not actively pointing out something. Speak slowly and clearly. The adrenalin circulating through you will almost always make your words come out faster. Speak distinctly, and try to project the words to the back of the auditorium.

It usually takes about 2 minutes to read one page of double-spaced text reasonably slowly and clearly. This means, if you have a 10-minute talk, your paper should be no longer than 4 1/2 to 5 1/2 pages at the very most. Regarding projections, recall that it takes varying lengths of time to get the projectionist's attention, turn off and on the lights, and show the material. Many presenters read their paper at the same time they show slides. However, quite often speakers ad lib when the slides appear. This then adds time to the presentation—about 5–15 seconds per slide, because it takes the audience at least that time to digest the material.

Do not hesitate to bring in props, or the real things that you used or found in your investigation. A can of tainted food or pesticide, or a piece of equipment that was associated with disease is very convincing, can be very useful, and "lightens" your presentation.[5]

Content

A 10-minute presentation should include most of the key components of a scientific article. There often will be acknowledgments at the beginning and then a brief introduction with a statement of background and purpose. Your materials and methods must emphasize the most important parts of your investigation or analysis. You cannot go into detail here—simply state the barest essentials so your audience will know exactly what you did. Avoid referring to methods that you do not have time to explain (i.e., there should be no "black box").

State the most important results, recalling that you cannot tell the audience everything you found. This part will be the longest of your presentation. This is where you may use tables, figures, and charts, which, if well used, will generally increase comprehension and minimize explanation. Discussion comes next, when, as in a written paper, you highlight what was most important, how it fits in with what is presently known, and your interpretation of the findings. Then state your conclusion: a very brief summary and what it all means including control and prevention, if appropriate.

When you are finished, say "Thank you." Do not simply stop talking at the end of your presentation. The audience does not know what to expect. Also, it is simple courtesy to thank them for listening to you.

How to alienate your audience

There are some relatively simple rules that, if broken, can seriously impair your ability to communicate with your audience and at the same time lose credibility and/or stature.

1. Probably the greatest offense is taking more time than you are allotted. This is selfish, it is unfair, and if there is a discussion period set aside for your paper, you are using time that is not yours. The discussion is time for the audience to react to your presentation. Exceeding your time will infuriate most moderators, and if grossly abused, you stand to suffer the major embarrassment of being asked to stop talking and sit down. Furthermore, taking more time than allowed implies you were not well prepared and did not know what were the important points to make. All of which boils down to the simple fact that you must not and cannot expect to present everything you did or found. You must be selective. Perhaps the discussion will touch on some areas that you could not present during your allotted time.

2. The next major problem concerns visual aids. You are responsible for the quality and order of your projections. If they are out of order or upside down or illegible, they will materially detract from your ability as a communicator and even your credibility as an investigator. For some strange reason, some people simply do not care about their visual aids. They seem to be above it all. Do not be one of them. If at all possible, bring your own slide carousel or laptop to the auditorium. Put your slides in the carousel yourself. Check them or the computer order at least two times before you make your presentation. Nothing can ruin a first-rate presentation faster than out-of-order, upside down, or backward visual aids.

3. Do not use projections that are illegible or have too much data on them. Avoid this simply by projecting the material in a room roughly the size of the room where the meeting is. If you cannot read them easily at the back of the room, you have no business wasting everyone's time showing them.

4. Do not talk down to the audience. This is hard to define easily, but avoid pompous attitudes, long words, or an air of superiority. Along the same line, remember that the moderator is your supervisor; do not disregard his or her requests. If you do not follow the moderator's instructions, this can cause great embarrassment and loss of credibility.

5. Do not become angry or upset in front of your audience. This is especially a hazard during the discussion period. Compliment the questioner on his or her

question; stay composed; say you don't know if you don't know; respect the opinion of others, even if they are outrageous; and remain calm and pleasant, even if you are furious underneath.

SUMMARY

Whether you are writing or speaking, your primary purpose is to transfer facts and ideas so your audience will understand and believe you. Keep your words simple, your logic clear and understandable, and your tone one of friendly persuasion. And, always remember: never tell your audience everything you know.

REFERENCES

1. King, L.S. (1991). *Why Not Say It Clearly. A guide to expository writing*, 2nd ed. Little, Brown, Boston.
2. Huth, E.J. (1987). *Medical Style and Format. An international manual for authors, editors, and publishers*. ISI Press. Philadelphia.
3. Berkelman, R.L., Martin, D., Graham, D.R., et al. (1982). Streptococcal wound infections caused by a vaginal carrier. *JAMA* 248, 2680–82.
4. Mandel, S. (1987). *Effective Presentation Skills. A practical guide for better speaking*. Crisp Publications, Los Altos, CA.
5. Heinich, R., Molenda, M., Russell, J.D. (Eds.) (1993). *Instructional Media and the New Technologies of Instruction*, 4th ed., pp. 54–57. MacMillan Publishing Co., New York.

SUGGESTED READING

1. *American Medical Association Manual of Style*, 8th ed. (1989). Williams & Wilkins, Baltimore.
2. Fowler, H.R. (1980). *The Little, Brown Handbook*. Little, Brown, Boston.

11

SURVEYS AND SAMPLING

Joan M. Herold
J. Virgil Peavy

A survey is a canvassing of people for the purpose of collecting information. Surveys are done when there is a question to be answered, and there is no existing data source to provide the needed information. A survey is a lot of work and should never be conducted when the information can be obtained more readily elsewhere. Therefore, it is important to investigate thoroughly the availability of existing data before undertaking a survey. A good place to start is to contact a national statistical office, census bureau, ministry of health, or other governmental organizations that would have knowledge of large data collection efforts and the availability of existing data.

Surveys can be classified in a number of ways. One distinction is between a census, or a complete population survey, in which every element in the target population is included, and a sample survey, in which only a portion of the target population is selected. Census or complete population surveys are extremely expensive and are rarely used to collect detailed information from large populations. Even the United States census does not collect detailed information from the total population. Instead it asks fewer than 10 questions of the total population and collects the more detailed census information from a sample of households. Large health-related surveys are also sample surveys. Only when the target population is small should you consider doing a complete population survey.

STEPS IN CARRYING OUT A SURVEY

1. Write a protocol.
2. Select a survey mode.
3. Develop a questionnaire.
4. Design and select the sample.
5. Train interviewers (or prepare for mail out).
6. Collect data (fieldwork).
7. Enter data into computer, edit, and process the data.
8. Analyze the data.
9. Write a survey report.

WRITING A PROTOCOL

Perhaps more than any other type of data collection, a survey cannot be undertaken without a protocol or detailed plan. The various steps in survey design are all interconnected and, therefore, must be thought out carefully prior to beginning any steps in survey preparation. For example, the budget influences the choice of the survey mode, sample design, sample size, and length of questionnaire. The analysis plan affects the format of questions, sample design, and sample size. The sample size influences the mode, analysis, and interpretation of results. The mode dictates length and format of the questionnaire. A protocol allows all these interrelationships to be considered—and they *must* be considered—before actually choosing a mode, designing a questionnaire, or selecting a sample. The protocol should include: Study Objectives; Methodology, including a list of information to be sought from the survey, survey design, sampling plan, and data editing plan; Analysis Plan, including the computer software necessary to analyze the data; Logistics for implementing the survey, including personnel and equipment needed; Budget; and Time Line. Once all these steps have been thoroughly thought through, you are ready to begin work on the survey.

SELECTING A SURVEY MODE

Surveys can be classified by their mode of data collection. There are mail surveys, telephone surveys, and face-to-face interview surveys. There is now also a newer method of data collection using the Internet. Prior to developing a questionnaire and choosing a sample, the survey mode must be decided. Each of these modes has its advantages and disadvantages.

Mail, or self-administered, surveys are seldom used to collect information from the general public because names and addresses usually are not available, and the response rate tends to be low. However, the method may be highly effective with members of particular groups, such as members of an HMO or members of a professional association. The principal advantages of mail surveys are that they may obtain more thoughtful responses, and they are the least expensive to implement. The biggest disadvantage of the mail survey is that it typically obtains a much lower response rate than a telephone or face-to-face interview. A response rate of 50% is not unusual for a mail survey. Questionnaires that are distributed and returned by computer share many of the advantages and disadvantages of the mail survey, including the principal disadvantage of a low response rate. Moreover, a computer survey is not a good choice for a general population survey in most countries because of the selectivity of persons who use or own computers. Sometimes survey data are obtained with self-administered questionnaires that are not mailed or sent over the Internet but are provided to respondents in person, such as at a clinic or at a group gathering. If sufficient time is allowed for response to the questionnaire, this method will have most of the advantages of a mail survey without the principal disadvantage of a low response rate.

Telephone interviewing is an efficient survey method and has become quite popular in the United States. Investigations of epidemics frequently rely on telephone surveys because they are quick, inexpensive, and sensitive (i.e., they quickly reveal whether a problem truly exists). Under good conditions, the response rate for a telephone survey is better than a mail survey but not as high as that of a face-to-face interview. Unfortunately, cooperation with telephone surveys by the public has recently begun to decline, particularly in large cities. Also, populations with and without telephones may differ, creating a possible important bias.

A face-to-face interview is often the preferred or only feasible method of survey data collection. Among its many advantages, the most important is its high response rate (70%–95%). It also has the advantage of permitting the collection of more complex and more sensitive information than a mail or telephone survey. It can tolerate a much longer time for questionnaire administration, thus allowing for more information to be collected. The principal disadvantage of the face-to-face interview is the cost: interviewers' salaries, their transportation, and, at times, their meals and housing have to be considered. Furthermore, it takes longer to locate respondents for face-to-face interviews, which extends the time that interviewers' salaries, transport, room, and meals must be covered. A second disadvantage is the potential for interviewer bias (also a risk in telephone surveys), but we will see later in this chapter that this can be considerably controlled with proper selection and training of interviewers.

Surveys may combine these various modes. The telephone may be used to "screen" for eligible respondents and then to make appointments for face-to-face interviews. Additionally, mixed mode surveys may use a less expensive method to start, then switch to a method that yields a higher response rate for those who fail to respond to the initial method. The most popular of the mixed mode survey is the combined mail and telephone mode. Caution is advised, however, in the use of mixed mode surveys. Questionnaire construction is usually different for different survey modes, and this difference creates a problem with mixed mode approaches. Moreover, potential biases vary depending on the mode, and this can create problems in interpreting the results. Therefore, it is highly recommended that you seek the assistance of a survey expert if you choose to use a mixed mode approach.

DEVELOPING A QUESTIONNAIRE

Writing Questions

The first step in developing a questionnaire is to define the problem and to list the information that you wish to obtain. A list of information or variables that you want will help you create the question that will give that information, as well as help you avoid writing unnecessary questions. You will also need to know the type of analysis you plan to use and the mode of data collection. Your analysis plan will determine the form of responses to questions. For example, if you plan to work with proportions, you will want to collect categorical responses. On the other hand, if you can work with means, you may collect scaled responses. It is also possible that you want to do a content analysis on qualitative data, in which case you may seek open-ended responses (see below). The mode of data collection (mail, telephone, or face-to-face interview) will affect how the question is written, what response categories are shown, the length of the questionnaire, and the overall format of the questionnaire. Here are some general rules on question writing and questionnaire format.

The question format can be of three types:

1. Structured or closed-ended questions. These are questions that have predetermined response categories to choose from. The respondent is told what the response options are and is asked to choose from among the options. Multiple-choice and true/false questions are examples of this format. The structured format is easiest to implement for large samples, for self-administered questionnaires with hand-written responses, and when the range of response possibilities is known. A fundamental rule for writing structured questions is that the response options must be exhaustive and mutually exclusive.

2. Unstructured or open-ended questions. This format allows the respondent to answer in his or her own words. The unstructured question is useful when the researcher does not know what the range of response options might be. It may also provide a more accurate response, as it prevents the respondent from guess-

ing or misinterpreting a response category that the researcher has constructed. However, coding and analysis of answers to open-ended questions can be very difficult and time consuming. Open-ended questions, therefore, are to be avoided in large-scale surveys and by researchers inexperienced with coding or interpreting qualitative data.

3. Precoded open-ended questions. Open-ended questions that are precoded are often used in interviewer-assisted surveys. These questions do not provide answer options to the respondent, but have options written in the questionnaire for the interviewer to circle or check.

The interviewer must always be aware that errors in response—both voluntary and involuntary, due to misunderstanding, misrepresentation, or faulty memory—can and will occur. To obtain the most accurate information from a respondent, several things should be taken into account: (1) questions should be written as unambiguously as possible; (2) the vocabulary used in question construction should be consistent with the vocabulary of the respondents; (3) if interviewers are involved, they must be trained to avoid influencing the respondent and to read the question exactly as written so that every interviewee responds to exactly the same question; (4) use as many questions as possible from previously used questionnaires for your target population; (5) field test the questionnaire to ensure that respondents understand the questions and concepts in the same way that the researcher does.

Questionnaire Format

The order of questions in the questionnaire varies depending on the mode of data collection. A questionnaire administered by an interviewer should have some easy and nonthreatening questions to start. Often demographic questions are asked first to give the respondent an opportunity to get comfortable with the interviewer prior to being asked more difficult or personal questions. On the other hand, a mail survey should get right to the point, with questions specific to the principal purpose of the survey at the beginning of the questionnaire. In this way the respondent's attention is immediately engaged, and he or she is more likely to complete and return the questionnaire.

Threatening or embarrassing questions should be kept to a minimum and placed toward the end of the questionnaire. If the respondent chooses not to answer these questions, you will at least have obtained other information asked earlier in the questionnaire that you can use in analysis.

Avoid asking questions that are not applicable to a particular respondent. This is done by using filter questions and skip patterns that direct the respondent to skip over questions that do not pertain to him or her. It is possible to lose the interest and thoughtfulness of respondents if they feel you are asking irrelevant questions. Skip patterns may be used frequently in a questionnaire administered by an interviewer. They are to be used sparingly in a self-administered questionnaire.

Avoid offering the respondent a "don't know" option. A questionnaire that is developed for a personal interview may have "don't know" categories for all questions in the questionnaire, with instructions to the interviewer not to read these options. A questionnaire that is developed for self-administration, on the other hand, should keep these options to a minimum.

Use transition sentences to prepare the respondent for a new topic. Remember that the data you collect are as good as your respondent's interpretation and memory. Transition sentences allow the respondents to adjust their minds for a shift in subject matter.

Above all, the questionnaire must be well spaced, clearly typed or printed, and easy to follow. The placement of response categories for questions should be consistent throughout the questionnaire. They should be listed vertically and not horizontally, so they are easily seen. Keep in mind that the easier it is for the eye to identify the response options, the quicker will be the completion of the questionnaire, the fewer will be the errors in selecting a response category, and the fewer will be the errors in reading the response category when entering the data into the computer.

The questionnaire will need to be reviewed numerous times, by both content experts and editors. A questionnaire with many errors will produce data with many errors.

Finally, a cover page is usually advisable for interviewer-administered questionnaires. The cover page to a questionnaire will have a place for the interviewer to code the final status of the interview—"completed"; "unable to locate household or respondent"; "refused"; and other useful categories. It may also have a place for the interviewer to record date and time of attempts to reach the respondent, which is helpful in scheduling revisits. Most important, the cover page will also contain information that will allow the interviewer to identify the correct member of the sample. It may contain an address or name or telephone number of the potential interviewee along with other identifying information. The purpose of having any identifying information on its own page is so that the page can later be removed from the questionnaire after data entry and fieldwork are completed. In this way, the respondent cannot be linked to the answers he or she has provided.

The Pretest

A newly developed questionnaire that has not been used previously in a population *must* be pretested. A pretest is a form of pilot study to check on the validity and reliability of the individual questions and the instrument as a whole. In a pretest, the final questionnaire is administered, using the mode that will be used in the actual survey, to a small (usually purposive) sample taken from the same population that the final sample is drawn from. It is very important, however, that the respondents for the pretest *not* be included in the final sample. Thus the pretest is usually not conducted until after the final sample has been drawn. Depending on the length and complexity of the questionnaire, the sample size for a pretest can vary from 25 to 100 individuals. The pretest should reveal any problem respondents may have in understanding the questions and whether or not there are any difficulties in following the questionnaire. If the pretest is of sufficient size, it may also be used to identify questions that may be removed from the questionnaire because of lack of variability in response to that item. The pretest of the questionnaire also affords an opportunity to test other aspects of survey procedures, such as ability to locate respondents, willingness of prospective respondents to consent to interview, the duration of the interview, and so forth.

SELECTING A SAMPLE

To Sample or Not to Sample

Seldom do public health budgets have the resources for complete population surveys. Therefore, sampling methods are used to obtain information from a smaller number than the total population. When a large population is involved, well-designed sampling will usually provide more accurate information than a census-type survey. A few reliable, well-trained investigators working on a properly selected sample of the population can usually obtain information more accurately than would be possible for a larger team of less well trained field staff interviewing all individuals of a population. With available resources concentrated on a sample of a large population, the increase in sampling error from surveying a smaller number of persons will be more than compensated for by the reduction of other errors caused by resources spread too thin.

Proper sampling techniques provide a measure of the amount of error inherently introduced by the sampling process. Any estimate made from a sample is subject to error, but sampling errors have the favorable characteristic of being controllable through the size and design of the sample. Sampling errors, even for small samples, are often the least of the errors present in a survey. (See below for a listing of other sources of error.)

However, it is important to keep in mind, that for a small, geographically concentrated population, it may be possible to do a complete or census-type survey. For example, an outbreak in a small village or at a church supper may be best studied by surveying everyone in those small populations and thus completely avoiding sampling error.

Types of Samples

Sampling error cannot be calculated for all samples. Our ability to calculate sampling error depends on the type of sampling employed. There are two broad types of sampling used in sample surveys: probability sampling and nonprobability sampling. Probability sampling uses statistical theory in the design of the sample and, consequently, permits the calculation of sampling error. Probability sampling is the selection of a sample such that every member in the population has a known and nonzero probability of being included. This type of sampling is unbiased and enables you to draw valid conclusions about the population from which your sample is drawn. Nonprobability sampling is not based on statistical theory. It is a type of sampling that is inherently biased and does not permit the calculation of sampling error. Nonprobability samples include judgment samples, convenience samples, and the like.

Judgment or purposive sampling is the selection of a sample based on someone's judgment and knowledge of the subject matter. This type of sampling is biased and generally used only when there is no time to define a probability sample. An example might be the selection of community leaders in a refugee camp in such a way as to try to get maximum representation of the various ethnic groups residing there. The community leaders would then be asked questions about the members of their community.

Convenience or chunk sampling is the use of a sample that is near at hand. Such a sample is inherently biased by the fact that it includes only persons that happen to be out and about or taking a specific route or engaged in a specific activity at the time of the survey. Route samples, street-corner political surveys, or a sample based on persons coming into a clinic are convenience samples.

On occasions when the goal of a study is not to make statistical estimates about a population but rather to explore ideas and opinions of people about a new topic that may not be ready for a quantitative investigation, convenience samples may be very useful. They can provide ideas about people's thoughts and opinions and can be used to generate hypotheses for further study. But any study that wishes to produce statistics about the total population must use probability sampling.

Probability Sampling

As stated before, a probability sample is one in which every member of the population has a known and nonzero probability of being selected into the sample. A special case of the probability sample is the random sample, where each member of the population has an equal chance of being selected. The vast majority of the statistical tests we use carry with them the assumption that the sample has been randomly selected. While the selection of a random sample may not always be feasible, if we know the probability of selection of every member of the population, we can make adjustments to the data (through computer programs) to account for the differences between our probability sample and a strictly random sample. If we do not meet the criteria of a probability sample, we cannot draw conclusions about the population using standard significance tests and confidence intervals.

To draw a random sample you need to have a list of all members of the population from which the sample is to be drawn. This list is called a *sampling frame*. It is important that this frame is current and accurate. For example, when drawing a sample of college students, you will want a list of current students and not a list of those attending the college a year ago. When drawing a sample of housing units in a town, you will not want to use a list of housing units identified at the previous census 8 years ago. We often neglect to realize that our sample is only as good as the sampling frame from which it is selected. It is, therefore, very important to obtain an updated sampling frame that lists all elements of the population as close to the survey date as possible. If none is available, it is up to you, the survey implementer, to add to your budget the personnel and materials necessary to create a current sampling frame. If you are in a situation where you have to create a sampling frame for your sample, pay close attention to cluster sampling, described below.

Probability Sample Designs

Simple random sampling gives every member of the population an equal chance of being included in the sample. It requires a listing of every member of the population. Once all members of the population are assigned a number, a table of random numbers may be used to select individuals for the sample. Simple random sampling is theoretically simple, but often unrealistic in practice, because it can be expensive and may present logistic difficulties such as geographic dispersion of the study sample. Since no control of the distribution of the sample is exercised in this case, the variables in some samples may be poorly distributed (not biased, but unrepresentative). Therefore, simple random sampling is not always desirable. The principle of simple random sampling, however, is the basis of all good sampling techniques and can be utilized in each of the following more specialized techniques.

Systematic sampling is often used when elements (e.g., individuals) can be ordered or listed in some manner. Rather than selecting all elements randomly, one determines a selection interval (n), by dividing the total population listed by the sample size. The sampler then chooses a random starting point on the population list, and selects every *n*th person (the length of the selection interval). Good geographic or strata distribution (according to size) can be assured if the population is listed according to geographic area or other stratifying characteristic. It is an easy method to apply and a popular one among public health professionals.

In *stratified sampling*, the target population is divided into suitable, non-overlapping subpopulations or strata. Each stratum should be homogeneous within and heterogeneous between other strata. A random sample can then be selected within each stratum. In this way, each stratum is more accurately represented, and since members are more alike within each stratum, the overall sampling error is reduced. Separate estimates can be obtained from each stratum, and an overall estimate can be obtained for the entire population defined by the strata. The sample selection for each stratum is further defined by whether it is proportionate or disproportionate across strata. Proportionate stratified sampling uses the same sampling fraction that is calculated for the total population (sample size divided by the total population size) for selecting a sample from each stratum. Disproportionate stratified sampling uses different sampling fractions across strata in an attempt to get sufficient *numbers* of elements to make separate statistical estimates for each stratum. Disproportionate sampling is the method used when "oversampling" of a particular stratum is done. This method frequently is used to get sufficient representation of minority ethnic groups and to enable independent estimates of characteristics by ethnicity. While disproportionate stratified sampling allows for sufficient sample size within each stratum to make stratum-specific estimates with relatively equal precision, it requires the extra step of weighting the data when estimates are made for the total population, or all strata combined.

Cluster sampling is of particular value to save resources in surveys of human populations when the population is geographically dispersed or when a sampling frame for the elements of the population you wish to study is not available. In this type of sampling, the units first sampled are not the individual elements in which we are ultimately interested but, rather, clusters or aggregates of those elements. For example, in sampling the population of a rural area that is widely dispersed and difficult to reach, a sample of villages may be selected, and then all of the households in the sampled villages may be included in the survey. It is apparent that such a sample involves less traveling than a simple random sample of households throughout the rural area. Another typical example is in a study of school children, when a list of all children attending schools in an area is not available. One would then use a list of schools, and select a sample of schools from the list. In this case, schools are the sampling unit or clusters. Once the sample of schools has been selected, all of the students in the sampled schools may be surveyed. This type of sampling almost always loses some degree of precision. To maintain the same degree of precision as in simple random sampling, one would have to approximately double the sample size that would be calculated for a simple random sample.

Multistage sampling involves sampling at different levels of population groupings. It is used in surveys where a list of the final sample units would be too large to survey. In the cases given in the previous paragraph, for example, if one were to sample the households in the selected villages, or sample the children in the selected schools, there would be two levels of sampling involved, and they would demonstrate a two-stage sample design. Both of these examples, however, may be converted to three-stage designs. If, in the example of the population of rural areas, we were first to select a sample of villages (clusters), then select a sample of households (clusters) in each village, and finally select one adult (final sampling unit) in each of the sampled households, we would have a three-stage sample design. With respect to the children attending school, our first stage would be the selection of schools (clusters), the second stage might be the selection of a sample of classes or grades (clusters) in the schools, and the third stage would be the selection of a sample of students (final sampling unit) in the classes. Again, we would have a three-stage design. An obvious advantage in the school example is that you need only a listing of schools, classes within the selected schools, and students in the selected classes. You have bypassed the need for a list of all children attending school!

Most national surveys involve multistage sampling, with geographically defined clusters being the first stage or the primary sampling unit. This is, in part, because of the prohibitive cost of dispersing interviewers across a broad geographic area, but more important, it is due to many countries not having a list of all members of its population. The United States is an example. The United States does not have a list of all members of its population. Instead it has a list of census tracts. To conduct a sample survey for the U.S. population, one would have to first select census tracts from a list provided by the Census Bureau, then update the sampling frame for the selected tracts by mapping out the number and location of housing units in those tracts (unless you were lucky and that had been done with a recent census or survey), then select housing units from the updated frame, and finally select people living in the selected housing units.

Sample Size

Ideally, the sample size chosen for a survey should be based on how reliable the final estimates must be. In practice, usually a trade-off is made between the ideal sample size and the expected cost of the survey. The size of the sample must be sufficient to accomplish the purpose but should not be larger than necessary, because it will draw resources from other aspects of the survey process. Sample size is determined by the desired confidence level and precision of your estimates and the variability of the characteristic being measured for the population. The formula for calculating the sample size needed to estimate a proportion is:

$$n = z^2 \, pq/d^2$$

where,

n = the sample size

z = the standard normal deviate (1.96 for a 95% confidence level)

d = the level of accuracy desired, or sampling error, or one-half the width of the confidence interval (often set at .05)

p = the proportion of the population having the characteristic being measured (if proportion is unknown, set $p = .50$, which is maximum variability)

q = the proportion of the population that does not have the characteristic (i.e., $1-p$)

If the total population from which the sample is to be drawn is less than 10,000, then the size of the population must also be taken into account. Thus, for a population of size 10,000 or greater, n, above, is the final sample size; for populations less than 10,000, the following adjustment must be made:

$$nf = n/1+(n/N)$$

where,

nf = the final sample size, when population is less than 10,000

n = the sample size for populations of 10,000 or more

N = the size of total population

The above formulas may be easily modified when the estimates of interest are means rather than proportions. As stated, these formulas are the basic ones for simple random sampling. However, we know that in reality we often use stratified or multistage sampling methods. Adjustments to these formulas are necessary for these more complex designs or for more complex analysis than estimating proportions and means. Under such circumstances it is best to consult a statistician. If one is not easily available, some rules of thumb that may come in handy are: (1) for cluster designs, you will want to double the calculated sample size for a simple random sample; (2) for disproportionate stratified samples, you will want to calculate a sample size for each stratum.

Once a sample size is calculated, it must be appraised to see whether it is consistent with the resources available to conduct the survey. This appraisal demands an estimation of the personnel, materials, and time required to pursue the proposed sample size. It often becomes apparent that the calculated sample size has to be reduced. The usual loss is through increasing sampling error and losing precision in your estimates. If this happens, you are faced with the decision of whether to proceed with reduced precision or whether to abandon efforts until more resources can be found. On the positive side, however, is that if you conduct the survey and find less variability in your characteristics of interest than you estimated for your sample size calculations, your precision will be improved.

PREPARING FOR FIELDWORK

This section focuses on procedures relevant to face-to-face surveys. In field epidemiology, this is the mode you are likely to use, and the training of interviewers is the paramount feature for putting this type of survey into motion. You have spent time and effort in developing a good questionnaire and a representative sample of your target population, but your work can be all for naught with a casually selected and poorly trained group of interviewers. Remember, the interviewers are collecting your data!

You will want interviewers that are most likely to elicit honest responses from the respondents. You do not want high-ranking people whose status may influence the respondent to respond favorably (and untruthfully) to questions. Instead, choose interviewers who interact well with people and who are empathetic and unthreatening to the respondent. For certain situations, it may be preferable to have interviewers with similar social or demographic characteristics to the respondents, such as gender, age, or ethnicity.

Interviewers should be thoroughly trained in the following matters:

1. How to find the correct households or sample points. Detailed instructions on the importance of keeping to the sample design and how to locate the selected households or persons must be given. Often maps of survey areas are involved, and interviewers must be well trained in how to read the maps.
2. How to approach the respondent to assure agreement to be interviewed. This includes introducing oneself, specifying the value of the survey, and the authority behind the survey.
3. How to inform the respondent of the anonymity and confidentiality of their participation. The fact that the respondent's identification will be eliminated from the data, if this is the case, is important to convey.
4. How to introduce a consent form, if applicable, and obtain a signature (see Chapter 14).

5. How to administer the questionnaire so that question wording is not changed from one interview to another. This is best done by strong instructions to read the question and to resist the temptation of stating the question in the interviewer's own words.

6. How to define the terms used in the questionnaire, so that all respondents receive the same explanation of terms.

7. How to deal with new situations. It is important for the interviewer to consult with a supervisor about any new situations that arise in the field, especially those involving errors in the questionnaire or the interview procedure. Decisions in such situations should be made by, or communicated to, a field supervisor, so that determinations can be standardized across all interviewers.

8. How to administer the questionnaire. Sufficient practice sessions are needed to ensure adherence to skip patterns and other issues related to filling out the questionnaire, as well as to other procedures listed above.

9. How to dress for interviewing so the respondent feels at ease in the presence of the interviewer.

10. How to review the completed questionnaire after the interview has taken place to check for accuracy, consistency, and completeness in the field. At this point, there still is the opportunity for the interviewer to return to the respondent if there are any errors that must be corrected. For large-scale surveys, it is best to have supervisors in the field with the interviewers, one of whose tasks would be to review questionnaires.

11. The importance of the information they are gathering, to adhering to the sample design, to finding the respondent, to minimizing refusals, and of their contribution to the overall survey effort. The few additional hours required to explain to the interviewers the use of the data, the work that has gone into the survey thus far, and the value of the representative sample, is time well spent.

Interviewer training should comprise both classroom and field training. It is critical that interviewers not practice on members of the actual sample. A day or two of practice interviews in the field can do much to assure quality data collection when the real fieldwork begins.

It is also recommended that a reference manual or interviewers manual be developed that contains all the interviewer instructions for the fieldwork, including how to locate the sample points, definitions, and such.

Preparation for fieldwork also includes instruction on revisits to households or other places where respondents are to be found, in order to keep to a minimum the number of members of the sample that are not located.

When fieldwork is about to begin, the following supplies will be needed for the interviewers:

1. Sufficient supplies of questionnaires, pencils, and pencil sharpeners. (Pencils are easier to use because of erasures that are often needed during the interview.)
2. Any cards or pictures that may accompany the questionnaire.
3. Identification of the interviewer via a letter and/or an ID card.
4. A clipboard to make it easier to fill out the questionnaire.
5. A copy of the reference manual.
6. Maps or instructions on how to locate the respondents.

RESPONSE RATE

A response rate needs to be calculated at the end of every survey. The response rate is simply the number of completed questionnaires divided by the number of people in your original sample. Often survey directors will report other rates, using a smaller denominator, such as the number of people from the original sample who were actually located or the number of people who answered their telephone or the number of mailed questionnaires that actually reached a correct address. These rates are not true response rates. They are simply ways of avoiding having to report the real response rate. Note that the response is not simply a function of the number of refusals obtained, but also the number of sample points that were never located. Therefore, the response rate not only reflects the compliance of the population contacted, but the skill of the survey personnel in finding the members of the selected sample.

ENTERING AND EDITING THE DATA

Depending on the duration of fieldwork, the collected data may be entered into a computer while data collection is taking place or at the completion of data collection.

Data entry is a stage of survey work when many errors can occur. In the past, the standard way of checking for data entry error was to require double entry. Double entry simply means the data are entered twice, by different enterers. Then the two sets of data are compared (by computer), and when any disagreement in the data is found between the two data sets, the original questionnaire is consulted and the correct code is kept for the final data set. Double data entry is both costly and time consuming. Fortunately, there is less need for it today because of the proliferation of data entry/edit programs.

As can be deduced from the previous paragraph, in the recent past, data entry and data editing were two separate activities. Today, there are numerous computer programs that accomplish editing of data entry error concurrent with data entry. One such program is *Epi Info*'s data check program (see Chapter 12). These programs usually reproduce the questions from the questionnaire onto the computer screen and allow movement from one question to the next only if an acceptable entry is made. An acceptable entry may be defined by allowable codes or by following the appropriate skip pattern. An example of allowable codes may be an age range of 15–49 for a reproductive health survey. If the data entry person attempts to enter a 52 as the response for age, the computer will not accept it. Or, if there are five response categories for educational level, coded 1 to 5, the computer will only accept an entry in the 1 to 5 range. If the computer entry person mistakenly enters a 6, the computer will not move on to the next question until it is corrected. Such a data entry/edit program can identify the majority of data entry errors and consequently obviate the need for double data entry. In the absence of an entry/edit program, double data entry may be called for.

The data entry/edit program, however, does not identify all errors, and it cannot correct all errors. A miskeyed code that falls within the range of acceptable codes will not be caught. Furthermore, any errors that are in the questionnaire, and not due to data entry, cannot be corrected by the data entry person. The latter errors can only be corrected by the interviewer and often not without returning to the individual respondent. This usually is only done if data entry is timed close to the original interview.

Once a sufficient amount of data has been entered into the computer, other edits can be done. Consistency checks that may not have been easily programmed into the data entry/edit program may be written and run on the data (see Chapter 12). And when all the data have been entered, a set of frequencies for all the items in the questionnaire should be produced for further scrutiny for previously undetected errors.

After all the data have been entered and edited and there is no possibility of returning to the field, the cover sheets with identifying information on the respondents should be destroyed, as well as any other material (such as lists) that can identify participants in the survey. The questionnaires, themselves, should be kept—at least through the initial stages of analysis. Consistency errors may still be discovered during the analysis phase, and it is always helpful to be able to return to the original questionnaires.

ANALYZING THE DATA

Principles of data analysis are described elsewhere in this book (see Chapter 8). The analysis consideration unique to survey data, however, is the importance of using the appropriate statistical techniques to adjust for the sample design and to calculate sampling errors. As mentioned earlier, when disproportionate stratified sampling is used, weights must be calculated and used when producing any statistics, including percentages, for the total sample. Most popular statistical packages, such as *Statistical Analysis System* (*SAS*), *Epi Info*, and *Statistical Programs for the Social Sciences* (*SPSS*) accommodate weights very nicely for producing descriptive statistics. When calculating sampling error, statistical significance, and confidence intervals, however, for any method other than simple random or systematic sampling, it will be necessary to use a statistical package that can adjust for the design effect. The most common package with this ability is *Survey Data Analysis* (*SUDAAN*), but others are available as well.

REPORTING THE RESULTS

As in all epidemiologic work, the survey should be described in a written report. The report should include the survey's objectives, methods, results, and your interpretation of the findings. The report serves two purposes: (*1*) to document the methods used to conduct the survey; and (*2*) to communicate to decision makers, such as policy makers, funding sources, and program managers, the findings of the survey. Thus, you should keep in mind that you are writing for two very distinct audiences. A detailed description of your methods is of paramount importance to demonstrate to other researchers and users of the data that your data collection was sound and your results are reliable. (Be sure to include the response rate!) Your description of findings, on the other hand, must be clear and appropriate for decision makers who may be neither epidemiologists nor statisticians. Percentages and means may be the best way to communicate to this audience. Bear in mind that the findings must be presented in a way that is understandable to nonresearchers.

SOURCES OF ERROR

All along the route of survey implementation there are places for error to contaminate the data. While it is not possible to eliminate all error, you must be cognizant of potential error, must attempt to keep it at a minimum, and when all else fails, be prepared to define the bias that error may cause in the data. When conducting a survey, the following broad areas for error must be foremost in your mind as the survey planner and implementer.

1. Coverage error. Coverage error occurs when the population from which the sample is drawn is not equivalent to the target population. This usu-

ally results from outdated or poorly constructed sampling frames. It can also occur from incorrect information included in the sampling frame, such as incorrect addresses; or from an incomplete frame, such as only those households with computers or telephones when the target population is the total population. Attention must be given to the quality of the sampling frame and its close equivalence to the target population before a sample is drawn. If coverage error is not discovered until after the survey is implemented, you should report the bias caused by coverage error and its effect on interpretation of findings.

2. Sampling error. Sampling error is the least problematic in field surveys in that it is quantifiable and unbiased. As stated earlier, sampling error is linked to both the design and size of the sample. All sample surveys have sampling error.

3. Measurement error. Measurement error may be the most difficult to avoid. It often goes undetected and is nonquantifiable. Measurement error arises from various sources in the data collection process and is the error that makes a single respondent's answer incomparable to another's. Questions that are not clear or not interpreted in the same way by all respondents may not be measuring what you intend to measure for all respondents. Interviewers who are not consistent in the way they present questions or in the definitions they provide to respondents will create error, in that different respondents will have a different understanding of the question. Questions that are embarrassing or threatening or interviewers who are authority figures can evoke untruthful responses from interviewees. Questions that ask about events in the past may lead to recall bias that varies directly with the length of time that has passed since the event occurred.

4. Error due to nonresponse. This may be the most serious and most easily avoidable error in performing field surveys. Ask yourself, "What is the value of a carefully selected sample, designed to be representative of the population, when a response rate of 50% is obtained?" If only 50% of your sample has responded, you are very likely to have lost the representative properties of your sample design. Nonresponse can be attributed to two major factors: (1) failure of the interviewer to locate the respondent; and (2) failure of the respondent to consent to the interview. Both of the factors are controllable to a large degree by good selection and training of interviewers. At least three revisits should be made to households or other locations before assigning the status of "unable to locate respondent" to the interview. Often five to six revisits are recommended. As for "refused to participate," when surveying during a field investigation, you should not expect the level of refusal rate you would likely see in political, marketing, or other types of surveys. If you explain the health value

of the survey to the prospective respondents, it is usually not difficult to obtain their consent. A face-to-face survey, the mode that typically obtains the highest response rate, should never result in a response rate lower than 70%. An 80% to 90% response rate is not unusual for a face-to-face public health survey. In the case of a response rate lower than 80%, you are obliged to consider whether nonresponse has created a bias in the data and the direction of that bias. Keep in mind that respondents who are easily located may have different characteristics than those who are never at home. Persons who refuse to participate in the survey are likely to be less compliant in other areas, including health behaviors, than those who readily consent to be interviewed. A low response rate does more damage in rendering a survey's results questionable than merely reducing the sample size alone, since often there is no valid way of scientifically inferring all the characteristics of the nonrespondent population.

5. Data processing error. In the past, data entry was another significant source of error in surveys. But today the use of data entry/edit programs has reduced data entry error substantially. Another source of processing error still needs attention: that of coding. In surveys with reasonably large sample sizes that have open-ended questions in the questionnaire, it will be necessary to code these responses in order to manage them. The coding of open-ended responses should never be left to an unsupervised assistant. Coding takes skill and often the experience of a veteran investigator.

SHORTCUTS TO AVOID

Conducting a successful survey entails scores of activities, each of which must be carefully planned and controlled. Taking shortcuts can invalidate the results or cause them to be seriously misleading. Four of the shortcuts that occur too often are:

1. Failure to use probability sampling procedures. One way to ruin an otherwise well-conceived survey is to use a convenience sample rather than one based on probability design. It may be simple and cheap, for example, to get some needed information by selecting a sample of patients attending a public clinic. However, this sampling procedure could give incorrect results if you try to generalize them to the entire community.

2. Failure to pretest to the questionnaire. No qualified investigator will accept your results if they are based on newly formulated questions that have not been pretested. The pretest not only demonstrates whether or not the

target population understands the questions in the same way as the person who created them but also offers an opportunity to identify errors in the questionnaire.

3. Failure to train the interviewers thoroughly. Interviewers not only need to learn to conduct the interviews in a standardized fashion but they must also be taught the importance of *locating* the correct respondent and *convincing* that person to be interviewed. A week of interviewer training is not unreasonable for a large-scale survey.

4. Failure to use adequate quality control procedures. You should build into your survey necessary checks on its different facets at all stages—review of sample selection procedures, supervision of interviewing, random checks that interviews have actually taken place, and oversight of editing and coding decisions, among other things. Insisting on proper standards in recruitment and training of survey personnel helps a great deal, but equally important are proper review, verification, and evaluation to ensure that the execution of the survey corresponds to its design. Without proper quality control of all steps in the survey process, errors can occur that can be irreversible, costly, and have damaging results.

REFERENCES

Survey Methods

1. Abramson, J.H. (1974). *Survey Methods in Community Medicine.* Churchill Livingstone, Edinburgh and London.

3. Dillman, D.A. (1978). *Mail and Telephone Surveys: the total design method.* John Wiley and Sons, New York.

4. Fowler, F. J. (1993). *Survey Research Methods*, 2nd ed. Sage Publications, Newbury Park, CA.

5. Rossi, P.H., Wright, J.D., Anderson, A.B. (1983). *Handbook of Survey Research.* Academic Press, Orlando, FL.

6. Salant, P., Dillman, D.A. (1994). *How to Conduct Your Own Survey.* John Wiley and Sons, New York.

Questionnaire Design and Interviewing

1. Beimer, P., Groves, R.M., Lyberg, L.E., et al. (1991). *Measurement Errors in Surveys.* John Wiley and Sons, New York.

2. Belson, W.A. (1981). *The Design and Understanding of Survey Questions.* Gower, Aldershot, England.

3. Converse, J., Presser, S. (1986). *Survey Questions.* Sage Publications, Beverly Hills, CA.

4. Fowler, F.J., Mangione, T.W. (1990). *Standardized Survey Interviewing: minimizing interviewer related error.* Sage Publications, Newbury Park, CA.
5. Sudman, S., Bradburn, N.M. (1982). *Asking Questions: a practical guide to questionnaire design.* Jossey-Bass Publishers, San Francisco.

Sampling

1. Cochran, W.G. (1977). *Sampling Techniques*, 3rd ed. John Wiley and Sons, New York.
2. Kish, L. (1965). *Survey Sampling.* John Wiley and Sons, New York.
3. Levy, P.S., Lemeshow, S. (1980). *Sampling for Health Professionals.* Lifetime Learning Publications, Belmont, CA.
4. World Health Organization (1986). *Sample Size Determination.* World Health Organization, Geneva.

12

USING A COMPUTER FOR FIELD INVESTIGATIONS

Andrew G. Dean

Microcomputers are important tools for epidemiologic field investigations. Epidemiologists routinely use computers in field investigations along with questionnaires, statistics, laboratory tests, and other more traditional epidemiologic tools.

Computers, whether laptop, desktop, or palmtop, are machines, and, like most machines, require an investment of technical skill and setup time that can be recovered through increased quantity and quality of output.

Computers are most useful for:

- Tasks that are clearly defined and that will be done many times in the same way
- Rapid computation or counting involving large numbers of similar records
- Tasks matching the capabilities of existing software
- Numerically intensive calculations
- Accurate retention of details
- Investigators who have used the same system before

Manual processing is still indicated for:

- One-time or occasional tasks
- Small numbers of records

- Complex or changing tasks
- Operators who are not familiar with computer use
- Situations where staffing for manual tasks is easier to obtain than computers or knowledgeable operators

Tasks that may be usefully performed on a computer during an outbreak investigation include searching for information, sample size calculation, questionnaire design, data entry, importing or exporting files in various formats, tabulation of results, statistical calculations, graphing, mapping, presentation graphics, and computer communication.

MICROCOMPUTERS

Progress in the miniaturization of computers has been nearly miraculous in the past three decades, and a description of microcomputer hardware is sure to be outdated as soon as it is printed. At present a portable computer and a printer can be carried to the field in a briefcase and operated either from batteries or standard electrical power. Palmtop computers that fit in a pocket and do not require a keyboard are becoming popular, although they are still limited compared with laptop models. A laptop or desktop computer may have a hard disk capable of storing millions of records. Portable modems make it technically possible to send files, access bibliographic databases, or search the Internet from any area with telephone service, although some countries place restrictions on modem use. Wireless connections are rapidly becoming available in some areas.

The most common type of microcomputer is the Intel-compatible computer with a Microsoft Windows operating system. Since microcomputers running Windows 95, 98, NT, 2000, ME, and XP are ubiquitous and also permit fairly easy development of software, most epidemiologic software is available for these models. Laptop computers are more expensive than desktop models of the same capacity but are fairly rugged and light enough to carry, and most models easily adapt to international electrical variations. Palmtop computers running Windows CE have partial compatibility with other Windows operating systems but still require special versions of most types of software. Others have entirely different operating systems, although data can often be sent from one computer to another. The overall issues in choosing a computer include compatibility with other computers in the home office and field environment; availability of epidemiologic and statistical software; and the usual factors of cost, capacity, speed, durability, and repair service. As the age of computer communication progresses, the types of connections and provisions for security and virus checking assume greater importance.

SOFTWARE

The type of software available for epidemiologic investigation is more important than the brand of computer or operating system. During a field investigation, software may be needed for word processing, data entry, database management, data analysis and statistics, communications, bibliographic searching, and miscellaneous functions such as scheduling and note taking. Commercial programs are available for word processing, scheduling, note taking, graphing, and other functions that are common business applications. Data entry and database management can be done with commercial programs such as Microsoft Access, but these programs do not offer statistics for epidemiology, and setting up databases and manipulating records may require more attention than investigators are able to spare in a busy field situation. Commercial database software can also be quite expensive if multiple copies are required. Statistical software is available commercially, the most popular general purpose programs being *Statistical Analysis System*, (*SAS*, www.sas.com), and *Statistical Programs for the Social Sciences*, (*SPSS*, www.spss.com). They perform a wide variety of statistical procedures for those familiar with the statistics and with programming in *SAS* or *SPSS*. Since their commands are different from those of the database programs, the use of both statistics and database programs requires learning two "languages." *SAS* and *SPSS* both offer facilities for data entry, and thus may be used without a database program, although data entry usually cannot be controlled to the extent that it can in a database program.

Epidemiologic fieldwork often requires statistics for categorical (coded or yes/no) data rather than continuous data. Mantel-Haenszel analysis of stratified data is important, and for those who know how to use and interpret it, logistic regression may be desirable after preliminary Mantel-Haenszel analysis. It is important that entry, checking, coding, and editing of data be easy to perform. Setting up a new questionnaire is almost always required in a field investigation, and this should be easy to do in the software that is chosen.

The Centers for Disease Control and Prevention (CDC) and the World Health Organization have developed a program called *Epi Info* for use in epidemiologic investigations that attempts to provide the best compromise between ease of use and flexibility. It is in the public domain and versions for both DOS and Windows may be downloaded from the CDC website, copied for use by others, or translated. In this chapter, we use *Epi Info* to illustrate many of the tasks to be performed with computers in the field. Other free and inexpensive software for use in epidemiology can be found by searching the Internet. A recent search turned up links to free calculators for purposes as diverse as estimating caloric intake, civil engineering, producing random numbers, and doing specialized statistics, many of which could be useful in epidemiology.

Whatever software is chosen, it is important that you be familiar with its use and limitations before leaving for the field. A tense field situation with high stakes and an insistent press leaves little time for learning about software or devising programs to solve new problems. The analysis does not have to be sophisticated, but it should be correct with regard to the totals obtained and the elementary statistics. Logistic regression analysis can be refined later, but the basic data must return from the field intact, properly backed up, and well documented.

THE WORKING AND TRAVELING ENVIRONMENT

To minimize problems in the field, hardware, software, and operator skills should have been used as much as possible before leaving the home office. A "dress rehearsal" should be conducted before leaving to be sure that all necessary elements are available.

Magnetic disks must be treated like fine phonograph records and protected from fingerprints, scratches, coffee, magnets, sharp bending, and denting by firm objects like ballpoint pens. They will not be harmed by a reasonable number of passes through a modern airport X-ray machine, but metal detectors and motor-driven moving belts do generate magnetic fields that could be harmful to diskettes. Diskettes should be protected from both heat and intense cold. They should never be left in a parked car in warm weather. If possible, a portable Compact Disk (CD-ROM) writer should be used to make permanent backups of data, as optical media, particularly the CD-R or write-once CD-ROMs, are not affected by magnetic fields and are more resistant to physical abuse than floppy disks. Extra copies can be made and mailed home by more than one route in case of loss or theft of luggage. CD-ROM drives are delicate, however, and should be treated gently.

When traveling to other countries it is important to be sure that the type of power (120 vs. 240 volts) and connecting plug are known and compatible with the equipment being used. Portable computers may be run from car batteries in remote locations with appropriate adapters. Whenever possible, the computer should be protected from voltage surges with a voltage spike protector. Increasingly, uninterruptible power supplies (UPSs) are affordable, and will protect against power interruptions for long enough to allow saving current work and shutting down the computer. The device used must be designed for local voltage levels, as voltage spike protectors designed for 110 volts perish with a puff of smoke when plugged into 220 volts. Battery power is much less subject to effects from voltage variations.

Some countries require prior clearance to bring a computer in or out. Others have restrictions on the use of modem communications. It is important to check on such regulations with appropriate embassies, scientific colleagues, or customs officials.

In the field, your work space should be shielded from direct sun and protected from dust. The power cord for a desktop computer can be fastened to the outlet with tape or other means so that power will not be accidentally interrupted.

Organization of a portable computer's hard disk can contribute greatly to ease of use. Some investigators recommend creating a new directory for each investigation, keeping all files pertaining to that investigation in the same directory. The 1.4 megabyte floppy diskette has become a universal standard, but for files larger than one diskette, it is important to have software such as PKZIP or WinZip, which compresses files and automatically spans more than one diskette. A number of higher-capacity removable-storage devices such as ZIP drives are available, but with the more proprietary formats, it is important that more than one compatible drive be available, and that both generating and receiving machines use the same drive format. Files can be transferred via Local Area Network (LAN) connections or the Internet if these options are available. Sending backup files to the home office can provide protection against loss of data through theft or loss of luggage during a trip. A colleague should be asked to verify that the files arrived intact.

WORD PROCESSING

Word processing is used for producing questionnaires, plans, and reports, and for recording miscellaneous observations during the investigation. A word processing package previously used by the investigator is preferred, since it takes time to adjust to a new package.

If collaborators in the investigation use different software for word processing, a common format such as "Rich Text Format" (RTF) files can be used, but compatibility should be tested in both types of software, as even standard formats are sometimes version dependent. Plain text or ASCII files can be used as the lowest common denominator if necessary.

DESIGNING A QUESTIONNAIRE FOR COMPUTER USE

A questionnaire is a tool or template for structuring data collection so that items to be tabulated by computer or by hand are all of the same type. An item called AGE, for example, will contain data expressing age in a uniform way, perhaps as a number representing years. A good questionnaire, like a computer program or written essay, begins with an outline of major topics to be addressed. Theoretically, it is even more desirable to begin with the type of output desired and work backward to define the necessary input elements. In practice, an iterative approach to consider both input and output is often used until a satisfactory "design" is achieved.

Often the objective is to explore correlations between an illness or injury and one or more exposures or risk factors. The large topics in an outline could then be:

- Identifiers and follow-up information
- Demographic information (age, sex, etc.)
- Outcome (Disease or injury)
- Exposures
- Possible confounders

Desired Outputs

- Graph of case onset over time (Time)
- Map of cases by residence and workplace (Place)
- Tables of exposure by outcome (Person)

If the database design begins with a questionnaire, a series of questions is identified within each major section. These are usually given names that can also serve as field or variable names in the computer file-names like FIRST NAME, SOCIAL SECURITY NUMBER, DIARRHEA, and POTATO SALAD. Each of these can be developed into a question intelligible to the subject or to the interviewer. Some, like DIARRHEA, may require several questions (ONSET DATE and TIME, FREQUENCY, CONSISTENCY, etc.) that may be summarized in a final yes/no conclusion for meeting the investigator's case definition of DIARRHEA.

In designing a questionnaire, it is useful to know what computer program will be used to enter and analyze the data. If *Epi Info* is used, the following computer terms will be useful in describing data entry and analysis.

A *Field* or *Variable* is one data item, such as FIRST NAME or AGE. Usually *Field* is used to describe the blank in which data items are entered and *Variable* refers to the field name that may be manipulated later during analysis. A *Record* is usually the information from one respondent to a questionnaire. Many records are stored together in a *File* or *Table*. *Epi Info* 6 data files end in .REC as in DATA01.REC and contain both data and a description of the questionnaire.

Epi Info 2000/2002 records are stored in Tables in Microsoft Access format within MDB files. "*Views*" in *Epi Info* 2000/2002 are separate tables containing data for displaying the questionnaire on the screen. A file may be recalled for analysis or data entry, stored on floppy or hard disks, or copied from one disk to another. A file compression program such as WinZip can be used to compress files too big to fit on a single diskette, or a CD-ROM writer can be used to store larger files.

In *Epi Info*, a field has a prompt or text question and a space for entering data. In *Epi Info* 6, the questions are typed into a text questionnaire in a word processor. In *Epi Info* 2000/2002, the MakeView program guides the design of a questionnaire through dialogs that appear after right-clicking a location on the screen. For each field, the dialog requires a prompt and a field type, such as Text, Number, or Date. A variable name is created automatically after a question or prompt is supplied, but can be edited if desired

Almost all data entry programs accept data of the specified type (e.g., numeric) and reject other entries (e.g., "Jones" in a numeric field). Many have sophisticated methods for evaluating entries and taking appropriate action to prevent erroneous entries. In *Epi Info*, for example, setting field properties or inserting commands in the Check Code scripting language for data entry allows specification of minima, maxima, legal codes, skip patterns, automatic coding, and copying of data from the preceding record. In Check Code command blocks, the user can set up more complex checks to issue an error message if a particular date precedes another date or a diagnostic code conflicts with the person's age or gender. Check Code can also be written to do mathematics or to call another program to perform complex calculations and put the results in other parts of the data entry form.

Complex checking on data entry has a cost in terms of setup time and skill required. During an outbreak investigation with *Epi Info*, most epidemiologists would insert a few checks, such as ranges or legal codes and would tell the program to skip questions shown to be irrelevant by previous answers (e.g., skip the section on symptoms if the person was not ill). If several different people will be entering the data, it may be worth spending extra time to set up checks for consistency and acceptability, but this may be less necessary if one person enters all the data and the number of records is small enough to allow manual checking after entry.

In some situations, it is preferable to enter data directly into the computer rather than using paper forms first. Direct entry has been used in door-to-door survey work and for abstracting records in medical record rooms. In most outbreak investigations, however, a paper form will be used for interviews and the results will be transferred to a computer later, perhaps in a health department office or in a motel room with a portable or laptop computer. In the future it is likely that palmtop hand-held computers will expand the possibilities for direct data entry in the field.

There are two styles of questionnaire images that may be used on the computer screen. The first is a telegraphic or "keypuncher's" form. It consists of field names and data entry blanks only, arranged on the screen to allow the fastest possible entry by a person thoroughly acquainted with both the paper and the screen forms. Such a questionnaire might begin as follows:

```
    Idnum  ####
     Name  _____
      Age  ##
      Sex  <A>
   County  <A>
  Disease  <Y>
  Chicken  <Y>
      Ham  <Y>
     Beef  <Y>
```

The second style is an extended format that resembles the paper form as closely as possible, complete with headings, questions, instructions to the user, and blanks. With slight editing, the same form may be used in an actual interview. This format is most useful if there are relatively few questionnaires, if there are several people entering the data who do not have time to become "experts" on the data format (entering 100 questionnaires might produce an "expert"), or if those entering data will be frequently interrupted.

In *Epi Info*, either format may be used, according to the investigator's preference. With either form, the screen prompts can be more extensive than the briefer name chosen for the variable to be manipulated during data analysis.

In using *Epi Info* and other programs, it is important to know how the program handles missing values before finalizing the questionnaire. *Epi Info* allows a missing value to be entered by pressing the <Enter> key to leave the field blank. Some programs record missing values as zero for numeric fields. In these programs the questions must be designed so that there is no confusion between a true code or value of zero and a missing value where this distinction is important. Zero glasses of water consumed and "unknown" glasses of water consumed, for example, are quite different, so a special code (often 9 or 99) should be assigned for the case of "unknown." Such codes are unnecessary in *Epi Info* and most current data entry programs, since missing data are stored as values distinct from zero.

In some investigations, particularly in research settings, it is useful to assign additional codes (e.g., 8's) to distinguish answers cited as "unknown" by the subject, those considered less accurate or unknown by the interviewer, and those somehow omitted during data entry. These extra codes can complicate the analysis considerably and should be assigned only after careful thought about the format of the table that will show the results. "Somebody might ask about it later" is not sufficient reason to burden the investigation with a series of extra codes unless they contribute meaningfully to the analysis. In a field investigation it is often sufficient to use only one kind of missing value, since the modest number of cases and rough-and-ready data-collection process may not permit analysis of bias that may have arisen due to more than one type of missing data.

To provide proper analysis of questions, codes should be assigned during data entry. Merely typing in the names of counties or diseases can result in a profusion of synonyms and misspellings that is impossible to analyze. Either numeric or text codes may be used. When producing tables during analysis, codes indicating the actual values are more useful than numeric codes, although numeric codes can be recoded to produce useful labels during analysis. Generally "Y" and "N" are less likely to produce errors in data entry than "0" and "1" and "URI" is more meaningful than "7002" for Upper Respiratory Infection.

A key issue in setting up data entry forms involves multiple-choice questions. The question:

> How many glasses of water do you drink per day (choose one)?
> >   0. None
> >   1. 1–2
> >   3. 3–4
> >   5. 5 or more
> >   9. Don't know
> >   Water #

has five mutually exclusive answers, and the entire question, therefore, has a single answer. A one-digit numeric field called WATER is enough to record the answer.

Another type of question is:

> What symptoms have you had in the past month?
> >   1. Diarrhea
> >   2. Fever
> >   3. Chills

Note that all three symptoms might have been present. Each part of what looks like a single question requires a yes/no answer, and this question should be set up as follows:

> What symptoms have you had in the past month?
> >   Diarrhea <Y>
> >   Fever <Y>
> >   Chills <Y>

The same would be true of a list of foods possibly eaten at a meal. Each item is really a separate question, since the answers are not mutually exclusive. In the Analysis program in *Epi Info*, the first question is summarized with the command FREQ WATER, to display the codes for each level and the number of times each code is represented.

The symptom question is more complicated, however. By asking for a frequency distribution of the variable DIARRHEA (FREQ DIARRHEA, in *Epi Info*), it is a simple matter to ascertain the number of persons with and without diarrhea. But discovering how many symptoms each person had takes more complex programming—complex enough so that it may be easier to add another summary question below the list of symptoms such as "Number of symptoms #," if this is important for the analysis. The person entering data can quickly scan the paper form, count symptoms, and enter this number rather than requiring the investigator to do extra programming during the analysis stage. The trade-off between intelligent data consolidation during data entry and having the computer do the work is evident at many points during design of computer entry forms and paper questionnaires. If you will be using both, consider simplifying as much as possible the data transferred to the computer from the paper form. Names, addresses, and other follow-up information may be omitted, and complex case definitions may be summarized with a single yes/no question. Field investigation usually results in scores or hundreds of questionnaires, and the human mind and eye may be a simpler processing alternative for some kinds of questions than having a busy investigator with modest computer skills try to write a program to condense the data electronically.

In the end, the investigator must decide what to collect, how much of a completed questionnaire to process by hand, and in what form to code it for computer use. Although experience plays a major role, pilot testing can be a good substitute. With modern systems such as *Epi Info*, it is quite easy to enter data from five or six sample instances of a questionnaire (preferably from people who will not be included in the final study). These are then processed to produce a model for the final analysis, saving the program that results. This procedure will often reveal gaps, inconsistencies, or ambiguities in the questionnaire and point out questions that do not contribute to the analysis, and is almost guaranteed to improve the final questionnaire design. Before finalizing the design, the investigator should examine each question with the additional questions, "What do I really want to know? " and "How am I going to process this variable?"

DATA ENTRY AND VALIDATION

Usually paper questionnaires from the field are far from ready for analysis after data entry. They contain misspellings, synonyms, abbreviations, upper/lower case mixtures, marginal notes, and missing data. Data entry is an opportunity for partial "cleaning" of the data set. It must be done with scrupulous dedication to preventing bias—the kind that could insert data favorable to a hypothesis or eliminate items detrimental to it. Since field investigations seldom have the luxury of "blind" coders and data entry personnel, only strict and literal attention to accuracy can prevent bias.

It is a good idea to alternate case and control forms during data entry to avoid bias from the small decisions and adaptations that occur during the course of entering forms. If there is more than one data entry person, each should enter the same ratio of case to control forms.

In most data entry systems, including *Epi Info*, a cursor on the screen indicates where entry will occur. The cursor jumps automatically from field to field. When an entry is made, the item is checked for correct type (numeric, date, etc.) and additional checks programmed into the check file are performed. If a problem is encountered, the program indicates this and waits for correction before going on to the next field. At the end of each questionnaire, the record is saved automatically or by answering an explicit question such as "Save data to disk? (Y/N)" In *Epi Info*, a power failure (or someone tripping over the power cord) will not result in loss of records already saved, although the partial record being entered may have to be reentered. If other programs do not have this feature, save your work frequently. It is a good idea to mark each paper questionnaire as data entry is completed to avoid accidental reentry.

When all records have been entered, the entries should be carefully validated to be sure that they represent the source documents accurately. One person can read the data entered aloud while the other verifies that the entries represent the source document accurately.

Further checking may be done by performing frequencies on each field. FREQ * will accomplish this in *Epi Info*. Examining the results will often disclose outliers such as "*Gf!" that crept in during a moment of distraction. These may be edited in the data entry program before beginning the actual analysis.

Some investigators prefer to have the same set of questionnaires entered in duplicate by two different operators in separate files. The two files are then compared, and differences are reconciled by a person authorized to make data entry decisions.

ANALYSIS OF DATA IN FIELD EPIDEMIOLOGY

Analysis of a descriptive study or survey usually begins with a simple frequency for each variable (in *Epi Info*, FREQ *). Then, for a study with two or more groups, such as cases and controls, ill and well, exposed and unexposed, you would want to compare the two groups. For categorical (coded) data the TABLES command in *Epi Info*, for example TABLES * ILL, will produce cross-tabulations of each variable by illness status (Y/N), with appropriate statistics for each.

Often in a case-control or cross-sectional study, a histogram or epidemic curve is needed. In *Epi Info*, the case group would first be selected before doing the histogram, for example, SELECT CASE = "Y". The histogram might be performed with: HISTOGRAM ONSETDATE. Continuous variables such as age or diastolic blood pressure are analyzed with the MEANS command, for example, MEANS SBP ILL if SBP is systolic blood pressure and ILL is case status.

In most analytic programs it is necessary to use names of variables to do an analysis. Unlike algebraic notation, computer notation usually allows a descriptive name for each field. In some programs the length of these names is limited to, for example, 8 or 10 characters. If transfer of data from one program to another is contemplated, be sure that variable names truncated to the length allowed in the most restrictive program are unique. For example, "ADDRESSLINE1" and "ADDRESSLINE2" might both emerge as ADDRESSLIN in a program with variable names limited to 10 characters. "ADDRESS1" and "ADDRESS2" would survive truncation to 8 characters, however.

After doing frequencies for each field, you will have an idea of how many records are in each group, and how many missing values there are for each field. If missing values are displayed, many of the tables may be three-by-three rather than two-by-two tables, and the statistics that result are not as complete as those that accompany two-by-two tables. Some packages allow you to suppress missing values (In *Epi Info*, SET IGNORE = ON). Repeating the analysis after giving this command will omit the missing values and focus the analysis solely on records that have data for the tables and frequencies being produced. Two-by-two tables in *Epi Info* are accompanied by chi-square tests, odds ratios, risk ratios, confidence limits, and, if indicated, Fisher exact tests.

Often one or more "significant" findings may be indicated by p values less than 0.05 or confidence limits that exclude 1.0 for odds ratios or risk ratios. Further analysis to consider confounding variables is indicated, at least for frequent confounders such as age and sex. This is done by stratifying the table of interest (say SALAD by ILL), producing a separate table for each value of the confounder.

In *Epi Info*, the crude table is produced by TABLES SALAD ILL and stratification by SEX by TABLES SALAD ILL SEX to produce separate tables for males and females. The Mantel-Haenszel summary chi-square and p-value for the stratified result may be compared with the results of the crude analysis. If the odds ratios in the two or more strata are similar, interaction is not present, and a difference in the crude and Mantel-Haenszel odds ratios may be taken as an indication that SEX was a confounder. Other potential confounders such as AGE, socioeconomic status, etc. can be evaluated similarly, either one by one or in combination (TABLES SALAD ILL SEX RACE).

Stratification does not work well for small data sets if there are many strata, and variables such as AGE may need to be recoded to produce fewer strata, such as

CHILD and ADULT. A number of examples of data manipulation, including automation of a complex case definition, are included in the *Epi Info* 6 manual in a chapter on epidemic investigation.

At this point the analysis may be complete enough for field purposes, if confounding has been identified and eliminated through stratification, and interaction has been addressed (perhaps recording the results for more than one stratum rather than the overall results, as in "For people up to the age of 18, the effect was–. . . ; those over 18 did not react the same way."). The significant findings must be evaluated from a biomedical point of view and distributed to interested parties.

Graphing of important findings may be helpful in visualizing or explaining results, particularly those pertaining to temporal variables. *Epi Info* offers bar, histogram, pie, scatter, and line graphs. Two variables are required for scatter graphs, and one variable for other formats. A second variable can be represented by plotting a separate graph for each of its values, as in showing date of onset in separate histograms for males and females, for example.

In cases where there are several significant risk factors or several confounders, logistic regression may be helpful. Logistic regression is offered as part of *Epi Info* 2000/2002, and a number of other programs are available for this purpose after exporting data from *Epi Info* for DOS.

GEOGRAPHIC INFORMATION SYSTEMS AND THE ANALYSIS OF "PLACE"

In some outbreaks, the place of residence, work, visitation, food or water consumption, or aerosol inhalation is important in the analysis. Geographic Information Systems (GIS) are used to link database information with maps or other graphics to provide opportunities for spatial analysis. Locations can be recorded in variables such as city, state, mail code, or census tract. Exact locations can also be recorded as longitude and latitude, obtained through geocoding or from field measurements with a hand-held geographic position sensor (GPS). Geocoding means obtaining exact longitude and latitude coordinates from street addresses or other location information. It is done through the use of special geocoding databases or services available commercially or provided on the Internet.

One or more geographic variables must match the geographic information in the "map," called a boundary file in *Epi Info* 6 and *Epi Map* for DOS, and a shape file in *Epi Info/EpiMap* 2000/2002. City names must be spelled the same way in both data sets, for example, or point coordinates must be in the same units, such as latitude/longitude in decimal degrees. The GIS software combines the map image with the database to show locations as colors, patterns, dots, or other symbols that represent spatial information. An entire science has developed around the analysis of geographic information, but the basic operations can be performed in *Epi Info* 2000/2002 with the *Epi Map* program, and refined if necessary in dedicated GIS software. Eng describes the use of dot maps in investigating an outbreak.[1] *Epi Info* uses software produced by the makers of ArcView (Environmental Systems Research Institute, Inc., www.esri.com) so that maps can be displayed by either system.

OBTAINING AND USING EXISTING COMPUTERIZED DATA

Sometimes useful computerized information already exists at the site of an investigation. For example, hospital computer systems may have laboratory values, diagnostic information, or operative schedules; a water treatment plant may have results of water analysis. Such files may contain more information than is relevant and may be in a variety of file formats. Selection of relevant information can be done by the person managing the data system. If you specify a time period or category of record to be selected, it may be relatively easy for the data manager to create a file containing only the desired items, perhaps with only certain fields represented.

The file format is also important. Most computerized database and statistics programs, including *Epi Info*, will accept an ASCII file in fixed-field format. This means that only the first 128 standard characters are included and each line represents a different record. A field is distinguished by its position on the line and always occupies a fixed number of characters. It is important to obtain a list of the fields, their types, and length.

Epi Info for DOS will analyze files in the DBASE format directly and will import files in the LOTUS 1-2-3, comma-delimited, DBASE, and fixed-field ASCII formats with a program called IMPORT. The Analysis program in *Epi Info* 2000/2002 will READ files in more than 20 different formats and can WRITE files in these same formats, allowing for extremely flexible data conversion.

Whenever external files of any kind are copied, the source disk should first be checked for computer viruses with a suitable program, no matter how reputable the supplier of the data. Reference data such as telephone lists or the *Epi Info* manual may be carried as files on hard or floppy disks, so that heavier paper copies are not needed.

COMPUTER COMMUNICATIONS

A computer equipped with a modem can be used to send files of any type to another computer over the telephone system. In many parts of the world, Internet access is available for modest charges in Internet cafes. If available, the Internet provides not only facilities for e-mail but also access to searches, guidelines, textbooks, calculators, reference data, and information (of variable quality) on almost any conceivable subject. Woodall provides a review of the use of computer networking in investigating disease outbreaks, with particular reference to biological and toxic weapon use.[2]

It is not always easy to connect a portable computer to a telephone line, as many businesses and hotels have digital telephones that do not work with standard types of modems. Hotels increasingly have made special provisions for e-mail connections, however, and asking about these facilities in advance is a good idea before traveling to a field site.

OBTAINING INFORMATION FROM THE WORLD ELECTRONIC AND PRINT LITERATURE WHILE IN THE FIELD

Unless the investigator is a specialist in the type of problem being investigated, bibliographic searching may be of great importance. In the United States (and many other countries where it is available), the *MEDLARS* database of the National Library of Medicine is the most comprehensive source of information. It contains references and often abstracts describing millions of articles in thousands of biomedical journals. Searches can be performed free of charge at the National Library of Medicine portal http://gateway.nlm.nih.gov/gw/Cmd or at other sites that allow *MEDLARS* searches.

One Internet search site, www.google.com, provides free-text searching, returning first the references most heavily cited by others, thus filtering out much of the chaff from billions of possibilities. Other search engines, such as www.yahoo.com, provide classification hierarchies that may be better for reviewing a systematic field of knowledge. In either case, the Internet is becoming more and more a reflection of the state of the world and of both episodic and cumulative information that cannot be ignored. A quick search of the Internet is often a practical way to obtain a grasp on a new field, such as air handling, plumbing, laws, lay medical advice, organizations dealing with relevant problems, and even telephone numbers or methods of locating people.

Most computer products are supported by websites, including *Epi Info*, and it is possible to download a free copy of *Epi Info*, or an update, from www.cdc.gov/epiinfo/. Many hardware companies such as printer manufacturers provide free downloads of current drivers for their products. Searching for statistical calculators turned up one site (http://www-sci.lib.uci.edu/HSG/RefCalculators.html) that links to over 16,000 calculators, many of which could be useful in epidemiology. Maps in great detail are available for downloading, and *Epi Info* contains an on-line reference chapter with links to hundreds of sites that provide resources for mapping.

OBTAINING TECHNICAL ASSISTANCE DURING A FIELD INVESTIGATION

Occasionally a computer problem arises in the field that requires more expertise than the investigator possesses. Computer breakdowns, unfamiliar file formats, access to special printers or other equipment, and difficulties with telephone connections may all require assistance. Technical expertise is available in most communities from a variety of sources. If calling your home base support staff does not solve a problem, a search of local health departments, technical schools, computer stores, and computer clubs may lead to a person with the necessary knowledge or piece of equipment. The Internet and e-mail provide sources of information that can be accessed at any hour of the day or night because of the differences in time zones.

COMPUTER VIRUSES AND DATA BACKUP

There is little satisfaction in having written a book whose only manuscript was lost in a fire, and, similarly, proper backup of computer data is essential. Whatever can go wrong should be expected to do so—perhaps more than once. In the past few years computer viruses have been added to the list of things that can go wrong, but they are only an additional cause for careful backup procedures that already were necessary to protect against hard disk crashes, power outages, theft, and late-night human errors.

Computer viruses are becoming more and more prevalent. They cause a variety of problems, but the most serious destroy all data on disks used in a particular computer. They may be acquired from a source outside a previously uninfected computer, either by copying files or through communication with another system.

Commercial programs are available to detect and often remove these viruses, and one of these should be used to check all disks inserted into the computer before copying any files, processing data, or running programs. A suitable virus protection program should be active at all times in a computer, and special care should be taken to check diskettes that may have been in other computers and become infected. Portable computers are attractive to thieves, and their hard disks—like all hard disks—may "crash," making data difficult or impossible to recover. More than one floppy disk or CD-ROM copy of all data should be made on a regular basis, and the backups should be carefully stored in places separate from the computer itself, to rule out the possibility of complete loss from theft, carelessness, or fire. Several well-verified disks, traveling by different routes, mailed home, and/or stored with different people are the best backup system. New backups should be made at intervals, perhaps every hour or two during data entry. It is also useful to have CD-ROM copies of important software in case a hard disk must be replaced in the field.

Generally in a field investigation it is practical to give new names to each new set of backup files so previous files are not written over. If anything goes wrong with a current file or disk, the previous set of files may provide a good copy of most of the data set. Although good commercial programs are available for backing up hard disks, they are usually not necessary in field investigations, since the data files are usually small. The files may simply be copied to floppy disks, maintaining several such carefully labeled disks to be used in sequence.

When things go wrong, a frequent reaction is to make the problem worse through panic. If difficulties in recovering files are experienced, first obtain technical help in diagnosing the problem. If you decide to restore files from the backup disks, be sure that the write-protect function (see previous section) is set on these disks to avoid having the backups destroyed by a virus or faulty procedure. If files have been accidentally erased on the hard disk, it is important to avoid entering further records or copying files until an attempt has been made to recover the lost files. Programs such as *Norton Utilities* can restore erased files and repair many corrupted files if they have not been written over by further manipulations.

DATA CONFIDENTIALITY AND LEGAL ISSUES

Maintaining confidentiality of data on a portable microcomputer is similar to protecting a stack of questionnaires. The best protection is through maintaining careful physical custody of any disks containing data, including the internal hard disk of the computer. With small data sets, files can be kept on floppy disks so the hard disk does not contain confidential data. In many investigations, names and addresses are not needed in data files, and such data should not be entered unless it . is absolutely necessary. Arbitrary identification numbers are adequate for most computerized data sets. Frequently names and other identifiers may be left with the local health department and only code-identified data transported to a more central site. Encryption programs or compression programs with password protection should be used to protect data in case CD-ROMs or diskettes are stolen, lost in the mail, or the computer itself is stolen.

Occasionally outbreaks lead to legal proceedings for negligence or even homicide. Records of the investigation may be subpoenaed or otherwise required for legal purposes. This possibility and scientific documentation make it important to keep good records of the investigation and to store them in such a way that they can be accessed by appropriate parties even if the investigator moves on to another job. Analytic programs may be written with comments explaining important steps, which also facilitates reuse of the programs in another investigation.

Computer disks should be carefully labeled, and after the investigation stored in an organized way so others can access the files. Paper copies of the data may be made for permanent documentation and ease of filing, since computer disks lose their magnetic data after a few years and for archival purposes should be copied to new disks annually or stored on CD-ROMs.

THE FUTURE OF COMPUTERS IN EPIDEMIOLOGIC FIELD INVESTIGATION

Future computers for field investigation will be smaller, lighter, and more powerful. Soon both voice and handwritten input will be practical. Medical and other records will be computerized to a greater extent, offering opportunities for capturing relevant information in detail for the investigator with the skills and tools to convert data from diverse formats. Eventually, perhaps, better programs will alleviate some of the compatibility problems between various types of software, but the competitive marketplace will insure that other types of incompatibility arise. Palmtop computers will extend direct data collection to environments such as earthquake sites, the bedside, or other field locations, and digital cameras will find more use in documentation.

The Internet has begun the process of providing access to the entire world from a portable computer as though all resources resided on a single hard disk. Search capabilities will be used eventually not only for information access but, perhaps, to provide data content for actual investigations.

Like most aspects of field investigation, computer use will continue to require ingenuity and adaptation. Those who have acquired the skills for using a portable computer, however, find that the rewards in quantity and quality of epidemiologic work accomplished make it an indispensable companion in field investigation, and that the communication and information access offered by the Internet are becoming more and more central to the epidemiologic process.

NOTE

Use of trade names is for identification only and does not constitute endorsement by the U.S. Public Health Service.

REFERENCES

Note: References to Internet addresses supplied in the text may change but can usually be recovered by searching for the topic of interest or a trade name with an Internet search engine.

1. Eng, S.B., Werker, D.H., King, A.S., et al. (1999) Computer-generated dot maps as an epidemiologic tool investigating an outbreak of toxoplasmosis. *Emerg Infect Dis* 5(6), 815–19.
2. Woodall, J. (1998) The role of computer networking in investigating unusual disease outbreaks and allegations of biological and toxin weapons use. *Crit Rev Microbiol* 24(3), 255–72.

FURTHER READING

Beck-Sague, C., Jarvis, W.R., Martone, W.J. (1997) Outbreak investigations. *Infect Control Hosp Epidemiol* 18, 138–45.

Bruce, J.C., Swan, A.V. (1991) Epi Info: the outbreak investigator's all-in-one computer toolkit. CDR (Lond Engl Rev) 1(7),R78–80.

Dean, A.G., Arner, T.G., Sangam, S., et al. (2002) Epi Info 2002, a database and statistics program for public health professionals for use on Windows 95, 98, NT, 2000, ME, and XP computers. Centers for Disease Control and Prevention, Atlanta. (Can be downloaded from www.cdc.gov/epiinfo/).

Dean, A.G., Dean, J.A., Burton, A.H., et al. (1991) Epi Info: a general-purpose microcomputer program for public health information systems. *Am J Prev Med* 7(3), 178–82.

Gerstman, B.B. (2000) Data Analysis with Epi Info. http://www.sjsu.edu/faculty/gerstman/EpiInfo/.

13

DEALING WITH THE PUBLIC AND THE MEDIA

Bruce B. Dan

Early in a field investigation, the variety of problems facing an epidemiologist can be daunting—sketchy information, wary local officials, long hours, and a looming crisis. Certainly the last thing the field team wants to add to their tasks is confronting the news media. But once the media learn of an investigation in the community, they will naturally insist on knowing what's happening in their own backyard. And while those charged with working up the problem are reticent to speculate on causes early in an investigation, it is precisely then that the public wants simple, direct, black-and-white answers. Every epidemic investigation has its own unique facets, and every local situation will have its own peculiarities, but this chapter attempts to provide helpful guidelines in dealing with an investigation under the spotlight of the news media.

BACKGROUND

Until recently, virtually the only way the public learned about medical information was by talking to their personal physicians. Now anyone can become educated about health and disease by reading newspaper articles, health magazines, and diet and nutrition books, or by watching television news, celebrity fitness tapes, and late-night infomercials.[1] In fact, the average time that a household spends viewing television is estimated to be almost 7½ hours each day, 30 minutes more than when surveyed a decade earlier.[2]

There are now in excess of 1800 commercial and public television stations in the United States, and their broadcasts reach 95% of the 100 million households with television sets. Another 9000 cable systems invade an additional 80 million homes. Add to that the 8000 AM and FM radio stations sending signals to 99% of households with radios, and the 13,000 newspapers with a combined circulation of more than 100 million, and you can see we are awash in information. Moreover, the Internet now provides access to an almost unlimited amount of medically related material.

Medical information may emanate from a variety of sources, for example, medical journals, scientific meetings, federal and state health bulletins, or hospital press releases. But no matter whence it comes, medical news is first filtered through and disseminated by the mass media. The public naturally wants to hear from medical experts during times of uncertainty. Indeed, their health may well depend upon the immediate advice of medical authorities during a serious disease outbreak, or they may just need to have their fears calmed during the almost annual occurrence of head lice in elementary schools.

Surveys have shown that the high volume of media coverage that medical reports invariably generate has not always brought clarity to health issues.[3] A large portion of the problem can be laid at the feet of health professionals themselves who often do not interact well with the media. Understanding how the media provide information to their audiences, and knowing how to deliver a message can determine whether or not the public takes effective action. The reality is that if health care providers want to improve public health, they must be as comfortable and skilled at appearing in the media as they are in taking a history, listening to the chest, or filling out a prescription. Health information is of little use unless it can be communicated effectively and clearly to those who will benefit from it most—the public.

The public health community confronted the reality of these issues on an enormous scale during the events surrounding the bioterrorism attacks with anthrax. While health officials must always be adept at communicating health information, they must be unerring when the situation has the potential of a national epidemic. Often, as in the case of the anthrax threat, the actual number of persons becoming ill may be small, but the consequences—cultural, financial, and political—may be immense. The missteps of public health officials during the early phases of the anthrax investigation were not the result of diagnostic errors, badly constructed case definitions, or imprecise laboratory techniques. The problems occurred because responsible health officials did not possess the necessary communication skills and strategies to deal with an epidemic of that order.

News

While everyone knows what news is when we see it or hear it, it's not so easy to define. When you read about new medical breakthroughs or new discoveries, you know that's news. But what exactly makes an event newsworthy? It helps to know how reporters define news. News happens when something strays from the ordinary—news, in its essence, is the unusual. Reporters and their media outlets are interested in change, change that has significance, change that appears threatening, anything that disrupts the status quo—new diseases, new victims. That's news!

As the person being interviewed, you actually have no way of controlling what reporters write—no more than they control how you conduct surveillance or choose a case definition. More problematic, you will not know what other interviews or elements are going into the story. What you *can* do is to ensure that the most favorable aspects, reflecting on you and your organization, are put into the mix. It takes communications skills and strategy, but once they are mastered you may even enjoy being part of the process.

Journalists and broadcasters divide news into two categories: *soft* news and *hard* news. Soft news (also called a *feature*) is the story behind the story. Features are not *the* events so much as the *background* behind them. Features can include a report on the issues of a particular story or trend, such as a television documentary on food-borne illnesses in America, a radio series on low-birth-weight infants, or an article on health-care budget cuts.

Hard news concerns the events that precipitate coverage by the media—they *are* the story. Many news outlets refer to hard news as "breaking" news. It's the plane crash, bomb explosion, or epidemic.

Deadlines

Each of the traditional media (print, radio, and television) suffers from a particular form of pressure—the deadline. Unlike most other enterprises, journalism runs under a continuous and unrelenting schedule. News reporters must get their stories in print or on the air under exacting constraints. For them, news a day late is no longer news. This pervasive pressure explains many of the quirks of the news business. When reporters seem curt or abrupt, it often merely reflects the conditions under which they must work.

Monthly magazines generally have long lead times, and reporters often have weeks to work on a story. And even newspaper reporters can work on a story for an entire day for the next day's edition. Even at deadline, a rapidly transcribed quote may be all that is necessary for the next morning's edition.

Radio news needs to conform to a much more precise broadcast schedule. Hourly news programs are the rule, but 10-minute updates are common during the early morning and late afternoon drive times. The emergence of "all news" radio stations means that they need to keep up on a minute-by-minute basis. However, even breaking medical news can be written rapidly and read over the air if need be. A quick phone call can provide a radio station with the information and voice it needs to make the story real.

Television correspondents work under the tightest deadlines. The reason that television news is the most rigidly constrained is because it is a visual medium. Obviously, it takes time to edit and put video images together in a logical and orderly sequence—and for TV, if there are no pictures then there is no story. For most afternoon and evening news broadcasts on commercial stations, interviews must be set up early in the day in order to schedule camera crews and reporters. With the proliferation of cable channels and 24-hour news programs, television news has become a hungry and competitive business looking for the latest breaking stories.

With the emergence of 24-hour news programming and the Internet, reporters and their editors are under even greater pressure to provide information to the public as quickly as possible. This really means that when reporters call about a story, they generally need it then (not tomorrow or next week), and they may need to talk to you at that moment, not later that day. While it is important that you respond when the news media call, it is also critical that you be prepared when they speak to you. We will discuss later the proper balance and timing of interviews.

The News Business

It's also of vital importance to understand the interplay between reporter and news source. Each has an agenda.[4] The media are part of a journalistic exercise in the principles of the First Amendment, and they are also part of the free enterprise system, that is, they are businesses. It is critical to understand that they are not in the business of public health. While it may seem that news organizations are doing a public service by communicating important health information, they do it only to sell more newspapers or charge higher rates for commercial time. The priorities for public health organizations and news organizations are different. Public health officials need the media to disseminate important information; the media need medical stories to sell news. But in the end, good relationships between these two diverse groups benefit the public at large.

THE INTERVIEW

All journalists share a common tool in their work: the interview. The interview is the most frequent interaction between you and a journalist, and it is also the most flexible format. A print or radio reporter may interview you on the telephone. A television reporter may ask you to participate in a videotaped interview arranged at a convenient place and time. Reporters will want to give their source of news some sort of attribution not only to identify the source but to give an air of credibility: "Dr. John Smith, epidemic specialist in diarrheal diseases." Develop a title that the audience you are speaking to will easily understand. Few lay people are familiar with terms such as "a nephrologist, neonatologist, or a hematologist-oncologist." And labeling yourself as a "medical epidemiologist" is certainly treading on unfamiliar ground.

In conducting an interview, journalists may visit you at your office or may even intercept you unexpectedly in the field (the dreaded "ambush" interview). Most reporters and news organizations use a combination of formats, depending on the nature of their story. News reporters, like health officials, vary in their characteristics and their backgrounds. Not surprisingly, the story reported by the science writer for a local newspaper may differ from that of the health correspondent for a major network, but all reporters are looking for the answers to the same six questions: Who/ What/ Where/ When/ How/Why. It is your job to have the answers to those questions ready and to present them in a clear and concise manner.

But before consenting to any interview, those same six questions should be asked of the interviewer. Who is going to do the interview and from what organization? What is the subject matter to be discussed and what questions will be asked? Where will it be done (in the comfort of your office) or in some strange TV studio? When will the interview take place and when will it appear (tonight's evening news or in next month's health magazine)? How will the interview be conducted (videotaped or live, one-on-one with the reporter or in a group)? And, perhaps, most important, why is it being done?

Unless you have all of those questions answered, the interview should not be conducted. There is a tendency to feel honored, important, and in the spotlight when asked to be quoted in *Time* magazine or appear on *Nightline*, but be wary of the temptation. An overeager and ill-prepared health official usually does more damage than good.

Additionally, it is imperative that you check with local, state, or national public information personnel about any prospective interviews. Each level may have its own rules of engagement with the press. Regardless, the media relations experts can give you sound advice on carrying out an interview, and it is imperative to keep them abreast of press inquiries. That knowledge will allow them to coordinate interviews, keep track of media attention, and prevent miscommunication with the press.

Interview Objective

By far, the most important thing to remember is that a news interview is solely an opportunity to deliver your message to an important audience. Despite its appearance, a news interview is not a venue to answer the reporter's questions or to make him or her happy. You are there to communicate an idea that you believe is critically important. An interview is not an intellectual exercise or a debate. It is certainly not an argument or a friendly chat.

Often reporters come to an interview with a mental story already written. The challenge to you is to make certain they have the *right* story. Too many people who are interviewed try to tell a reporter everything they know about a subject, and their basic point gets lost in the clutter. Your primary duty is to make a comment that captures the reporter's attention and gets your point across. That task is accomplished by constructing a single critical message and learning how to deliver it.

That unique message has been referred to as the Single Overriding Communication Objective (SOCO), pronounced *SOCK-oh*. It is by definition the single, most important message you can deliver about your topic. In fact, it is fair to say that your goal is to turn each and every question during an interview into an opportunity to relay your SOCO.

Here are some rules of thumb:

- Construct a single cogent idea and write it down (your SOCO)
- Find a means for getting your SOCO across in the interview
- Get your SOCO across early (the interview may end abruptly)
- Get your SOCO in as many times as possible
- Learn to relate your SOCO in a language the audience will understand

Exercising this art of good communication requires a great deal of preparation. Avoid the temptation to "wing it." Remember that no professional goes to a performance without a script.

Language

In attempting to get a single message delivered, you will be most successful if the words you use are understandable to the greatest number of people. Avoid medical jargon. It works well in a clinical setting but not with the lay public. Learn to say it simply, for instance:

- Instead of "communicate," try "say"
- Instead of "disseminate," try "send"
- Instead of "metastasize," try "spread"

Stay away from potentially confusing words and phrases like "atypical," "subclinical," "negative test results," or "positive cultures." Avoid esoteric terminology such as "relative risk," "odds ratio," "controls," "sensitivity," and "specificity."

Try to find alternatives to prefixes such as "pre-," "post-," and "pseudo-." Leave Latin and Greek to the textbooks.

Interview Techniques

Bridging

You can prevent reporters from straying from your message or turning the interview into an interrogation by anticipating the tough questions and using the technique called *bridging*. Bridging is simply transitioning—forming a bridge between one point and another. In other words, moving from where the reporter is going to where you want the interview to go. Rather than ignoring or evading the question you simply recognize it briefly and then move or *bridge* to your SOCO. Rather than having to develop answers to dozens of potential questions, you merely need a few transitional phrases to bridge to your SOCO. These are some very simple bridges to use:

- *Don't know* to *do know*—"I don't know the answer to that, but I can say . . ."
- *Time*—"That was true in the past, but now we know that . . ."
- *Importance*—"That's a factor, but what's more important is . . ."
- *Affirmation*—"Yes, but in addition to that . . ."
- *Contradiction*—"No not really, let me explain . . ."
- *Contrast*—"That's the number one cause in women, but for men . . ."
- *Focusing*—"In general that's true, but let's take a closer look at . . ."

You can construct innumerable ways to get back to the main point: "You alluded to something else I should mention . . ."; "Let me put that into perspective . . ."; "What that means is. . . ." Find comfortable phrases that fit easily into your own style of conversation. But the important point is to take the subject back to your message. Do not attempt to answer a question about which you are not knowledgeable. You can easily lose your credibility, but more important, you may misinform your audience.

Flagging

You can punctuate your message and make it more memorable to the reporter and the audience by calling attention to your SOCO using the technique called flagging. It is simply using a phrase to *flag* your comment as the major component of the conversation. Flagging statements include:

- The most important thing I could say about frostbite is . . .
- If a woman who is sexually active asked me . . .
- The bottom line for people living near nuclear plants is . . .

- The single fact a food handler needs to remember is . . .
- The take-home message for people with tuberculosis is . . .

Handling Difficult Interviews

In dealing with a potentially troublesome or even hostile interview, just make certain that your responses bridge to your messages. Because professionals in many occupations have a natural tendency to defend their positions when questioned, clever reporters will use this to lead you from curious questions to what often seems like a heated debate. Your opportunity to deliver your message gets lost in the intellectual fisticuffs. However, you are not required to justify your thoughts or actions, and you are not on the witness stand. Simply use the interviewer's statements to bridge to your SOCO. Do not repeat negative phrases. Pause and give thoughtful positive responses. Take control, have conviction, and do not wait for permission to tell your side of the story.

Interviews may be on-the-record, off-the-record, or something in between, called "background." If you cannot give an interview that is "on-the-record" (meaning that everything you say or do can be used and attributed to you), then you probably should not be talking to the press. Never agree to an off-the-record interview. You have no guarantee that it will remain so. Do not say anything to a reporter that you would be uncomfortable seeing in the next morning's headlines.

Planning for an Interview

Interviews should not be hit-or-miss affairs but carefully planned encounters. Before you agree to do any interview, the following guidelines should be followed:

Screening

- All media contacts should be first screened by a media relations staff, or failing that, by yourself.
- Get a clear understanding of why the reporter wants to interview you. What is the precise topic? Is it to your advantage to take part? Is it in your area of expertise or is someone else more suitable?
- Establish the reporter's deadline and how much of your time is required.

Preparation

- An ill-prepared interview serves neither the reporter's nor your interests. Getting ready for an interview is as important as doing one.
- Make it clear to the reporter that you want to confine the questions to the prearranged topic. Set a time limit for the interview.

- If possible, send fact sheets, background information, and photographs to the reporter before the interview.
- Prepare for the interview. Plan your strategy. Write out your primary public health message and practice it. Draft some colorful quotes and anecdotes that illustrate your point.

The interview

- When the reporter arrives, reconfirm the topic and the length of the interview.
- Give him or her your business card with the correct spelling of your name and organization.
- When you are both seated, ask the reporter, "How much do you know about (the interview topic)?" Since you are the expert, take control and lay out the situation as you see it—your SOCO.
- Briefly bridge through the negative or irrelevant questions and move the conversation back to your message. You can prevent "fishing expeditions" by reminding the reporter that you are prepared to be interviewed on the agreed-upon topic for that day. You are, of course, happy to set up an interview on another subject on another day.
- Stick to your agreed-upon time limit (you may want to have an assistant call you when the time limit has elapsed). Bring the interview to an orderly close with a summary, which should be a crisp and concise version of your message.
- Arrange a follow-up procedure so that any last minute or verification questions can be handled.

Post-interview

- Each interview, whether for the print or broadcast media, should be an opportunity to learn and improve.
- Keep an index card for every interview, jotting down the date, the reporter's name, the subject discussed, and where it appeared. Grade yourself on the interview. Did you get your SOCO in? Grade the reporters and file the card for future reference. Were they knowledgeable or uninformed? Are they friends or foes?
- If you discover you have given a reporter erroneous information, correct it immediately—even if the story has already appeared. If reporters have misstated facts, alert them so the story can be corrected. If your statements have been distorted, and you feel that the interview has been unfairly conducted, let the reporter know. If there is not a satisfactory response, inform the reporter that the issue will be brought to the attention or his or her editor.

There are not any prescribed formulas for the "correct" interview. However, there are some helpful hints in conducting yourself with each of the media. Below is listed some brief advice for each type of interview you may encounter.

Print Interview

The print interview is probably the most common and perhaps the least threatening. It usually involves a one-to-one conversation with a newspaper reporter either in person or on the phone. Most of us are reasonably comfortable talking to another person about a subject in which we feel confident. The danger is in feeling too comfortable and saying too much. Make it clear to the reporter that you want to confine questions to the prearranged topic.

Reporters may tape the conversation to have exact quotes on hand, but they may simply note some important points. If the reporter calls on the phone (and you have already been cleared to speak with him or her), remember that you do not have to speak at that moment. It is perfectly acceptable to tell the reporter that you will call back in 10 minutes. Hang up, collect your thoughts, jot down some notes, get comfortable, and call back when *you* are ready to be interviewed.

Beware of inflections. Tongue-in-cheek remarks, a sarcastic tone, and even humor do not translate well in print. The exact opposite of what you meant may come through. In addition, your comments may be characterized: a statement with a condescending tone or with a smirk may be reported as such.

Try to speak in even, succinct, declarative sentences, but try to be natural and informative. Do not talk too fast. The reporter may be frantically trying to scribble down your message, so slow down and ask the reporter if you should repeat it more slowly. The print interview is the one place where you can use exact medical terms (if you explain them) because the reader can pause, reread, and study a word or phrase. The same is not true for the electronic media.

Remember that the interview is not over when the reporter stops the recorder or puts down the pen. Any comments you make during the time spent with the reporter are on-the-record. The interview is over when the reporter is out of earshot.

Radio Interview

Here you must be sharply aware of inflections. The only thing the listener hears is your voice. Learn to modulate your voice in pitch, volume, and cadence. A deadpan monotone is as dreary and uninformative on the radio as it is from the podium. Use your hands and make facial gestures when expressing yourself on the radio. They will not appear themselves, but their effect will carry emotion and inflection to your voice. Use short, preferably monosyllabic words ("give" instead of administer, "make" instead of fabricate). They are easier to pronounce and easier to understand.

Many radio interviews are done by telephone. Again, do not engage in an interview either live or taped until you are ready. You are not required to carry out the interview while seated at your desk. It is permissible to stand up, walk around, do anything else that makes you comfortable (but do not tap your fingers on the desk or chew your pencil). Talk to your interviewer as you would talk to the people whom you meet on the street or someone you would meet in a super-market—simply, directly, and interestingly.

TV Interview

As with print and radio, television requires information and an articulate delivery. But additionally, TV interviews require two other vitally important factors—appearance and appeal. In particular, television has the peculiar property such that it is far more important how you say something than what you say. This may seem heretical to some and "unprofessional" to others. But it is perhaps the most critical aspect of the television medium and one that must be understood and accepted, if you have any desire to transmit information through this medium.

This unique aspect of "seeing" is what also gives television its powerful impact, but if not used properly, results in the media manipulating the message giver rather than the other way around. Television in the end does not deliver information, it gives perceptions; it does not deliver facts, it leaves impressions. As illogical as it may seem, your appearance and demeanor carry more weight than your command of information.

TV segments usually only contain a few 10–15 second quotes (called sound bites) from the interviewee. That means that you must be able to relate your entire message in a very short sentence and do it in an interesting and appealing way. You must also speak in short easily understood words. If the viewers misunderstand you, they do not, as with newspapers, have the ability to go back and "reread" the story.

Even if what you say is technically correct, TV reporters are looking for catchy sound bites (like good one-liners). If your message is dull, but you also happen to mention some other extraneous, but media grabbing statement, you can imagine what will make the air. Your job is to make your message so exciting, the reporter is virtually obligated to put it on. The following, again, is a brief listing of tips to enhance your ability to get your message across on television:

- Be calm and relaxed. TV cameras and strange studio lights and microphones tend to make anyone uptight. Viewers will be turned off to what they perceive as stiffness and formality. This only comes with practice; there are no secrets.

- Use natural eye contact. Unless told otherwise, always look at the person to whom you are speaking. That is a natural disposition. Do not look briefly at the cameras or studio monitors, it will give you a shifty appearance.
- Dress conservatively. For men, wear a dark jacket (gray or navy blue), and avoid checks and plaids. Wear a tie with small patterns of red (darker shades), whites, and blues. Shirts should be light colored (try to avoid bright white) with a straight collar (not buttoned down). Women should wear a simple dress or business suit; stay away from large brightly colored prints. Reflective and jingling gold jewelry, large distracting earrings, and bizarre hairdos will take the viewers attention away from what you are saying.
- Facial expressions should be pleasant and natural. Avoid the natural tendency to look numb and stiff. *Smile*! It is not only all right, it is preferred— it gives your countenance a look of warmth and friendliness.
- Your body and posture should be straight but relaxed. Even a small slump looks terrible on TV (if you feel comfortable, you probably look bad). Feel free to move naturally, and use your hands when you talk (just stay away from wild gestures especially in front of your face). Sitting forward toward your interviewer lends a sense of interest and confidence; leaning back, one of indifference and aversion.
- Speak in words of few syllables. They are less likely to be mispronounced, more likely to be understood, and you can get a lot more of them in the conversation in 15 seconds. Use Anglo-Saxon words; they carry emotion and add vitality to your speech: words like "live," "die," "love," "hate," "make," "save," "get," "find." People "get sick and have heart attacks." They do not "acquire illnesses and suffer myocardial infarctions."
- Speak in declarative sentences. Avoid answering questions with a simple yes or no.
- Do not quote exact figures from medical journals. Do not bother letting everyone know that exactly "53.2% of the case-patients taking 325 mg of aspirin daily significantly decreased their relative risk of suffering a re-infarction during the study period." Simply respond, "More than half the people taking an aspirin a day greatly reduced their chances of a second heart attack." Get used to using terms like "most of," "the majority," "almost all," "very few."
- Be a good listener. Nothing sounds worse than trying to answer what you thought was the question when the reporter actually asks something else. Do not assume you know what the reporter is getting at and jump over his or her lines. Hear the reporter out.
- Lastly, project conviction and confidence. Speak to your questioner with a real sense of interest and caring. It will come across to the viewer that way as well.

EPIDEMIC MANAGEMENT

The best way to learn how to handle an epidemic is on-the-job training, but there is value in learning from those who have already been through the process. Every epidemic is different; every local situation will have its own peculiarities; but the following may prove helpful:

- Stay away from the media. This advice may seem contradictory after talking about the importance of communicating with the public, but your number one job on an investigation is to assist the local health officials, not appear on a morning talk show. If you are spending time before the cameras, you are not working up the problem.
- If accosted by the media as you arrive at the locale (and it is not uncommon to be met by a phalanx of reporters as you get off the plane) do not stop but calmly keep walking to your destination. Answer any questions with a smile and the obvious response, "I'm here at the request of (the local authorities) to assist in their investigation, I'll be glad to talk to you after I have conferred with them." If pressed further, simply repeat your SOCO in any interesting way you wish, "As I said, I'm here to help, and I'll be happy to chat with you after I've gathered some information."
- Designate a single spokesperson. The underlying and inviolable rule is, "One messenger, one message." If the epidemic involves several agencies, attempt to have one person speak for the group effort. When differing viewpoints from competing agencies simultaneously appear in the media, it merely breeds confusion, and more damaging, signals to the public that those in charge of protecting their health are in disarray. Local and state health agencies have public relations specialists who are trained and get paid to talk to the press. Those communications experts probably know all the media people, have already established a good working relationship with them, and know the ins and outs of the local scene. Let them handle the press. They will have to do it anyway after you have gone.
- Try to have your spokesperson seek out the media first in a proactive informational manner. It not only demonstrates responsibility but it also lets you set the agenda and control events. If the media find out first, it becomes, "What did you know, and when did you know it?"
- Set a regular press briefing time. It establishes a routine; the media are not caught by surprise; and it offers you, again, the chance to make prepared statements and control events.
- Try to keep technologists and other allied people behind the scenes; they can give potentially confusing and contradictory information to the press. There must be one messenger delivering one cogent message. The press likes

nothing better than controversy. Even something as simple as two different totals for the number of cases can give the media grist for unnerving criticism. Along that line, try not to get into a numbers game with the press. Refrain from "upping" the numbers everyday. Even with no news, an increasing number becomes in itself a news story and reason for headlines.

- Above all else, coordinate information with the local, state, and national officials. Not only will you keep the team players happy but you will also avoid creating controversies—since the press likes nothing better than to find that the state has facts that the local health department does not have, and vice versa. To paraphrase the late Mayor Richard J. Daley of Chicago, "The field epidemiologist is not there to create disorder, the field investigator is there to preserve disorder."

PRESS CONFERENCES

The news conference increases your control in getting your message out to the media. But in the question-and-answer period that control can be snatched way by an aggressive reporter. Suddenly, a quiet give-and-take session can be turned into a feeding frenzy. To make sure that you do not end up with a negative situation, learn to shield yourself.

- Have a spokesperson open up the news conference by introducing the participants and stating the ground rules. Handouts should be distributed at the beginning of the conference. The spokesperson should tell the assembled reporters what areas will and will not be covered and for what reasons.
- Make sure you introduce yourself when you step to the microphone. Spell your name and give your position and affiliation.
- Your first sentence should be your key message (SOCO). Make it one that will be memorable and mentioned. If done well, it will be the first sound bite carried on all networks that night.
- Keep your opening statement brief and tightly focused. If it is concise, it reduces the chances that a reporter will misunderstand, interrupt, or even walk out. Speak in headlines; save the details and documentation for the handout.
- Do not just read your statement—communicate it. Look at the audience; speak with enthusiasm or concern; gesture.
- Set some ground rules for the question-and-answer session. For example, "Now I'd like to open it up briefly for a few questions. So that everyone gets a turn, I'll take one question from each of you. I'd appreciate it if you'd raise your hand when you have a question and identify yourself."

- If no questions arise, ask yourself the first question. That might break the ice and trigger other questions.
- Do not allow yourself to be bullied. When a reporter tries to interrupt you, tell him or her nicely that you would like to finish your answer. Use your hands—signaling to one reporter that you are ready to take his or her question, while gesturing with the other hand to tell another reporter that he or she is up next.
- Sum up. When you feel your topic has been sufficiently covered in the Q & A session, give notice that you will take one more question. Then do precisely that. Finally, briefly restate your key point, thank the audience, and leave.

SPECIAL PROBLEMS

It is not possible to cover every twist and turn of dealing with the media, but several special situations often come up that require thinking about in advance.

- Personal opinion vs. local/state policy: If asked what the official local policy is on a certain subject, you should probably refer the question to the public information officer (unless in the rare instance you have been given the authority to be the spokesperson). You should feel free, in good conscience, to give your opinions on matters of science as a physician, veterinarian, nurse, or other health personnel. But policy matters are best left to those who know the policy and can take responsibility for it. If you feel foolish saying that you do not know the policy when you feel you should know it, simply say that you would like the reporter to meet with the person who can best answer that question.
- Press embargoes: Many releases of information to the press (including medical journal publications) have dates specified as to when that information can be disseminated to the public, the so-called press embargo date. The purpose of the embargo is to allow all media outlets to have an equal opportunity to cover the story. No one will have an edge due to the vagaries of the mail or access to the press release. If *everyone* has the written material in hand before the story is broadcast, then its health message can be disseminated in a coordinated, logical fashion.

Most medical reporters will receive the press release or medical journal before the release date and begin working with the story. If you are called before the release date, simply remind the reporter of the embargo and say that you are speaking with the understanding that the story will not be published before that time. If you have any particular questions, check with the publisher of the press release or journal's editorial office.

SUMMARY

In contrast to past decades, the American public now gets most of its medical information from the media: newspapers, magazines, radio, and television. You may be asked by the media to report and comment on your findings either during an investigation or afterward. Although your mission is to protect and maintain the public's health, the primary mission of the media is not public health but to sell their product or their time. Despite these somewhat opposite objectives, the media can and should be your ally. Learn how the media operate, and cultivate some simple practices of interviewing so you can communicate effectively with the public.

Be prepared for the interview, know what you are going to be asked about, and know the subject. Have a message to get across and do it simply, directly, and with conviction. Tell the truth, do not be afraid to say you do not know, and do not field questions in an area that is not yours. If possible, avoid the media in the field and refer them to the local health authorities. They, rather than you, should report the results of the investigation to their constituents. They, too, should comment on health policies and issues. Keep the appropriate media relations specialists informed of your press contacts. And, lastly, be sure that all levels of government have the same information. Nothing destroys confidence in our health structure more than conflicting facts.

REFERENCES

1. Survey by Roper Starch Worldwide in The National Health Council Report (1997). *Americans Talk About Science and Medical News*. National Health Council, Washington, D.C.
2. Survey by Galaxy Explorer 2000/Nielson Media Research (2001). The medium is the message. In *Red Herring: the business of technology (2000)*, 85.
3. International Food Information Council (1998). *Improving Public Understanding: Guidelines for Communicating Emerging Science on Nutrition, Food Safety, and Health*. International Food Information Council Foundation, Washington, D.C.
4. Jeffres L.W. (1986). *Mass Media: processes and effects*. Waveland Press, Prospect Heights, IL.

III

SPECIAL CONSIDERATIONS

14

LEGAL CONSIDERATIONS IN A FIELD INVESTIGATION

Verla S. Neslund

The purpose of this chapter is to provide an overview of the legal considerations affecting an epidemiologic field investigation. Applicable federal laws and regulations are discussed. Because of the differences in state and local laws in the various jurisdictions in which such investigations are conducted, however, the discussion of nonfederal laws and regulations is necessarily generic. The chapter covers four basic legal issues: the legal bases for investigating public health problems, for gaining access, for collecting data, and for applying intervention strategies.

LEGAL BASIS FOR PUBLIC HEALTH INVESTIGATIONS

Federal and state governments both have inherent powers to protect the public's health. Article 1, Section 8 of the U.S. Constitution gives Congress the authority to impose taxes to "provide for the general [w]elfare of the United States" and to regulate interstate and foreign commerce. The U.S. Public Health Service (PHS) and CDC are both examples of federal agencies established under the authority of the welfare clause. Under the authority of the commerce clause of the Constitution, the federal government oversees such health-related activities as the licensure and regulation of drugs, biological products, and medical devices. Although

255

the provisions in the federal Constitution are broad, the activities of the federal government relating to public health and welfare nonetheless must fit within the enumerated powers.

By contrast, the public health powers of a state are very extensive, rooted in its inherent powers to protect the peace, safety, health, and general welfare of its citizens. Unlike the federal government, the states have public health powers that are not limited to specific constitutional provisions. The state's police power includes its intrinsic right to pass laws and to take such other measures as may be necessary to protect the citizenry. In many instances, states have delegated their public health responsibilities to county or municipal governments who, likewise, exercise the state's broad authority to examine, treat, and, in the case of certain contagious diseases, even to quarantine citizens in order to protect the public's health. The state's public health laws include not only the established statutes of the state but also regulations, executive orders, and other directives from health authorities that may have the force of law.

The courts have consistently upheld the state's exercise of its police powers to protect the public's health. The court decision usually regarded as the seminal case in the exercise of public health police powers is *Jacobson v. Massachusetts*, 197 U.S. 11 (1905). In *Jacobson*, the Cambridge, Massachusetts, city Board of Health had issued a regulation requiring that all citizens be vaccinated for smallpox. Mr. Jacobson was arraigned and prosecuted by law enforcement officials after he refused to be vaccinated, maintaining that the regulation violated due process because vaccination was contrary to his religious beliefs. Mr. Jacobson further argued that compulsory vaccination deprived him of the fundamental right to care for his own health. In a strongly worded opinion, the United States Supreme Court upheld the health board's exercise of its police power in mandating the smallpox vaccinations, providing the following rationale:

> [I]n every well-ordered society charged with the duty of conserving the safety of its members, the rights of the individual in respect of his liberty may at times, under the pressure of great danger, be subjected to such restraints, to be enforced by reasonable regulations, as the safety of the general public may demand [197 U.S. at 29].

The exercise of the state's police powers with respect to public health matters has limitations. The U.S. Constitution provides procedural safeguards to ensure that the exercise of these powers is not excessive and unrestrained. The Fifth Amendment prohibits the federal government from depriving—without the due process of law—any person of life, liberty, or property. The Fourteenth Amendment imposes similar due process obligations on states. Due process demands that the government use even-handed and impartial procedures in the exercise of its police power. The basic elements of such due process include notice to the person involved, a hearing or similar proceeding, and the right to representation by counsel. In addition, the exercise of the state's police power should incorporate the principle of using the least restrictive alternative that would still achieve the state's interest, particularly when the exercise involves limitations of the individual's personal liberty.

Similar to the public health activities enumerated above, the inherent powers to protect the public's health provide the general authority for laws and regulations that empower health officials to conduct epidemiologic investigations. Although cooperation of institutions and individuals in epidemiologic investigations is usually voluntary, the intervention of state or local officials is within the scope of governmental legal authority. Furthermore, the police power of the state provides the necessary authority to compel cooperation in such investigations in instances in which individuals or institutions are reluctant to grant access to certain properties, records, or individuals associated with information essential to the investigation.

GAINING ACCESS

As mentioned previously, institutions and individuals generally cooperate voluntarily in epidemiologic investigations. However, if investigators meet with resistance, local or state public health officials may take legal actions such as applying to a court with jurisdiction over the agency (individual) for a subpoena or court order to compel the agency to grant investigators access to the premises or records at issue. An individual can be compelled by court order to provide the information necessary for the public health investigation.

Institutions or individuals being investigated may question the legal authority for requiring such access. The general constitutional underpinnings discussed above provide the foundation for federal and state statutes and regulations that govern the conduct of health officials directing an epidemiologic investigation. For epidemiologists employed by the federal government, the laws relating to the general powers and duties of the PHS for research and investigation are found in Title III of the Public Health Service Act. The general statutory authority that is applicable to federal epidemiologic investigations is Section 301(a) of the Public Health Service Act, 42 U.S.C. § 241(a):

> The Secretary shall conduct in the Service, and encourage, cooperate with, and render assistance to other appropriate public authorities, scientific institutions, and scientists in the conduct of, and promote the coordination of, research, investigations, experiments, demonstrations, and studies relating to the causes,

diagnosis, treatment, control, and prevention of physical and mental diseases
and impairments of man . . . [42 U.S.C. § 241(a)]

In addition, subsection 6 of Section (a) indicates that the Secretary is authorized to "make available, to health officials, scientists, and appropriate public and
other nonprofit institutions and organizations, technical advice and assistance on
the application of statistical methods to experiments, studies, and surveys in health
and medical fields." Although these provisions of Section 301 are broadly worded
and are permissive rather than compulsory, they nonetheless give legal authority
for intervention by federal epidemiologists in disease outbreaks and other instances
in which such assistance is requested.

Individual states and local jurisdictions will have various laws and regulations that authorize or relate to the conduct of public health investigations. However, state laws in regard to compelling access to facilities and records are generally
more specific, and likely have provisions that compel cooperation, within the
boundaries of due process.

COLLECTING DATA

The process of collecting data during an epidemiologic field investigation involves
a number of legal considerations, including the following: (*1*) protection available under state or federal law during and after the investigation for the records
collected and generated in relation to the investigation; (*2*) special confidentiality
provisions for medical or other information; (*3*) required reporting of particular
diseases or conditions; (*4*) status of information in investigative files under the
federal Freedom of Information Act (FOIA) (5 U.S.C. § 552) or state FOIA counterparts; and (*5*) the applicability of federal or state human subjects research regulations, including the need for review of study protocols by institutional review
boards and the need for informed consent for participation in the investigation or
for procedures related to the investigation.

Protection of Investigational Records

To determine what records will be kept or generated and where and how such
records will be stored, you need to know what legal protection is in place for the
documents and other records that will be examined, extracted, and compiled in
association with the investigation. Most states provide specific statutory and regulatory confidentiality protection over medical and public health records. In general, the confidentiality protection prevents the disclosure of a name-identified
record without the consent of the person on whom the record is maintained. Ac-

cordingly, such medical records in the hands of an investigator generally are protected by state law. Furthermore, such state laws frequently require that only certain authorized personnel have access to such confidential records, and that such records be maintained in a secure manner. You would usually be authorized access to such records but would be bound to maintain the records in a manner that would protect the confidentiality of the identifiable information from unauthorized or inadvertent disclosure.

In the course of an investigation, you may create or compile a number of documents (e.g., questionnaires, forms, investigative notes, copies or extractions of patient or other records, letters, reports, memoranda, drafts, manuscripts, and final reports). Depending on the nature of the records and the status of the investigation, these documents may not be protected from disclosure to the public by state or federal laws. Except for records afforded specific protection by state or federal laws (such as state laws protecting medical records), you should probably assume that all records collected may at some point be open to public scrutiny.

Investigators who are federal employees need to be aware of the provisions of the Freedom of Information Act (FOIA), 5 U.S.C. § 552. In general, the FOIA provides that all documents in the hands of federal employees, on federal premises, or within the control of federal employees are available to the public unless specifically exempted by the act. The act contains nine exemptions. In general, four of these exemptions may affect epidemiologic investigations:

- Inter-agency and intra-agency communications: Exemption (b)(5) permits the federal government to withhold from disclosure inter-agency and intra-agency memorandums or letters that would not be available "to a party other than an agency in litigation with the agency." An example of the use of this exemption would be to protect from disclosure a draft memorandum written by the investigator to his supervisor describing the early findings of the investigation.
- Personnel and medical records: Exemption (b)(6) permits the federal government to withhold from mandatory disclosure "personnel and medical files and similar files the disclosure of which would constitute a clearly unwarranted invasion of personal privacy." This exemption may be invoked by the federal government to protect confidential medical information on an individual contained in a record collected by a federal investigator.
- Information otherwise exempt from disclosure by statute: Exemption (b)(3) provides that a federal agency may withhold from disclosure information "specifically exempted from disclosure by statute." If an epidemiologic investigation is conducted under an assurance of confidentiality authorized by a federal statute (such as § 301(d) or § 308(d) of the Public Health Service Act), the information collected pursuant to the confidentiality assur-

ance is protected from disclosure under the FOIA in a manner that would contravene the statutory provision. You should be aware that such assurances of confidentiality are not commonly used. Instead, with legal counsel and on a case-by-case basis, such assurances are limited to exceptional circumstances in which the sensitivity of the information demands additional confidentiality measures or when the cooperation of the study subjects would be impeded in the absence of such an assurance.

• Trade secret and commercial or financial information: Exemption (b)(4) permits the federal government " to withhold from disclosure commercial or financial information obtained from a person and privileged and confidential." Although this exemption may be less commonly applicable than the other three outlined above, it would be relevant to an epidemiologic investigation that involved, for example, a commercial product on which the investigator has records containing trade secrets or confidential information on the components of the product. Likewise, confidential financial information may be contained in investigative records, even records that might otherwise be disclosed under the FOIA.

Disease Reporting

Within the realm of collecting information, you must be aware of the public health responsibilities regarding disease reporting to appropriate authorities. While the diagnosis of reportable diseases more commonly occurs in the treatment setting, it is possible that the investigation may identify a reportable disease or a previously diagnosed condition that has not been reported. Accordingly, you should be knowledgeable about the requirements for disease reporting in the jurisdiction in which the investigation is being conducted and should be prepared either to make such reports, if appropriate, or to see that the report is made by the responsible person or institution.

Research Involving Human Subjects

Federal employees and those supported by federal funds for an investigation should be aware of the provisions of the federal regulations governing the Protection of Human Subjects, 45 C.F.R. Part 46. Although you may question whether your investigation constitutes "research," the definition for research under Part 46 is specific: "'Research' means a systematic investigation designed to develop or contribute to generalizable knowledge." This definition is very inclusive of activities that may be termed surveillance, outbreak investigations, and other public health interventions. However, Part 46 also provides certain exceptions for "research involving survey or interview procedures," including an exception if the responses are recorded without identifiers. Accordingly, when you plan your field investigation, be aware of the provisions of 45 C.F.R. Part 46.

The requirements regarding informed consent of individuals who are interviewed or studied in a field investigation are usually a matter of state law in the jurisdiction in which the investigation takes place. However, 45 C.F.R. 46.116 outlines the circumstances that require written or oral informed consent if Health and Human Services (HHS) Administration funds support the research activity. The Part 46 regulations also describe the basic elements of informed consent, including information on benefits and risks of participation that must be disclosed to research subjects.

Privacy Act

The federal Privacy Act, 5 U.S.C. § 552a, is applicable to any investigation conducted by a federal employee and to the retention of personally identifiable records within a federal "system of records." The Privacy Act generally allows individuals to have access to their records held by a federal agency. Certain national security and criminal law enforcement records are exempt from the Privacy Act.

In addition, federal agencies must publish notices describing all systems of records and must make reasonable efforts to maintain accurate, relevant, and timely information. Information collected for one purpose must not be used for another purpose without notice to or the consent of the individual on whom the record is maintained. The Privacy Act applies only to records containing personal indentifiers. Accordingly, you should consider whether there is a valid need to retain identifying information. For example, the CDC pledges that records that contain names and other identifiers will be retained only when necessary, and only with identifiers as long as necessary. Violations of the Privacy Act are punishable by civil and criminal penalties.

Department of Health and Human Services Privacy Regulations

Congress acknowledged the need for minimum national health-care privacy standards to protect against inappropriate use of individually identifiable health information by passing the Health Insurance Portability and Accountability Act of 1996 (HIPAA), Public Law 104-191, which called for the enactment of a privacy statute within 3 years of the date of enactment on August 26, 1996. In the law, Congress addressed the opportunities and challenges presented by the health-care industry's increasing use of and reliance on electronic technology. Sections 261 through 264 of HIPAA are known as the Administrative Simplification provisions. Pursuant to various parts of these sections, HHS published proposed standards concerning electronic exchange of information regarding financial and administrative transactions and security of electronic information. (See 63 Fed. Reg. 43242 [Aug. 12, 1998]; 63 Fed. Reg. 32784 [June 16, 1998]; and 63 Fed. Reg. 25272 [May 7, 1998].)

In addition, Section 264 of HIPAA called for the secretary of HHS to develop and send to Congress recommendations for protecting the confidentiality of health-care information. On September 11, 1997, the secretary presented to Congress recommendations for protecting the "Confidentiality of Individually-Identifiable Health Information." In those recommendations, the secretary called for new federal legislation to create a national floor of standards that provide fundamental privacy rights for patients, and that define responsibilities for those who obtain identifiable health information. These recommendations are available on the HHS website at http://aspec.os.dhhs.gov/admnsimp/pvcrec.htm

Within the provisions of HIPAA, the Congress further recognized the importance of such standards by providing the secretary of HHS with authority to promulgate health privacy regulations if Congress did not enact a privacy statute prior to August 21, 1999. In the fall of 1999, after extensive consultations with other federal agencies, professional associations, and representatives of state and national organizations, the secretary of HHS published in the Federal Register draft health privacy regulations that included many of the secretary's 1997 recommendations (64 Fed. Reg. 59918-60065 [Nov. 3, 1999]). To the extent permitted under the HIPAA legislative authority, this new regulation, which became effective April 14, 2001, is an elaboration of the secretary's recommendations, including new restrictions on the use and disclosure of health information, the establishment of new consumer rights, penalties for misuse of information, and redress for those harmed by misuse of the information.

Proposals to Protect Privacy of State Public Health Records

In 1998, CDC, working in collaboration with the Council of State and Territorial Epidemiologists provided funding for Georgetown University Law Center to draft a model state public health privacy act. The purpose of the model privacy act project was to develop a model state law addressing privacy and security issues arising from the acquisition, use, disclosure, and storage of identifiable health information by public health agencies at the state and local levels. While the model law project was initiated at the time CDC announced that it would begin comprehensive human immunodeficiency virus (HIV) surveillance, the model act was intended to protect all health-related information.

The model act was finalized in August 1999 and was posted on a special website sponsored by Georgetown. The model act includes regulation of the acquisition, use, disclosure, and storage of identifiable health-related information by public health agencies without significantly limiting the ability of agencies to use such information for legitimate public health purposes.

While most states have not significantly revised their state public health statutes for decades, public concerns about the privacy of medical information and questions about who can have access to such information have prompted some states to reexamine their laws and regulations governing public health and medical information. Accordingly, epidemiologists need to stay abreast of any changes in state laws that may affect their access to medical and public health records.

THE EPIDEMIOLOGIST AND LITIGATION

Occasionally, you may conduct an investigation that results in the need for intervention by federal or state law enforcement authorities. In this circumstance, you must be aware of other legal considerations. For example, epidemiologic investigations of clusters of deaths of hospitalized patients have led to homicide and assault prosecution of nurses who had cared for the deceased patients. Studies of deaths in a pediatric intensive-care unit led to action by the Food and Drug Administration against the manufacturer and distributor of an infant feeding formula.

The realm of enforcement actions will place you in somewhat unfamiliar territory. For the epidemiologist trained to collect and analyze data objectively and quantitatively, the partiality of the advocacy role of attorneys can be frustrating. Although epidemiologists are more comfortable with probabilities, associations, and confidence intervals for populations, attorneys usually seek cause and effect for an individual. While the epidemiologist seeks to retain the appropriate terminology for the conclusions, prosecutors may hope to portray the findings as definitive rather than circumstantial. The enforcement arena likewise places the epidemiologist in a potential new role—that of a witness. The scrutiny you are subjected to in the peer review process may be comfortably familiar, but the scrutiny of the same scientific data in an enforcement proceeding is less predictable.

Attorneys are advocates who take an oath to pursue vigorously the case of their client. Understandably, then, the situations that involve formal encounters with attorneys for either side in a controversy are seldom impartial or dispassionate. Whether in administrative hearings, depositions, or court proceedings, witnesses are questioned by one side, and then they are cross-examined by the attorney for the other side. The purpose of cross-examination is generally to minimize, discredit, or at least limit the effect of the testimony given on direct examination. The prospect that a nonscientist will scrutinize the data in a manner that appears more to be twisting, stretching, and perhaps even misconstruing is usually disconcerting to the epidemiologist as a witness. If you believe you can provide an impartial, independent third-party view to a legal forum, you may find yourself ensnared by adversaries, legal objections, judges, and rules of procedure. However, the unfamiliarity of the forum does not obviate your responsibility to assure the public's health.

INTERVENTION

Compulsory Measures

The state's ability to carry out its role in protecting the public health strongly depends on the cooperation of citizens in voluntarily complying with the various disease control standards and good public health practices. Nonetheless, the state's broad police powers also include the power to compel persons in certain circumstances to undergo medical examinations, immunizations, testing, and to require quarantine or isolation of persons who may pose a threat to the public because they have a particular communicable disease. Most states have general public health laws and regulations that enumerate the compulsory powers and the procedures associated with the exercise of those compulsory powers. In addition to the general compulsory public health statutes and regulations on compulsory powers and duties, however, most states also have laws that are specific to the control of tuberculosis and sexually transmissible diseases.

The following are examples of compulsory procedures that have been upheld by the courts: requirements for immunization prior to school attendance; pre-employment screening for communicable diseases such as tuberculosis or in occupations where the individual will have contact with the public; compulsory treatment of persons with active tuberculosis; mandatory examinations or screening of marriage license applicants; laws or ordinances mandating compliance with sanitation standards in public and private buildings; closing of bathhouses to prevent high-risk sexual activity; and the authority to involuntarily institutionalize individuals in certain situations (most often mental illness or drug abuse).

Isolation and Quarantine

As indicated previously, state laws have provisions for stricter methods of disease control than are generally used in current public health practice. Federal law and laws in all states still provide authority for quarantine for certain communicable diseases. In addition, some states have enacted laws that provide specific authority for quarantine and isolation of persons with HIV or AIDS. Quarantine usually involves complete restriction of the patient and the household contacts of the patient to the location where the patient is receiving care. These laws, written decades ago, usually still contain enumeration of such requirements as posting of a placard to warn other persons against entering the quarantined area.

Federal and state courts have upheld quarantine statutes as a valid exercise of the state's police power. The U.S. Supreme Court in the case of *Jacobson v. Massachusetts* (discussed previously) held that states have the authority to enact quarantine and other health laws as a means of protecting the community against communicable diseases. Likewise, other state and federal courts have followed the rationale of the *Jacobson* case and have uniformly upheld state quarantine statutes in the context of communicable disease control.

Quarantine of persons with venereal disease and HIV have also been upheld. The U.S. Court of Appeals for the Tenth Circuit in *Reynolds v. McNichols*, 488 F.2d 1378 (10th Cir. 1973) ruled that quarantining and compelling treatment of persons with venereal disease was a proper exercise of the state's police power. State courts in Florida, California, and Nevada have used quarantine statutes to detain HIV-infected prostitutes. In one case in Florida that received significant press coverage, an AIDS-infected female prostitute was ordered to stay in her home and was forced to wear an electronic device that would signal police if she traveled more than 200 feet from her telephone. In 1983, a New York State court held that the state could quarantine prisoners who had AIDS, because the actions by corrections authorities constituted a reasonable measure to stop HIV transmission in the prison population (*LaRocca v. Dalsheim*, 120 Misc.2d 697, 467 N.Y.S. 2d 302 [N.Y. Sup. 1983]).

The exercise of the state's public health powers, including quarantine and isolation, is limited by constraints that are part of the federal and state constitutions. These provisions place both procedural and substantive safeguards that put limits on the state's exercise of police power. The courts have mandated that the state exercise its police power using the "least restrictive alternative" when depriving an individual of liberty while pursuing a valid state interest. The concept of the "least restrictive alternative" is a principle of Constitutional law that provides when a citizen is being deprived of a fundamental right in order to further a legitimate governmental end, the government must use a means that is the least restrictive of the individual's personal liberty while still accomplishing the government's purpose. For example, if a state takes action to confine an individual to a hospital or treatment facility to prevent the spread of a contagious disease, this confinement should not be more extensive or intrusive than is necessary to reasonably control the spread of the disease. The use of the least restrictive alternative represents a balancing of the public health interests with the individual's deprivation of personal liberty. Most notably, the use of the least restrictive alternative has developed in situations involving civil commitment proceedings, such as involuntary commitment of mentally retarded or mentally ill individuals who present a threat of danger to themselves, family, or others, who can reasonably benefit from the available treatment. Similarly, application of this principle to quarantine law enforcement may provide for compliance with a regimen of care under the supervision of a physician rather than mandatory hospitalization.

Use of State Public Health Powers in Response to a Bioterrorism Threat or Emergency

In 1999, federal government initiatives designed to improve national public health capabilities to respond to acts of chemical and biological terrorism raised questions about the adequacy of state quarantine, isolation, and other compulsory public health powers. A preliminary review of state quarantine, isolation, and other critical agent laws showed that most of these laws had not been revised since the 1940s, probably because voluntary cooperation of the public and advances in medical interventions have made use of compulsory actions less frequent. However, in the context of potential bioterrorism events, the infrequency of use also suggested that public health officials may be inexperienced or unfamiliar with the proper procedures for invoking the compulsory powers. In the event of bioterrorism, an effective and lawful response is essential to ensure public safety and ward off the panic and dread that a terrorist may hope to cause. Accordingly, CDC and other federal officials began to strongly recommend that states examine public health laws that affect the ability to effectively respond to potential chemical and biological threats, including quarantine and isolation powers, to insure that the laws give public health officials the ability to act promptly while still providing adequate due process protections for individuals who may have been detained as part of the bioterrorism response. In addition, bioterrorism initiatives were increasingly focusing on the need for advance coordination, planning, pharmaceutical stockpiling, and training that involves the various law enforcement, emergency response, civilian and military intelligence experts, and public health officials (see Chapter 20).

To assist in the process of reviewing and revising state public health statutes, CDC initiated a project in collaboration with appropriate state and local officials to develop draft model legislation. Released for review and use in the aftermath of the September 11, 2001 bombing and subsequent anthrax attacks, this legislation, known as the Model State Emergency Public Health Powers Act, was intended to provide states with strong public health powers to rapidly detect and respond to bioterrorism and other emergency health threats. The Act requires the reporting of suspect illnesses or conditions; provides standards for a Governor's declaration of a public health emergency; allows a public health authority to access and use private facilities during an emergency; and contains provisions for mandatory medical examinations, isolation and quarantine, as well as access to patient records. The Act also immunizes from legal liability the Governor, public health authority, and other state executive agencies or actors for actions taken during a public health emergency. The goal of the Act is to provide a public health authority with those powers that would be needed to respond adequately to a public health emergency while protecting an individual's right to liberty, bodily integrity, and privacy to the fullest extent possible. State legislatures may adopt any or all of the provisions of the model law or tailor individual provisions to meet their needs. Many states have already begun to use portions the Act to draft legislation to revise their public health and emergency response laws.

SUMMARY

The field epidemiologist should understand that the basic authority of public health officials to conduct investigations of diseases or epidemics is the state's inherent police powers. Federal and state laws that govern the health and safety of the public are enacted pursuant to this broad authority. These laws provide not only for the state to have access to medical and other records for purposes of public health investigations but also for protection of the individual's interest in privacy by placing strict limits on access to medical, hospital, and public health records. While public health investigations and activities usually rely on the voluntary cooperation of individuals and institutions, federal and state laws provide authority for the use of compulsory measures when necessary for the protection of the public health and safety.

Field epidemiologists are certainly not expected to know every facet of public health law. Yet they should have an appreciation of the legal issues that pertain to surveillance, to confidentiality of medical records, and to the legal responsibilities of both federal and state governments. The quality, quantity, and ease of collecting epidemiologic data can be enhanced materially by an awareness of these issues and, if necessary, consultation with the legal profession.

REFERENCES

1. Gostin, L.O. (1989). The politics of AIDS: compulory state powers, public health and civil liberties. *49 Ohio State Law Journal 1017.*
2. Gostin, L.O. (2000). *Public Health Law: power, duty, restraint.* University of California Press, Berkeley, CA.
3. Grad, F.P. (1990). *The Public Health Law Manual,* 2nd ed. The American Public Health Association, Washington, D.C.
4. Wing, K.R. (1990). *The Law and the Public's Health,* 3rd ed. Health Administration Press, Ann Arbor, MI.

15

INVESTIGATIONS IN HEALTH-CARE SETTINGS

William R. Jarvis
Stephanie Zaza

The term *health-care setting* refers to hospitals, rehabilitative centers, transitional care, ambulatory care, outpatient, private physicians' offices, free-standing clinics, long-term care facilities, and homes where health care is being delivered (Table 15–1). Investigations of outbreaks in these settings require special attention and differ from community outbreaks in several ways.

This chapter prepares you for field investigations in health-care settings. It highlights the differences between conducting a community investigation and one confined to a health-care facility or setting where health care is being delivered. The emphasis is on how to find the information you need and how to use data and resources that are generally readily available only in health-care settings.

BACKGROUND CONSIDERATIONS

Community versus Hospital-based Outbreaks

This section describes four of the most important and distinctive characteristics of infections in the hospital setting as compared to community acquired infections. First, hospital-acquired infections (e.g., bloodstream, respiratory tract, urinary tract, or surgical site infections) are common, occurring in approximately

Table 15–1. Health-Care Facilities

Hospitals
Private physicians' offices
Freestanding clinics
   Dialysis
   Ambulatory surgery
Long-term-care facilities
   Nursing homes
   Rehabilitation centers
   Institutions for the mentally or physically handicapped

6% of hospitalized patients or nearly 2 million infections per year in the United States.[1,2] Of these, urinary tract infections occur in an estimated 24 of every 1000 hospitalized patients; pneumonia in 6–10; bloodstream infections in 3; and surgical site infections are estimated to occur in 28 of every 1000 operations performed.[1,3] Although it has been estimated that approximately 32% of hospital-acquired infections may be preventable by fully implementing current recommendations, only 6% are actually being prevented.[3]

Most hospital or health-care-associated infections are endemic; epidemics of infection are infrequent.[4] When they do occur, outbreaks cover a wide range of infectious agents and sites—including outbreaks of noninfectious diseases. For example, recent outbreaks investigated by state health departments and the Centers for Disease Control and Prevention (CDC) included such problems as gram-negative bacteremia and endotoxin reactions in dialysis patients associated with the pooling of single dose erythropoietin,[5] toxic reactions—decreased hearing and vision—in dialysis patients associated with the use of old dialyzers,[6] vancomycin-resistant enterococci (VRE) in a community of acute and long-term care facilities,[7] vancomycin-intermediate resistant *Staphylococcus aureus* (VISA) infections in inpatients and a person on home therapy,[8] bloodstream infections in home infusion therapy patients,[9,10] and potential community acquisition of methicillin-resistant *S. aureus* (MRSA). Other examples include *Serratia marcescans* infections associated with narcotic use in a health care worker, transmission of VRE and other multidrug-resistant pathogens in long-term care facilities,[11] Malassezia or Aspergillosis spp. infections among immunosuppressed patients,[12] surgical site infections after cardiac surgery, tuberculosis among patients and health-care workers (HCWs),[13,14] anaphylactic reactions to latex among pediatric surgery patients, and aluminum toxicity among dialysis patients.[15]

Second, patients receiving health care, for example, patients in acute or rehabilitative care settings, residents of long-term care settings, ambulatory care patients, and those receiving chronic hemodialysis or home care have underlying diseases that make them significantly more susceptible to infection than their healthier community cohorts. Other risk factors for development of infection include invasive devices, such as intravenous catheters, indwelling urinary catheters, and endotracheal intubation; or invasive procedures, such as surgery. These numerous, interacting, intrinsic host and external exposure factors add complexity to the investigation and may require multivariate analyses to reduce or eliminate the effect of confounding variables and to identify the independent risk factor(s).

Third, pathogens associated with health care, such as multidrug-resistant pathogens, *Mycobacterium tuberculosis*, MRSA, VRE, VISA; viral pathogens, such as hepatitis B and C viruses, respiratory syncytial virus, or rotavirus; fungal pathogens, such as Malassezia, Aspergillus, or Candida spp; and other microorganisms pose a much greater risk to patients and HCWs in these settings than members of the surrounding community. Transmission of pathogens in health-care settings is often only appreciated after infections appear in patients or HCWs, and the transmission of the pathogens causing colonization—the unrecognized iceberg effect—is not detected.

Finally, any outbreak in the health-care setting poses a risk for litigation against that facility. This adds to the pressure to rapidly identify the problem and institute effective control measures during the investigation.

Overall Purposes and Methodology

As with community outbreak investigations, the primary purpose of your investigations in health-care settings is to determine the source of the outbreak and the mode of spread, and to prevent further spread of disease. Investigation in these facilities also provides you with the opportunity to identify new or re-emerging agents or complications,[7,8,11,13–15] previously unrecognized human or environmental sources, and new or unusual modes of transmission.[5,6,8,9,12] Furthermore, investigations in health-care settings may help determine risk factors for acquisition of disease in patients and HCWs and facilitate development of prevention interventions.

Pace and Commitment of the Field Investigation

Like all other epidemiologic investigations, your work must be conducted quickly, thoroughly, and responsibly. Pressure from a variety of sources may add to the sense of urgency to complete the investigation quickly. Health-care professionals will be looking to you for answers and recommendations to prevent further spread of disease to their "healthy" patients or to HCWs. The hospital administrator(s) may have already stopped admissions to the affected unit, so every day that unit stays closed means loss of income for the hospital. Finally, the health-care industry is a common target of the media, and outbreaks in a health-care facility may lead to adverse publicity. However, these added pressures should not affect the conduct, thoroughness, or organization of your investigation. Although you can make preliminary recommendations based on sound infection control practices, such as patient isolation and hand washing, collect your data carefully; analyze it appropriately; and then make specific recommendations based on your findings. Whoever made control recommendations *before* you arrived, such as closing a certain ward to all admissions, discontinuing surgery, or relieving a health-care worker from duty, should be the one who reverses these decisions.

RECOGNITION AND RESPONSE TO A REQUEST FOR ASSISTANCE

The Report

There are a variety of ways you may learn of adverse events or outbreaks in the health care arena. First, the Joint Commission on Accreditation of Healthcare Organizations (JCAHO) requires that health-care settings maintain an active infection control program, including surveillance for health-care-associated infections, as a part of their standard for accreditation.[16] So surveillance data can serve as a source for the identification of infectious disease (and noninfectious disease) outbreaks and as a measure of the intensity and efficacy of the facility's infection surveillance and control program. With caution (if similar definitions, surveillance methods, and numerator and denominator are used for rate calculations), these data also can be used to monitor and benchmark infection rates by comparing the facility's rates to itself over time (intra-facility) or with others in similar settings (inter-facility comparison). You must be sure that you are comparing your rates to others with a similar case mix and distribution of underlying diseases and procedures.

Second, professionals trained in infection control techniques monitor infections in hospital settings. These infection control professionals, or ICPs, also may work in free-standing clinics or long-term care settings and may work for home care companies. ICPs conduct routine surveillance for health-care-associated infections, usually using uniform definitions developed by CDC.[17] Cases most frequently are found by review of records from the microbiology laboratory; medical, pharmacy, radiology, and Kardex-medical records; nursing, surgical service, physician reports; and discharge summaries. Detection of outbreaks in health-care settings often results from analyses of these surveillance data. Possible outbreaks may also be uncovered when an ICP calls a local or state health department or

CDC for information on possible sources or modes of transmission of certain pathogens or for advice on prevention and control of infections. Reports of a possible outbreak may also come from the microbiology laboratory, physicians, the employee health department, or directly from employees, patients, patients' families, or the news media.

Lastly, an outbreak in a health-care facility may be recognized when laboratory support is requested from the state health department or CDC. When inquiring about the underlying problem you may identify an outbreak that the facility would like help investigating.

The Request

Requests for epidemiologic assistance usually come from the ICP, the hospital epidemiologist, the facility's administrator, the company owning the facility or agency, or a private physician who has an outbreak in her or his practice. Health-care facility personnel may simply need laboratory support, such as culture confirmation, assessment of intrinsic product contamination, and molecular typing of isolates to determine clonality. The laboratory may lack epidemiologic expertise or simply be too busy or understaffed to conduct an investigation on its own while still performing its usual duties. Inquiries about possible assistance may be guarded because of concern about potential future litigation or adverse publicity. This concern applies particularly if the federal government (e.g., CDC) is involved, where data obtained during the investigation are available through the Freedom of Information Act (FOIA). However, patient identifiable information is protected through the Privacy Act, but institution identity and nonidentifiable data on patients are not similarly protected by the Privacy Act. Thus, not infrequently, to protect privileged information health-care personnel prefer on-site assistance from the local or state health department or a private consultant, rather than the federal government.

The Response and the Responsibilities

Not all requests to investigate presumed outbreaks in a health-care setting require on-site visits. Because infections and other complications are so common in these settings and personnel resources are limited, you should obtain additional background information before agreeing to initiate an investigation. Quite frequently the problem can be solved by mail or telephone consultation. For example, if you receive a call requesting assistance to determine the source of surgical site infections among open-heart surgery (OHS) patients during the previous 2 months, try to get additional information that may be useful in evaluating the need for assistance. This information might include current and background OHS-surgical site infection rates; the pathogens causing the infections; the availability of isolates; changes in personnel performing OHS or the surgical or other methods performed; and a line-listing of "cases" and their characteristics, exposures, and risk factors. Always ask if the "outbreak" isolates are available; this is particularly important to confirm the identity of the infecting strain(s) and to determine clonality of the strains, both of which are essential for conclusive epidemiologic investigations.

Next, ask the contact person to determine the OHS-surgical site infection rate among patients for several months to years before the suspected outbreak. From the background and current surgical site infection rates, determine if an outbreak may, indeed, be occurring or if the health-care facility actually has a high endemic rate. In other words, are background and current rates similar and are both above national median benchmark rates? Determine if the increased OHS-surgical site infection rate could be due to surveillance artifact. For example, has there been an increase in the surveillance staff or training of a new ICP? Have there been additions to the OHS staff or changes in OHS procedures or practices, such as new techniques, changes in procedures (like preoperative shaving), or changes in antimicrobial prophylaxis? Are there any changes in the laboratory that would have increased recognition of the pathogen(s) (e.g., introduction of a new diagnostic test used on surgical specimens)? If an increase in the rate of these infections can be temporally linked to one or more of these factors, a full on-site investigation may not be necessary. Finally, ask the contact person about any interim infection control measures that may have been put into place. If good infection control practices have been implemented and the problem persists, an investigation may be warranted.

Before beginning an investigation, the participants need to discuss several critical issues, such as organization, personnel, resources, and responsibilities— all of which are discussed in Chapters 4 and 5.

PREPARATION FOR THE FIELD INVESTIGATION

Collaboration and Consultation

Investigations of outbreaks in health-care settings usually require substantial laboratory support. In addition to identifying the agent (which may already have been done), further typing of the organism may be necessary. For example, since many serotypes of *Pseudomonas aeruginosa* exist as common environmental organisms in hospitals, outbreaks of *P. aeruginosa* may require genotyping to link patient and environmental isolates. In addition, for some multidrug-resistant pathogens, such as MRSA, their prevalence in the facility may be so high that genetic typing, using pulsed-field gel electrophoresis or protein A sequencing, may be necessary to determine if the outbreak is caused by one or more strains. Also, serologic testing of numerous blood specimens may be required in outbreaks of health-care-associated viral infections, such as hepatitis A, B, or C, or cytomegalovirus. Typing methods vary from organism to organism (see Table 15–2). Except for antimicrobial susceptibility testing, most genetic typing methods are available only in reference laboratories (private, state health department, or CDC). Before accepting an invitation to start an investigation on-site, contact your reference laboratory to request its assistance; to identify a contact person; to ask what capabilities the laboratory has for this particular investigation; and to determine what types of specimens should be collected and how they should be shipped. The laboratory personnel also should be able to estimate a time frame for results. In some investigations, it may be warranted and more efficient for one or more laboratory personnel to join the on-site epidemiologic team. A more comprehensive discussion of the laboratory's role in investigating outbreaks can be found in Chapter 22. For outbreaks involving medical products, devices, biologics, or blood products, the Food and Drug Administration (FDA) should be notified (http: www.FDA.Medwatch; Phone: 1-800-FDA-1088: Fax: 1-800-FDA-0178) and consulted for laws requiring the reporting of adverse effects. In addition, the FDA may know of a similar occurrence in other settings, indicating a problem of potentially greater scope. The FDA can help reduce the extent of the outbreak by issuing alerts or initiating a voluntary or nonvoluntary recall. Similarly, for outbreaks primarily involving HCWs or physical plant problems like potential toxic exposures, state agencies responsible for occupational health and/or CDC's National Institute for Occupational Safety and Health (NIOSH) can lend assistance with industrial engineering evaluations (see Chapter 17).

In some contrast to many community outbreak investigations, in a health-care facility you will often have assistance from personnel, such as ICPs and hos-

Table 15–2. Types of Organisms for Which Typing Method Can Be Used

TYPING METHODS	TYPES OF ORGANISMS
Antimicrobial susceptibility profiles	Bacteria (except *Pseudomonas cepacia* and *Staphylococcus epidermidis*), fungi, occasionally viruses
Serotyping	Some bacteria and viruses
Pulsed-field gel electrophoresis	Bacteria and fungi
Ribotyping	Bacteria
Phage typing	Bacteria (i.e., *Staphylococcus aureus*)
Plasmid analysis	Bacteria
Restriction fragment length polymorphism	*Mycobacterium tuberculosis*

pital epidemiologists who are knowledgeable about the health-care facility and trained in infection control practices. These ICPs are an invaluable resource for background information about infection rates in the facility and the location of other resources that may be available to you. In addition, the ICP's staff may be available to be a part of the investigative team and assist you in the design of the study, the abstraction of data from medical records, the analyses, and the development of recommendations for prevention and control.

Personnel in the health-care facilities want to minimize the potentially negative impact that an investigation at those settings may generate. Often, disgruntled employees or those with a particular agenda may alert the media about the outbreak. You should anticipate public inquiries, and arrangements should be made early in the investigation—or even before the team arrives on-site—for such inquiries to be directed to and handled by administrative, public relations, or risk management personnel at the facility. In outbreaks that involve considerable media attention, it is essential that the media expert for the facility be included in frequent updates about the investigation. In this way, he or she will be knowledgeable and current and can determine what information to release to the media. In addition to permitting you to conduct the investigation unhindered by the media, this allows the facility to maintain control of this very delicate aspect of the investigation.

THE FIELD INVESTIGATION

Health-care settings lend themselves to outbreak investigations because of easy access to many kinds of records (see above). Documentation is very important in these settings, but it varies; hospitals and free-standing clinics (surgery or dialysis centers) generally have more complete documentation than long-term care facilities or private physicians' offices. Computerized records are often very valuable, and obtaining large amounts of data from a computer record is much more efficient than reviewing the medical records for this information. To the extent possible, attempt to obtain as much of the data as you can from the computer records; however, before fully depending upon this source, be sure that the data are complete and valid. Often, the personnel recording such data are not familiar with the importance or the meaning of the information and incorrectly enter or misinterpret the data they are handling. Use your imagination to identify other sources of documentation, and do not be afraid to ask if other types of records exist. Outbreaks predominantly involving HCWs often are more difficult to investigate because not all of the HCWs will be treated at the health-care facility. Employee health department records can be used, although medical students, house officers, private physicians, outside agency personnel, volunteers, and other nonpaid hospital personnel are often not included in hospital employee health programs. Time cards (to determine absenteeism possibly due to illness) and interviews with affected employees also are helpful.

Immediately upon your arrival at the health-care facility, arrange a meeting with all of the key personnel involved with the outbreak. This meeting should include the hospital administrator, chief of service, physicians who have patients involved in the outbreak, the hospital epidemiologist, the infection control staff, risk management personnel, appropriate public health authorities, and the field team. Also, invite any other key personnel who may be involved, such as the operating room manager, the head nurse from the affected unit, or the heads of the microbiology and medical records departments. At this meeting you should outline your initial plan for the investigation, indicate the time frame this will require, and request any resources you need immediately, such as: an office with a telephone, phone numbers of key personnel, a map of the facility, and directions to the laboratory and medical records department. If security is strict, request a temporary identification badge to allow freer movement around the facility. Also, ask for any additional information you may need to start the investigation, for example, policy and procedure manuals, any recent changes in them, and the opinion of the involved personnel about the potential cause of the outbreak. It also is important to confirm to all involved that you will maintain the strictest confidentiality for the patients and will work with all personnel to conduct the investigation quickly and efficiently with as little disruption of usual business as possible.

Determine the Existence of an Epidemic

This step may have been started during the preparatory stages of the investigation. In the field, determine the background rate of the adverse event for yourself (see Chapter 5). Start with the appropriate records, often the microbiology and infection control records. Outbreaks involving blood products will require examination of transfusion reaction records; those involving dialysis patients require examination of dialysis session records. Be creative—what you need is not always computerized but often is systematically collected and recorded somewhere. You may have to look back at several years of data to calculate accurate background rates. If the data suggest a hyper-endemic rate rather than a true outbreak, the problem still may be worthy of investigation. Occasionally, only or no periodic surveillance will have been conducted in the "outbreak area." If this occurs, it may be very difficult, time consuming, or impossible to determine the background or current rate. In those instances, it may be necessary to estimate the rate of infection or adverse reaction using a sampling method.[18] Remember to look at other changes that may have occurred that will affect the rates you are calculating, for example, the ICP hired six new assistants one year, or four new surgeons or a new infectious disease specialist were added to the medical staff. New procedures may have been implemented before or during the outbreak, new diagnostic tests may have become available, or new units opened in the hospital—all of which might lead to an increased infection or illness rate.

At the same time, start looking closely at procedures around the patient care areas that are relevant to the outbreak. Look at everything and ask questions about every aspect of patient care no matter how seemingly trivial. See for yourself what is actually happening rather than relying on others. Written policies may or may not reflect what is really occurring on the patient care ward. Observe practices for yourself! After your initial review of the procedures occurring around the patients, create your initial case definition and determine what data you want to collect for each case. For example, patient demographic information, hospital locations, underlying diagnoses, date of onset of illness, and dates of invasive procedures should be collected. Other important data might include severity of illness indicators (e.g., the Acute Physiologic and Chronic Health Evaluation [APACHE] score, the Pediatric Risk of Mortality [PRISM] score, or the National Nosocomial Infections Surveillance surgical site infection risk index).[19-21] You very likely will want to get information on possible exposures such as operating rooms, surgeons, operating room team members, nursing and other patient contact personnel, and medications.

Confirm the Diagnosis

In an infectious disease outbreak, contact all laboratories where the patient specimens initially are being processed and ask them to save all relevant isolates for possible further study. If the outbreak strains have been isolated or sent to an outside or private laboratory, obtain the isolates for possible confirmation or further testing. If possible, confirm that the cases are related by reviewing the microbiology laboratory data for species identification and/or antimicrobial sensitivity testing results. If you need typing of organisms beyond the capability of the microbiology department at the facility, consult a private laboratory, the state health department, or CDC. Remember, some typing techniques are research tools that may not be performed rapidly or may not be practical to apply to large numbers of isolates. Maintain communication with your laboratory colleagues to inform them of the progress of the investigation, what isolates are available and being sent to them, and to discuss what other specimens or samples they may want. At the same time, you can discuss with them the reasonable time frame for notification of results.

Define a Case and Count Cases

The case definition(s) should start with the clinical aspects of the disease. Try to include laboratory and clinical data in the case definition and inclusionary characteristics that relate to time, place, and person. For example, a case definition might include persons who developed a staphylococcal surgical site infection between November 1 and January 1; who were located on surgical floor, 3-West; and who had an orthopedic procedure. If the clinical case definition is confirmed by laboratory methods, you can call this a *Confirmed Case*. A patient with similar symptoms but lacking laboratory confirmation will then be called a *Possible Case*. This distinction may be useful later on when you analyze all your cases. Remember, start with a broad case definition; you can refine it as you continue the investigation.

Methods for case finding depend on the type of disease (infectious or noninfectious) causing the outbreak. Sources that may be useful include records from the infection control surveillance system, microbiology laboratory, clinic patients, emergency room, blood bank, or dialysis sessions. Case finding can be done by reviewing the entire cohort of patient charts, if the cases are limited to a single ward or unit, or if the health-care facility has a reasonably manageable number of patients to review. Dialysis outbreaks may require you to count each dialysis session, rather than counting each patient. This is because a patient may have more than one exposure at a single session, thus allowing each dialysis session to be treated as a single exposure.

At the same time you are ascertaining cases, collect the basic information you have already deemed important during your initial procedure review of the first identified cases. Again, after you have determined your case definition and found cases, compare the attack rate with the background rate to assure yourself that an outbreak is, indeed, occurring.

Orient the Data in Terms of Time, Place, and Person

Descriptive epidemiology in health-care settings differs from that of community outbreak investigations only in that all of the cases are already hospitalized (in acute or long-term care facilities) or each patient has an available medical record (outpatient, ambulatory, or home care). As with community outbreaks, organizing the data in terms of time, place, and person allows you to postulate who was at risk and who may still be at risk for developing the disease or adverse reaction.

Time

The "epidemic curve" gives you a picture of the scope of the outbreak over time. It may give a clue as to whether the outbreak was due to a common source, person-to-person transmission, or another mode of transmission (see Chapter 6). For example, a common source outbreak with subsequent person-to-person transmission is well illustrated by a food-borne outbreak in a retirement community

(Fig. 15–1).[22] A high initial peak of onset of illness, suggestive of a single point source of infection, is followed by the continued occurrence of cases due to secondary person-to-person transmission, typical of outbreaks of viral gastroenteritis. The epidemic curve of an outbreak caused by contaminated patient equipment or poor infection control techniques also may span long periods of time until the recurring problem is corrected. For example, an *Acinetobacter baumannii* outbreak, traced to reuse of intravascular pressure transducers that were not adequately sterilized, continued for over a year until the problem was recognized and the decontamination/disinfection technique corrected (Fig. 15–2).[23] If HCWs and patients are both affected by the outbreak, the date of onset of disease for patients and HCWs should be plotted together and then separately to help determine how transmission may have occurred, that is, from patient to patient, patient to HCW, HCW to patient, or HCW to HCW.

Place

At times, the location of the outbreak will be limited to a certain floor, unit, or operating room; at other times to a certain type of floor (e.g., all of the general surgical units because only surgical patients are being affected). The location of the outbreak may provide a clue to the mode of transmission or to certain risk factors due to patient placement or exposure. For example, during the initial phase

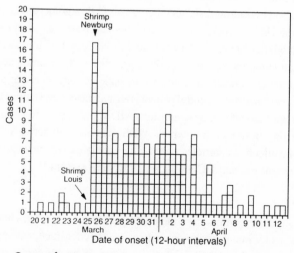

Figure 15–1. Cases of gastroenteritis originating from a common source with subsequent person-to-person transmission, by date of onset—California, March 20–April 12, 1988. [*Source*: Gordon et al., 1990.[22]]

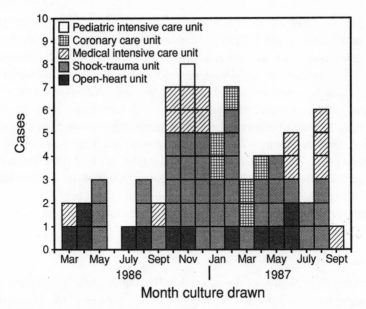

Figure 15–2. Cases of *Acinetobacter baumannii* bacteremia caused by contaminated patient-care equipment, by month that culture was drawn—New Jersey, March 1986–September 1987. [*Source:* Beck-Sague et al., 1990.[23]]

of an investigation in a hospital of an outbreak of tuberculin skin test conversions among HCWs and multidrug-resistant tuberculosis (TB) among patients, it was noted that most of the HCWs worked and the patients had been treated in the outpatient human immunodeficiency virus (HIV) clinic. Further investigation documented that air in the examination rooms was at positive pressure to the central patient area and that the air from the examination rooms, where patients were receiving aerosol treatments, was recirculated to the central patient area and the nurses station. Thus, HCWs and acquired immunodeficiency syndrome (AIDS) patients were being exposed to the air originating from rooms in which AIDS patients with active TB were being treated, and the infectious particles were being circulated via the ventilation system to areas where patients and HCWs without TB were present.[13,24]

Person

In investigating communitywide epidemics, you will often characterize the affected persons by many attributes such as age, gender, race, occupation, socioeconomic level, and the like. In general, however, in health-care settings, you do not need to classify cases by so many variables. Most often, age, gender, and underlying disease are the most often used attributes that help you define the "at-risk" population. In contrast to community outbreaks, in many hospital outbreaks one must control for severity of illness or birthweight, because many exposures the patients have are linked to how sick they are. Once one controls for severity of illness or birthweight, many factors that look important are no longer significant.

Determine Who Is at Risk of Becoming Ill

As discussed in previous chapters (see Chapters 5 and 6), the purpose of characterizing the ill persons by time, place, and person is to give you an idea of who is at risk of disease and whom to study further. Therefore, in these settings you can either examine the entire population in a cohort study or you can randomly select controls from this population for a case-control study (see Chapter 7). If, for example, you find that patients located on all general wards of the hospital over a period of one year developed pneumonia, you may want to take a random sample of all patients admitted to the hospital during that same year as controls for a case-control study. If, however, you determine that the only patients in the facility who are at risk were located on a particular ward during a specific time interval and had a particular underlying diagnosis (e.g., appendectomy patients on a general surgical ward during the months of April and May 2001), you may want to select *all* appendectomy patients located on that ward from March 1 through June 30, 2001, and review their charts as a "retrospective" cohort study.

Selection of controls is exceedingly important, because the wrong control group can easily lead to erroneous conclusions. For example, if, during case finding, you discover that patients undergoing general anesthesia for a variety of surgical procedures developed surgical site and bloodstream infections, several possible control groups for a case-control study could be selected, as well as several different cohorts.[25] If the study group (controls or the cohort) is selected from all patients undergoing surgery, there is a good chance that many of the non-ill patients will have undergone local, spinal, or epidural anesthesia, while all of the ill patients will have undergone only general anesthesia. Since the ill patients were previously known to have undergone only general anesthesia, specific exposures related to general anesthesia (e.g., particular injectable anesthetics or intubation equipment) probably will not be identified with this group of controls. A better study group would include patients undergoing general anesthesia for surgical procedures during the correct time frame. This will allow analysis of each individual injectable and inhalational agent, respiratory equipment, anesthesiologist, and other possible risk factors.

Developing and Testing Hypotheses

It is inefficient to test only one or two hypotheses at a time. You can test several hypotheses at once by collecting data on cases and controls, or the cohort, that examine a variety of risk factors. For example, if the disease is predominantly spread by the respiratory route, and all of the cases were intubated, you may want to examine all respiratory therapy practices and exposures, including the type of ventilator used, duration of ventilation, which respiratory therapist(s) took care of the cases each shift, which nurses suctioned the patients' endotracheal tubes, which medications were administered through the endotracheal tube and who prepared them, and how often the ventilator reservoirs were changed.

An excellent example of an outbreak investigation in a hospital is the investigation of surgical site infections caused by an unusual human pathogen, *Rhodococcus bronchialis*, after open-heart surgery.[26] This outbreak provided an opportunity to assess risk factors for infection with *R. bronchialis*, mode of transmission of the organism, and potential sources for this unusual nosocomial pathogen. Logical hypotheses for the source of surgical site infections after open-heart surgery included three possible exposures: preoperative (e.g., nurses, physicians, wards), operative (e.g., operating room environment or personnel), and postoperative (e.g., recovery room or intensive care unit personnel) exposures. By retrospective cohort analysis, the investigators analyzed a large number of variables as measures of potential risk for infection and possible exposures as the source of infection (Table 15–3). The only factor significantly associated with infection was the presence of one operating room nurse, Nurse A, during the operative procedure. Examination of Nurse A's intra-operative practices revealed that she could potentially contaminate the sterile field after performing an activated clotting-time test that involved the use of a water bath for incubation of a tube of the patient's blood. A revised hypothesis was that Nurse A contaminated the sterile operative field after performing the test; this would account for all of the cases of *R. bronchialis* surgical site infections during the epidemic period.

Compare the Hypothesis with the Established Facts

Environmental and personnel cultures can help support the results of an epidemiologic investigation. Because many organisms are ubiquitous in health-care environments and are part of the normal environment or human flora, performing cultures of the environment or personnel without epidemiologic implications can be quite costly, waste precious time, and lead your investigation astray. However, when performed to determine if your epidemiologic data are pointing you in the right direction, environmental and personnel cultures can be very valuable.

To continue with the previous example, in order to establish that Nurse A was, indeed, responsible for all of the cases of *R. bronchialis* at the hospital, the investigators performed numerous cultures as indicated by the epidemiologic data. These included cultures of Nurse A's and Nurse B's hands before and af-

Table 15–3. Potential Risk Factors for Rhodococcus Sternal Wound
Infection—May 1 through December 31, 1988[a]

POTENTIAL RISK FACTOR	CASE PATIENTS (N = 7)	CONTROLS (N = 28)	ODDS RATIO	P VALUES
Categorical Variables				
Male sex	7 (100)	24 (86)	NC	0.6
Underlying conditions	6 (86)	22 (79)	1.6	1.0
Diabetes	1 (14)	6 (21)	0.6	0.1
Obesity	3 (43)	4 (14)	4.5	0.1
Smoking	4 (57)	9 (32)	2.8	0.4
Cancer	1 (14)	0 (0)	NC	0.2
Renal insufficiency	0 (0)	0 (0)	—	—
Treatment with steroids	1 (14)	1 (4)	4.5	0.4
Chronic lung disease	2 (29)	3 (11)	3.3	0.3
Presence of nurse A	7 (100)	6 (21)	NC	0.0003
Coronary artery bypass graft	7 (100)	28 (100)	—	—
Saphenous vein	6 (86)	26 (93)	0.5	0.5
Mammary artery	6 (86)	25 (89)	0.7	1.0
Transfusion	4 (57)	13 (46)	2.2	1.0
Continuous Variables				
Preoperative stay (days)	1.8±1.3	1.9±1.8	—	0.7
Postoperative stay (days)	6.2±1.3	7.5±3.7	—	0.4
Age (years)	59.4±5.4	58.5±11.0	—	0.9
Number of underlying conditions	2.2±1.9	1.1±0.9	—	0.2
Duration of operation (min)	284±64	292±87	—	0.9
Duration of bypass (min)	119±38	128±44	—	0.7
Duration of aortic clamping (min)	67±43	70±27	—	0.8
Amount of blood reperfused (mL)	903±236	901±317	—	1.0
Cardiac index[b]	2.8±0.6	3.0±0.5	—	0.6
Duration of treatment (days)				
Stay in cardiac ICU	2.2±0.4	2.9±2.2	—	0.8
Swan Ganz catheter	1.8±0.4	2.2±1.0	—	0.6
Arterial line	2±0	2.3±1.0	—	0.6
Mediastinal drains	2±0	2.2±0.8	—	0.6
Pacer wires	4.8±0.4	5.0±1.6	—	0.8
Ventilation	1±0	1.6±2.7	—	0.6
Antimicrobial prophylaxis	4.2±2.2	3.7±1.0	—	0.9

[a]Plus-minus values are means ±SD. NC denotes not calculable; ICU, intensive care unit.

[b]Cardiac index was defined as cardiac output in liters per minute per square meter of body surface area.

[Source: Richet et al., 1991.[26]]

ter each performed the activated clotting-time test; nasal swabs from all cardiac surgery operating room personnel; swabs from Nurse A's scalp, pharynx, vagina, and rectum; swabs of Nurse A's operating room closet and its contents; her home; the neck-scruff skin, mouths, rectums, and paws of two of Nurse A's three dogs; and environmental swabs and air samples while Nurse A was present in or absent from the operating room. Only cultures of Nurse A's hands after performing the activated clotting test, Nurse A's nasal swab, settle plates from the operating room while Nurse A was present, Nurse A's scalp and vaginal cultures, and cultures of the neck-scruff skin of Nurse A's dogs were positive for *R. bronchialis*. Antimicrobial sensitivity testing, plasmid analysis, and restriction fragment length polymorphism analysis showed that all of the outbreak isolates (patient, Nurse A, and Nurse A's dogs) were identical and distinct from nonoutbreak stock isolates.

The role of the water bath used to incubate blood samples for the activated clotting-time test was analyzed by using a colorless fluorescent dye. After simulating the beginning of an open-heart surgery procedure, eight of eleven circulating nurses had "contaminated" the sterile field with fluorescent dye from the water bath. In addition, all of the nurses' hands; some of the nurses' wrists, forearms, and scrub suits; the outer surface of the water bath container; the table surface; and the floor around the water bath were "contaminated" with fluorescent dye. This experiment showed that, although the bath water was culture-negative for *R. bronchialis*, the water bath provided the mechanism for the organism to be spread from Nurse A's hands to the sterile field. Because Nurse A was epidemiologically implicated in the investigation, cultures were obtained from a variety of sources highly likely to yield positive results. Culturing of the operating room environment and other personnel earlier in the investigation would have been unfocused, increasing the work load on the laboratory without significantly aiding the investigation and very likely missing the ultimate implicated source.

Plan a More Systematic Study

Once the source and mode of transmission have been determined and you can make specific recommendations for control of the outbreak, you may want to perform additional studies. For example, after establishing by a case-control study that a certain group is at risk, such as hematology–oncology patients at risk for bacteremia, you may want to analyze that group further for other risk factors. Using a cohort study model, for example, you could analyze the duration of chemotherapy, the specific chemotherapeutic agents, or the duration of neutropenia. You might also want to perform sero-surveys of patients and HCWs to further define the population at risk after an outbreak of hepatitis B or anaphylactic reactions to certain drugs or products.

Evaluation of the efficacy of control measures that may have been undertaken before or during the investigation, and of recommendations that the field team makes to the hospital personnel, should also be conducted. It is imperative that you or members of the field team document that the implemented interventions terminate the outbreak and prevent further episodes of disease.

Prepare a Written Report

Before departing from the field site, you should hold a meeting with staff of the health-care facility and local or state health department representatives to appraise them of what you did and your results. The health-care facility administrative director and infection control personnel are primarily interested in your recommendations for control measures. In fact, the legal department may ask you for recommendations from the first day of the investigation. As described earlier in this chapter, you can give preliminary recommendations based on previously documented guidelines for isolation, hand washing, hospital environmental control, and disease-specific prevention guidelines[27–38] at the beginning of or during the investigation. Additional recommendations based on the epidemiologic and laboratory data should be given to the facility at this debriefing. Your written report should describe any of the interim measures that were initiated and your final recommendations.

The written report for the facility, the state and local health department, and your supervisor should describe the problem as it was presented to you, the background information that you collected before and during the investigation, the methods and results of your investigation, and your final recommendations to the facility. The written report provides documentation of your investigation and, therefore, should thoroughly and accurately describe your approach or methods, your results, your recommendations, and any follow-up activities either you are planning or that you recommend that facility personnel conduct. Often, it is helpful to write the report (or at least keep detailed notes) as you do the investigation. For example, write the background information before you arrive at the outbreak site, document your methods as you decide each step of the process (this is extremely important for case definitions, which may change during the course of the investigation), and compile a file of results as they become available. You should be able to leave a brief written report, which includes your recommendations for control measures, with health-care facility personnel at your departure. This report should be clearly marked as a *Preliminary* document as it will become part of the permanent record that could be used in court. After returning to your home office, a final report with "clean" data, final laboratory results, and more sophisticated statistical analysis can be written.

Medico-legal Aspects

Outbreaks of disease in health-care settings may lead to litigation against the facility. *Resist* all attempts by the facility administration to force you into making recommendations that your evidence and other relevant scientific data do not support. In addition, do not get caught up in interdepartmental politics and make recommendations without supporting data. The request for assistance in investigating an outbreak gives the health-care facility an excellent defense in court, especially if the recommended control measures were instituted and the problem stopped. By requesting assistance, the facility personnel have documented that they have taken the problem seriously and have sought a solution. Your final report may be one of the most important defense documents the facility may have for establishing that a thorough investigation was done and that recommendations by outside experts have been made. Furthermore, if the facility personnel can show that they fully implemented the recommendations with subsequent prevention of further diseases, they will have confirmed that they have controlled the outbreak.

Confidentiality and medical malpractice laws vary from state to state, therefore, conduct your investigation so that confidentiality of patients and employees is ensured (see Chapter 14). Therefore, you should not collect identifying data that are not absolutely essential; if you must collect identifying data to link records, a convenient method is the hospital identification number (if it differs from the patient's Social Security number) or the patient's birthdate and last four digits of the Social Security number. If possible, put this information on your data collection form where it can easily be removed by a paper cutter, that is, the top right hand corner of the first page. This will also allow you to easily remove identifying data months later if a request for your information is made by a litigant. If an agency of the federal government conducts the investigation, the data obtained are available under the Freedom of Information Act (FOIA) as are the name of the institution and related correspondence. However, the Privacy Act prevents the release of patient or HCW names or other identifying information by United States government workers. If state health department personnel conduct the investigation, it is important for them and the facility personnel where the outbreak is occurring to know what data/information are recoverable during possible litigation.

SUMMARY

Investigating outbreaks of disease in health-care settings is both similar to and different from investigating outbreaks in community settings. Both types of investigation involve a sick, frightened population who want immediate answers and solutions to the problem. Health-care settings have the advantage of multiple types of on-site records and a built-in professional staff of health-care workers, both of which are invaluable resources during an outbreak investigation. And, health-care settings provide the opportunity to study many aspects of disease in a closed, fairly well controlled setting. Cases of disease in health-care settings involve complex patients, and multivariate analysis of data may be necessary to control for host and device-related risk factors. On the other hand, health-care settings have the disadvantage of a fairly stressful work environment due to the legal implications of outbreaks.

Each state health department has state-specific regulations with which health-care settings must comply. Also, the CDC has published guidelines relevant to the control of infectious diseases in health-care settings.[27–38] These guidelines are meant to be a framework for individual health-care facility staff to use when writing policy and procedure manuals for the facility. The Occupational Safety and Health Administration (OSHA) writes the federal law that mandates certain practices in health-care settings (e.g., Blood-borne Pathogen Standard, Proposed TB Standard); many of these laws incorporate CDC guidelines. In addition, the CDC guidelines and OSHA regulations are references that should be used during the course of outbreak investigations in health-care settings.

REFERENCES

1. Haley, R.W., Culver, D.H., White, J.W., et al. (1985). The nationwide nosocomial infection rate. *Am J Epidemiol* 121, 159–67.
2. Jarvis, W.R. (2001). Infection control and changing healthcare systems. *Emerg Infect J* 7:170–173.
3. Haley, R.W., Culver, D.H., White, J.W., et al. (1985). The efficacy of infection surveillance and control programs in preventing nosocomial infections in U.S. hospitals. *Am J Epidemiol* 121, 182–205.
4. Haley, R.W., Tenney, J.H., Lindsey, II J.O., et al. (1985). How frequent are outbreaks of nosocomial infection in community hospitals? *Infect Control* 6, 233–36.
5. Grohskop, L.A., Roth, V.R., Feikin, D.R., et al. (2001). *Serratia liquefaciens* bloodstream infection and pyrogenic reactions at a hemodialysis center traced to extrinsically contaminated epoetin alfa. *N Engl J Med* 344:1481–1497.
6. Hutter, J.C., Kuehnert, M.J., Wallis, R.R., et al. (2000). Acute onset of decreased vision and blindness traced to hemodialysis treatment with aged dialyzers. *J Am Med Assoc* 283, 2128–34.
7. Ostrowsky, B.E., Trick, W.E., Sohn, A., et al. (2001). Successful control of vancomycin-resistant enterococcus (VRE) colonization in acute and long-term care facility patients: working together as a community. *N Engl J Med* 344:1427–1433.
8. Smith, T.L., Pearson, M.L., Wilcox, K.R., et al. (1999). Emergence of vancomycin resistance in *Staphylococcus aureus*. *N Engl J Med* 340, 493–501.

9. Danzig, L.E., Short, L.M., Collins, K., et al. (1995). Bloodstream infections associated with a needleless intravenous infusion system in patients receiving home infusion therapy. *J Am Med Assoc* 273, 1862–64.

10. Do, A.N., Ray, B.J., Banerjee, S.N., et al. (1999). Bloodstream infections associated with needleless device use and the importance of infection control practices in home health-care setting. *J Infect Dis* 179, 4442–48.

11. Trick, W.E., Kuehnert, M.J., Quirk, S.B., et al. (1999). Regional dissemination of vancomycin-resistant enterococci resulting from interfacility transfer of colonized patients. *J Infect Dis* 180, 391–96.

12. Chang, H.J., Miller, H.L., Watkin, N., et al. (1998). An epidemic of *Malassezia pachydermatis* in intensive care nursery associated with colonization of health care worker pet dogs. *N Engl J Med* 338, 706–11.

13. Beck-Sague, C., Dooley, S.W., Hutton, M.D., et al. (1992). Hospital outbreak of multidrug-resistant *Mycobacterium tuberculosis* infections; factors in transmission to staff and HIV-infected patients. *J Am Med Assoc* 268, 1280–86.

14. Edlin, B.R., Tokars, J.I., Grieco, M.H., et al. (1992). An outbreak of multidrug-resistant tuberculosis among hospitalized patients with the acquired immunodeficiency syndrome. *N Engl J Med* 326, 1514–21.

15. Jarvis, W.R. and the Epidemiology Branch, Hospital Infections Program (1991). Nosocomial outbreaks: the Centers for Disease Control's Hospital Infections Program experience, 1980–1990. *Am J Med* 91(suppl 3B), 101s–6s.

16. Joint Commission on Accreditation of Healthcare Organizations (1990). Standards: infection control. In JCAHO, *Accreditation Manual for Hospitals*. Joint Commission on Accreditation of Healthcare Organizations, Chicago.

17. Garner, J.S., Jarvis, W.R., Emori, T.G., et al. (1988). CDC definitions for nosocomial infections, 1988. *Am J Infect Control* 16, 128–40.

18. Cookson, S.T., Ihrig, M., O'Mara, E., et al. (1998). Use of an estimation method to derive an appropriate denominator to calculate central venous catheter-associated bloodstream infection rates. *Infect Control Hosp Epidemiol* 19, 28–31.

19. Knaus, W.A., Draper, E.A., Wagner, D.P., et al. (1985). APACHE II: A severity of disease classification system. *Crit Care Med* 13, 818–29.

20. Pollack, M.M., Ruttimann, U.E., Getson, P.R. (1988). Pediatric risk of mortality (PRISM) score. *Crit Care Med* 16, 1110–16.

21. Culver, D.H., Horan, T.C., Gaynes, R.P., et al. (1991). Surgical wound infection rates by wound class, operative procedure, and patient risk index. *Am J Med* 91(suppl 3B), 152s–57s.

22. Gordon, S.M., Oshiro, L.S., Jarvis, W.R, et al. (1990). Foodborne snow mountain agent gastroenteritis with secondary person-to-person spread in a retirement community. *Am J Epidemiol* 131, 702–10.

23. Beck-Sague, C.M., Jarvis, W.R., Brook, J.H., et al. (1990). Epidemic bacteremia due to *Acinetobacter baumannii* in five intensive care units. *Am J Epidemiol* 132, 723–33.

24. CDC (1990). Nosocomial transmission of multidrug-resistant tuberculosis to health-care workers and HIV-infected patients in an urban hospital—Florida. *Morb Mortal Wkly Rep* 39, 718–22.

25. Bennett, S.N., McNeil, M.M., Bland, L.A., et al. (1995). Multiple outbreaks of postoperative infections traced to extrinsic contamination of an intravenous anesthetic, propofol. *N Engl J Med* 333, 147–54.

26. Richet, H., Craven, P.C., Brown, J.M., et al. (1991). A cluster of *Rhodococcus*

(Gordona) bronchialis sternal-wound infections after coronary-artery bypass surgery. *N Engl J Med* 324, 104–9.

27. Garner, J.S., Hospital Infection Control Practices Advisory Committee (1996). Guideline for isolation precautions in hospitals. *Infect Control Hosp Epidemiol* 17, 53–80.

28. Pearson, M.P., Hospital Infection Control Practices Advisory Committee (1996). Guideline for prevention of intravascular device-related infections. *Am J Infect Control* 24, 262–93.

29. Mangram, A.J., Horan, T.C., Pearson, M.L., et al. (1999). Guideline for prevention of surgical site infection. *Infect Control Hosp Epidemiol* 20, 247–80.

30. Wong, E.S., Hooton, T.M. (1983). Guideline for prevention of urinary tract infections. *Am J Infecti Control* 11, 28–33.

31. Tablan, O.C., Anderson, L.J., Arden, N.A., et al. (1994). Guideline for prevention of nosocomial pneumonia. *Respir Care* 39, 1191–1236.

32. Bolyard, B.A., Tablan, O.C., Williams, W.W., et al. (1998). Guideline for infection control in health care personnel. *Infect Control Hosp Epidemiol* 19, 407–63.

33. CDC (1995). Recommendations for preventing the spread of vancomycin resistance. *Infect Control Hosp Epidemiol* 16, 105–13.

34. CDC (1997). Interim guidelines for prevention and control of staphylococcal infection associated with reduced susceptibility to vancomycin. *Morb Mortal Wkly Rep* 46, 626–28, 635.

35. CDC (1991). Recommendations for preventing transmission of human immunodeficiency virus and hepatitis B virus to patients during exposure-prone invasive procedures. *Morb Mortal Wkly Rep* 40(RR-8), 1–9.

36. CDC (1997). Immunization of healthcare workers. Recommendations of the Advisory Committee on Immunization Practices (ACIP) and the Hospital Infection Control Advisory Practices (HICPAC). *Morb Mortal Wkly Rep* 46(No. RR-18), 1–42.

37. CDC (1987). Recommendations for prevention of HIV transmission in health-care settings. *Morb Mortal Wkly Rep* 36(2S), 3–18.

38. CDC (1990). Guidelines for preventing the transmission of tuberculosis in health-care settings, with special focus on HIV-related issues. *Morb Mortal Wkly Rep* 39(RR-17), 1–29.

16

INVESTIGATIONS IN OUT-OF-HOME
CHILD CARE SETTINGS

Ralph L. Cordell
Margaret Swartz

Each weekday morning in the United States, millions of adults go to work in offices, factories, and stores while their preschool children go to some form of out-
of-home child care. These facilities range from child care homes, which may care
for fewer than five children of various ages in one group, to chain-affiliated child
care centers, where hundreds of children may be cared for in classes or secondary
groups segregated on the basis of age. Regardless of their size or structure, these
facilities all provide an opportunity for children to contribute the current strains
of microbes circulating within their respective households to a microbial potluck
and to acquire new infections that may be brought home and shared with other
family members. One result of this process is that child care facilities amplify the
prevalence of certain pathogens such as Giardia, Shigella, or hepatitis A within
communities. Attempts to control this process by excluding obviously ill children
from child care costs billions of dollars in lost productivity each year. Exclusion
often drives parents to pressure health care providers to prescribe inappropriate
antimicrobials, which contribute to increased antimicrobial resistance. Furthermore, a child excluded from one facility due to illness may be enrolled in another,
thus spreading the infection to a new care center.

Nonetheless, there are very real, positive public health aspects to child care.
The enforcement of immunization requirements, especially at the center level, has
resulted in higher immunization levels among children in out-of-home child care

than among children cared for at home. Quality child care programs also provide training in hygiene and reinforce healthful behavior. Knowledgeable providers are important sources of information on child development and parenting skills, and providers are often the first to recognize developmental problems and to recommend further follow-up.

You and other professionals representing the local health department may interact with child care providers in a number of different capacities. Public health personnel frequently serve as resources for health recommendations and consultation for child care providers. Public health professionals often respond to questions about health and hygiene requirements and practices; assist in developing health and safety policies, programs, and strategies; interpret recommendations and regulations governing exclusion and communicable disease prevention; and provide training to child care staff on health and safety issues. Unfortunately, outbreaks of communicable diseases in child care facilities are a common reason for interactions between local health workers and child care providers. Because of this interaction and the epidemiologist's role in an investigation, you should be aware of some of the unique aspects of the child care environment. This chapter focuses on the detection, response, and control of outbreaks in this setting.

SURVEILLANCE

As discussed in Chapter 3, surveillance is defined as the ongoing collection, collation, and analysis of information on illnesses in a given population coupled with timely feedback to those who use it to guide policy and prevention strategies. One of the best descriptions of this system was written almost 50 years ago:

> Our system of notification of individual case reports is a haphazard complex of interdependence, cooperation and good will among physicians, nurses, county and State health officials, school teachers, sanitarians, laboratory technicians, secretaries, and clerks. It is a rambling system with variations as numerous as the individual diseases for which reports are requested and, as numerous as the interests and individual traits of the administrative health officers, epidemiologists and statisticians in the 48 States and several Federal agencies concerned with the data. It is a system that depends on persuasion, education, and, in some instances, alarm. *And the variables cannot be eliminated by regimentation and fiat* (emphasis added).[1]

Although disease surveillance in the United States as a whole has vastly improved since then, those variables still have an impact to a greater or lesser degree—particularly in the day care setting.

The most immediate local use for surveillance in child care facilities is the rapid identification of child care–associated outbreaks or clusters of illness: additionally, children in child care provide an important sentinel for the health of the community at large. A call from a child care center director concerned about the large number of cases of diarrheal illness among children in her facility was one of the earliest indications of the massive outbreak of milk-borne salmonellosis in northeastern Illinois in 1985.[a] Calls from child care facilities also provide an important insight into the incidence of nonreportable conditions in the community, such as fifth disease, hand-foot-and-mouth disease, and respiratory infections.

Kinds of Surveillance

Surveillance for illness in out-of-home child care facilities may be *indirect* (information about child care–associated illness is obtained from another source—usually through individual case investigations) or *direct* (child care facilities are part of the reporting system).

Indirect reporting (notifiable disease case investigations)

In many areas, reports made to health departments by hospitals, laboratories, and other health care providers result in a minimum collection of additional information by local health officials. These often take the form of telephone interviews of ill persons or, in the case of children, their parents. The purposes of these investigations is to collect basic demographic and descriptive information; identify sources of infection; provide indications for follow-up activities, including isolation or restriction of infected persons or prophylaxis of potentially exposed persons, such as household contacts; and provide health education.

These single-case investigations are the cornerstone of effective public health surveillance and disease control activities within the child care environment. While they are usually conducted by well-trained staff at local health departments, we would offer the following observations. Parents may be reluctant to discuss specifics of child care arrangements with strangers over the telephone. These fears can often be reduced by explaining the reason for the information and how it will be used. Concerns about the interviewer's affiliation (e.g., "Are you really with the health department?") may be addressed by suggesting the person call the health department and then be transferred back to the investigator. Also, the structure and sequence of

---

[a]One of us (RC) was working with the Cook County Department of Public Health and took this call during the last week of March 1985. The director of a local day care center expressed concern that several children in her facility had an illness diagnosed as "stomach flu" by local physicians. Stool cultures were collected from a sample of ill children. These came back positive for *Salmonella typhimurium*. The director later reported serving a contaminated lot of milk. Subsequent phone calls indicated that staff were also infected and the facility director eventually voluntarily ceased operations temporarily because so many of her staff and children were ill.

questions may minimize respondent discomfort and contribute to the accuracy of information. Appendix 16–1 is a composite script drawn from hundreds of interviews conducted by the authors over a period of years and illustrates a sequence and phrasing that we found to be professional, nonthreatening, and productive in terms of obtaining sensitive information about child care arrangements.

Local health departments should develop a system for keeping track of information from these individual case investigations. This is especially important in programs where several persons are conducting investigations or where information is coming from multiple sources, such as complaints, case investigations, and relicensing inspections. The system should be simple, easy to maintain, readily accessible, and timely. If electronic systems are used, data should be accessible immediately after completion of interviews or investigations. Weekly data entry is of little use in detecting explosive outbreaks such as those caused by shigellosis in child care centers. We have found a note card system that lists the name and address of the facility, illness or problem involved (e.g., Giardia infection), and a record number that allows linkage with the complete case file to be useful. It is a good idea to follow facilities by both name and address as, in the case of chain centers, there may be multiple facilities with the same name and, as may be the case with child care homes, multiple names may be given for the same facility.

Direct reporting (child care provider–based reporting)

While indirect surveillance involves information from sources other than child care facilities, direct surveillance involves reporting from facilities themselves. The key to effective direct surveillance is maintaining positive working relationships with child care providers and making sure that providers know what to report and how to report it. Studies have shown that child care providers are often unaware of reporting requirements and mechanisms.[2] Follow-up studies to this work found that provider knowledge of reporting requirements was greatest in those states where reporting to health departments was required by both public health and licensing statutes (RLC, unpublished data). Periodic contact through training programs (preferably conducted by health department staff and held either at the child care facility or during weekends or evenings), through mailings, or during contacts for other reasons (e.g., licensing inspections) is needed to ensure that providers are aware of the need to report.

Reporting requirements should be worded in language appropriate for child care providers. Vague terms such as "outbreaks" or "unusual occurrences" should be linked with specific examples such as "two or more children with diarrhea in the same classroom within a 2 week time period." The average worker in an infant or toddler class probably has more contact with feces in a week than most pediatricians or public health workers experience in a year, and it may be useful to make sure that they realize "diarrhea" includes "the runs," "the loosies," "teething," "food allergies," and all the other euphemisms and explanations that are given for this condition. Time-based criteria such as "three or more loose stools in 24 hours" may be of little use as providers rarely observe children for 24 continuous hours. Two loose stools in the 10–12 hour period in child care may represent four or more loose stools in a 24 hour period These definitions may also be misinterpreted or disregarded, and we have had at least one provider tell us that diarrhea was three or more loose stools in an hour.

Lists of notifiable diseases should include instructions on how and when to report specific conditions and include the telephone number of local and state health authorities who can provide information and assistance, if needed. Diseases should be identified by names familiar to laypersons as well as those used by health care providers. Child care staff often do not have access to specific diagnoses and may need to be encouraged and empowered to obtain this information from parents. However, parents do not always provide accurate information, and we know of more than one instance where health professionals with children admitted they intentionally gave their child care provider inaccurate information about a health condition involving their child.

OUTBREAK INVESTIGATIONS

Probably the major reason to investigate outbreaks and clusters of illness involving children in child care facilities is to limit the spread of illness in the facility and among household contacts. Other reasons include gaining additional knowledge; training staff in skills and techniques of outbreak investigation; program evaluation and input; and public, political, or legal concerns. The nature and extent of investigative and control activities are also influenced by the severity of the illness, the risk to others, and the likelihood of meaningful intervention. Investigation and follow-up will always be necessary in outbreaks of severe illness such as shigellosis or *Escherichia coli* O157:H7 infections. At the other extreme, investigating outbreaks of hand-foot-and-mouth disease may have little impact with respect to control but provides significant results in terms of understanding factors involved with the prevention and spread of this infection.

You should have a broad understanding of the variations of clinical expression of the more common diseases seen in day care settings as well as their mode of transmission. The most common organisms spread by the fecal–oral route are: Shigella, Salmonella, Giardia, hepatitis A, rotavirus, and the enteroviruses. Rhinoviruses, influenza and parainfluenza viruses, *Haemophilus influenzae*, and streptococci are transmitted via respiratory secretions. Some conditions, like shigellosis, usually cause clinical signs and symptoms and spread easily to contacts in the facility as well as at home. Others, like hepatitis A in children, usually cause no or only mild clinical illness but more frequently cause overt disease in adults. Bacteria, such as *H. influenzae* and *Neisseria meningitidis*, can be carried by children in their nasopharynx, but only rarely will children develop overt disease.

Be aware that outbreak investigations can quickly become emotional, especially in those cases where children are being excluded or illness is severe. Parents of children who are not ill want assurance that their child will not be exposed, and parents of convalescing children want to return to work as soon as possible. Also pediatricians may be giving conflicting advice, thus making providers feel they have lost control and, therefore, concerned about losing the confidence of the parents of children in their care. In such a setting, your arrival as a confident, presumedly competent public health official can easily seem like the cavalry coming over the hill to those in charge of the child care facility.

Finally, one of the best tools in your arsenal is a well-developed protocol for dealing with the situation. Although outbreaks are unique events, and it may be difficult to develop a detailed protocol for every possibility, there are a number of general features and considerations in outbreak investigations that benefit from the structure provided by an established protocol. Chapter 5 details a logical progression of investigative steps for most situations, and they are outlined below. However, local conditions will determine their relative importance and order. In some instances, considerable time and resources may be devoted to a particular phase of the investigation, while, in others, the same step may receive very little attention.

Prepare for Fieldwork

Consider creating a general protocol that would specify those situations when field visits will definitely be made, situations where field visits may not be necessary, and the administrative personnel and process involved in making those decisions. The protocol should identify the tasks to be undertaken, personnel taking part in the field visit, their respective roles, and persons or groups to be notified prior to the visit. For initial visits involving outbreaks of significant infections, you may find it useful to include a public health nurse and a sanitarian besides yourself, as the epidemiologist, on the field team. Your role would be to interview the director and other staff to obtain the descriptive aspects of the problem—the time, place, and person information. The public health nurse should evaluate child care practices in classrooms involved in the outbreak; and the sanitarian should evaluate the environmental aspects, including food service and the physical plant. This approach focuses multiple talents and skills and allows staff to ask the same questions from different child care employees without seeming distrustful. Before the visit is completed, all three of you should meet, discuss your findings, and agree on follow-up activities. Representatives of child care licensing agencies should always be notified of potential field visits and invited to participate. Materials for specimen collection, sample notification letters for parents (see below), and educational materials for parents and staff should be assembled. It is a good practice to leave educational materials with the facility each time a field visit is made. Facilities do not always have photocopying capability; and misunderstanding can be reduced by using pressure-sensitive paper to document groups to be screened, follow-up activities, and recommendations.

Establish the Existence of an Outbreak

If criteria for an outbreak have been previously defined in writing, this phase of the investigation would not likely be a major concern, as circumstances either will or will not meet the criteria. Examples of such criteria might include: two or more reports of children with a given illness (e.g., giardiasis) in the same classroom in a 2 week period or more than 50% of children with a respiratory illness at any one time. However, it is often important to look for cases of similar disease in the patients' siblings, as child care cases may only represent intra-familial spread, not intra-facility transmission.

Generally, the best sources to help establish the existence of an outbreak include facility records and interviews with parents. While most child care facilities maintain records on attendance, they often do not give reasons for an absence and seldom indicate the nature of any illnesses involved. Information from parents is often unreliable, especially when it involves very mild illness or events more than one week prior to the interview. Moreover, despite the utility of having ready-made protocols and definitions, unusual situations or unpredictable circumstances are bound to arise. Perhaps you may have to create for yourself or others an epidemic curve to show that cases represent an unusual increase. Or you may have to inform parents and facility staff that a single case of a particular disease reflects just the tip of the iceberg and really represents many more unrecognized cases within the facility or possibly elsewhere. In such situations, creativity will be rewarded.

The creation of a clear, well-defined case definition is essential to demonstrating the existence of an outbreak and planning interventions. Case definitions should be written and included in the field notes and final report of every investigation. Case definitions should include time and population criteria as well as clinical or laboratory criteria.

Verify the Diagnosis

Verifying the clinical diagnosis of a child care–associated illness may be straightforward or may take considerable time and effort. Outbreaks identified through reports from health care providers usually involve at least one or two laboratory-confirmed cases of the illness in question. Your major task in this instance, then, is to implement effective control measures. Depending on a variety of factors unique to the outbreak, you may need to find and confirm additional cases, so that prevention and control measures can be extended to other groups or households. Outbreaks reported by child care providers and parents are often based only on symptoms. In these instances, determining a specific etiology can be labor intensive and require specimen collection and laboratory support. The purpose and extent of laboratory testing (e.g., whether it will be restricted to particular classrooms or be facilitywide, or whether it will be restricted to children or include staff) and plans for follow-up of persons found to be infected need to be determined before the first specimen is collected. When the causative agent is not known, the laboratory may have to screen for multiple pathogens. In these instances, a two-stage scheme may be used to initially screen a small, representative group of no more than 10 cases for multiple pathogens to identify the responsible pathogen. Clinical data should be obtained concerning these same 10 children. A larger group can then be screened for the causative agent. Follow-up surveillance may be undertaken to evaluate the effectiveness of these measures.

Informed consent should be obtained before collecting specimens from children in child care settings. Sending consent forms home with children is usually nonproductive unless it is tied with a requirement that children be either screened or excluded from child care. An alternative is to ask providers, often the director, to get consent from parents or to have field staff on-site to get consent from parents during the morning when children are dropped off and in the evening when they are picked up.

Information on types of specimens to be collected, timing, transport media, and other parameters should also be included in the basic protocol. As has been emphasized before, consult the laboratory staff prior to specimen collection and give them information on clinical histories. Although providers can often collect stool specimens from very young children in diapers, specimens from older children may need to be collected by parents at home. In this instance, parents should be provided with written instructions and materials (e.g., specimen containers and swabs) for specimen collection and submission. While it is very difficult to collect blood specimens from children, the process can be made somewhat easier with parental support and by using phlebotomists experienced in drawing blood from children. When available, molecular subtyping of isolates of bacterial pathogens may be helpful in defining links between illness in child care facilities and illness in the general community.

Orient the Data in Terms of Time, Place, and Person

You should be aware of some problems inherent to the day care setting that make history taking difficult and that can compromise the validity of your data. Try to get clinical histories from at least a sample of children who are ill. When interviewing a parent about a child's food history or past activities, you may find it advantageous to have the child present during the interview because children have first hand knowledge of the historical events. Mothers are generally better historians than fathers when it comes to the health of children in the household. In instances involving teen mothers, grandmothers are often the best historians.

With respect to time, dates of onset are often difficult to determine. Facility records may not be detailed or accurate. Providers are often not aware of illnesses, because parents may keep ill children at home or illnesses may take place during weekends, vacations, or other periods when children are not scheduled to be in attendance. Precision is nice, but be flexible in your expectations. Onset dates by 2 or 3 day intervals or even by week, depicted on an epidemic curve, can help in assessing the magnitude of the outbreak and even the mode of transmission.

If there are distinctly different classrooms or locations where cohorts of children spend several hours or more, consider drawing a map, locating each ill child as a spot on the map to help identify areas of high or low risk. It is always a good idea to have a floor plan available so you can get a good idea of the location and movement of children. Even knowledge of airflow patterns can help explain illnesses easily transmitted via the airborne route.

Equally as confounding as the issues just described can be those relating to age, class, movement, and individual contact with cohorts of other children—more key information for determining who is as risk. Data from child care–associated outbreaks are usually expressed in terms of classroom-specific attack rates, because age-specific rates will often include children from multiple groups and locations in the center and, thus, be a less useful epidemiologic marker. Groupings are often only loosely associated with age, and their structure depends on facility policies and licensing restrictions. For example, children in a 4-year-old classroom are probably not all 4 years old, and this group may also not include all 4-year-old children in the facility. Facilities commonly pool children from various classrooms early in the morning and late in the afternoon into "drop-off" groups. These groups need to be identified and their attack rates and group characteristics determined separately from classroom groups during regular operating periods. Sibling clusters may also be significant, as they may represent transmission outside the facility and provide a means for illness to spread from one classroom to another.

All these combinations and permutations of the children's attributes in the day care setting behoove you to dig deep for useful descriptive data and to be imaginative as well.

Determine Who Is at Risk

At this time in the investigation you should have a firm diagnosis, a good idea of when and where illness occurred, and who were primarily involved. In the majority of outbreaks this information will give you ample evidence to identify the group primarily at risk of getting sick. The relatively straightforward review of the descriptive data will lead you to those you need to study more and to analyze. Only rarely will you have to resort to analytic methods to identify those at risk (see Chapter 7).

Develop a Hypothesis that Explains the Outbreak and Test It

With a good grasp of who is at risk and how the disease in question is normally transmitted, an epidemiologist should be able to create a scenario of how and why the outbreak occurred. In many instances the explanation is simply common sense and requires no further analysis or thought. Indeed, public health officials frequently act on common-sense hypotheses and limited descriptive data whenever control measures are implemented. However, there will be times when your hypothesis will require more analytic techniques. For example, an outbreak of *E. coli* O157:H7 might be due to contaminated ground beef served at lunch, to exposure to a farm animal at a petting zoo, to spread of pathogens in a wading pool, or to fecal–oral spread from child to child. The control measures for each of these are obviously different. Analytic methods for most outbreaks are fairly straightforward and can easily be handled with spreadsheets or programs such as *Epi Info*. Staff should be familiar with whatever software packages or methods are used in tabulating or analyzing data. The white heat of a significant outbreak is no time to implement a new software package or data entry systems.

Information on the risks associated with specific exposures can be useful in future outbreak investigations. Your hypotheses might include questions about which groups have the highest attack rates and the effectiveness of control measures. For example, it may be useful to compare attack rates among children in drop-off groups with those among children who are not in those groups. While infants and toddlers generally have higher attack rates than older children, comparisons of age-specific or group-specific rates may indicate where control activities should be focused.

Evaluate the Hypotheses

Whenever possible, try to evaluate and/or confirm your hypotheses. Common-sense premises as well as hypotheses supported by statistical analyses in the field may all seem logical and persuasive; however, if practical, they should be evaluated by both observational and quantitative methods. The demonstration of higher attack rates in a particular classroom is enhanced by observations of inadequate equipment or poor hygiene practices. The importance of direct observation of child care practices cannot be overemphasized. Although caregivers may be especially careful when they know they are being observed, glaring problems can often be detected through observation. In the midst of a Giardia outbreak we have seen providers contaminate sinks with fecal material—sinks that were used for a variety of purposes besides washing diapers. Observations should include how equipment and facilities are actually being used rather than just what is present or absent. When observing operations in infant and toddler rooms, there is a tendency to focus on diaper-changing areas. While this is an obvious source of contamination, interactions among staff, children, and toys in other parts of the room may be more important and should receive as much if not more attention than the diapering table.

Post-intervention surveillance is probably the most critical evaluation of hypotheses generated and tested in conjunction with child care–associated outbreaks. Both parents and providers should be alerted to the need to maintain vigilance and be provided with information on how to report subsequent problems. Public health officials should make periodic contact with the facility for several weeks or months, depending on the nature of the problem, after the completion of interventions and other activities.

Refine Hypotheses and Carry Out Additional Studies

Post-intervention surveillance may suggest other leads that need to be pursued. This activity may extend the scope of the current investigation by implicating family groups, other classrooms, or other facilities. In other instances, continued surveillance may suggest avenues to follow in future investigations of similar problems. For example, isolation of bacteria from fomites such as toy plastic foods may suggest that these be investigated in more detail in subsequent investigations. In the context of child care outbreak investigations, this step suggests that you should make use of experience and knowledge gained from past investigations and that emergent problems be viewed as opportunities to refine interventions and control strategies.

Implement Control and Prevention Measures

Implementing control and prevention measures is the goal of a successful outbreak investigation. Most outbreaks resolve of their own accord once the number of susceptible children and staff has been reduced to the point where transmission no longer occurs. Your challenge is to end the outbreak before that point is reached. In many instances, how an intervention is implemented has as much impact on success as which interventions are implemented. Be sure to bring the providers into the decision-making process and keep the parents informed of the progress and findings. A summary list of control measures is presented in Appendix 16–2.

Informing

Control measures are those steps undertaken in response to a particular problem, while prevention measures are those that should be in place at all times as part of normal operating conditions. Minimal control activities usually involve informing parents about the situation at the facility. While this is often done using posters or notices placed throughout the facility, a better method is through notices or letters given to parents. Also, these notices or letters often also serve as sources of information for health care providers who may be queried about the situation. These materials should identify the illness, indicate the dates of exposure and groups exposed, describe signs and symptoms of the illness, and give parents recommendations on follow-up activities. The latter may range from keeping ill children at home and notifying the facility to seeking immediate medical attention. Notices or letters should include phone numbers and names of individuals who may be contacted for additional information. In serious situations, specified in protocols, parents may be contacted by local health officials to verify that they were notified and are taking appropriate action.

Educating

Control measures often include staff education, changes in policies and procedures, and modifications of the physical environment. Depending on the seriousness of the situation and available resources, health department staff may play a role in this training (e.g., by giving on-site training on hand washing or diapering). Specific examples of problem behaviors along with an explanation as to why such behaviors pose a problem are useful training tools. Supervision and enforcement of existing policies and procedures are necessary follow-up activities, and post-intervention observation should demonstrate the effectiveness of training. Staff can be asked to explain changes in policies and procedures in order to determine their understanding as well as their implementation of changes. Observations can also verify that recommended physical changes have been made, such as moving diapering surfaces closer to hand washing sinks, installation of towel and soap dispensers, or elimination of wading pools or communal floor mats.

Cohorting

Except for a few situations, such as those involving mild respiratory illnesses and fifth disease, symptomatic children are generally excluded from child care attendance. Criteria for readmission may range from resolution of symptoms to negative cultures. In situations where multiple children are involved, it may be possible to establish separate cohorts of infected and uninfected children. These are generally groups of children whose symptoms have resolved but who are still excreting a pathogen, most often an enteropathogen, and who are cared for in a group isolated from other children who are not excreting the pathogen. Although its effectiveness has only been systematically evaluated for giardiasis,[3] cohorting has been used to control outbreaks of other enteric illnesses including shigellosis.[4,5] Guidelines for establishing cohorts should be part of the outbreak investigation protocol. One of the first steps in establishing cohorts is to determine the feasibility of dedicating staff and at least one classroom to the care of these children. Staff and rooms involved in the care of cohorts should not be used for noninfected children until the cohort is dissolved. Special attention should be given to care patterns early in the morning and late in the day when children are often pooled and to minimizing interactions between children in nonclassroom areas during the day. Screening is normally used to identify children infected with a pathogen. A goal should be to screen all children in the affected group and set up the cohorts in as short a period of time as possible. This can be extremely frustrating and requires cooperation from providers and parents. It may be helpful to collect samples on a Friday and have results available on the next Monday. One advantage to the cohort process, however, is that the facility can serve as a focal point for specimen collection and drop-off. Children are generally removed from the cohort and returned to their normal group one at a time once it has been demonstrated that they are no longer excreting the enteropathogen of interest. Eventually only a few children may remain in the cohort. Management of this situation needs to be discussed up front with providers and parents, as it will be difficult for providers to devote resources to one or two children.

There are several reasons why child care facilities are almost never closed by health officials during the course of an outbreak investigation and subsequent control measures. Parents of children in closed facilities may place their children, who may be incubating an infection or asymptomatically excreting a pathogen, in other facilities and thus spread the problem further. As long as they remain open, child care facilities can serve as foci for specimen collection, post-outbreak surveillance, and information dissemination. Once a facility has been closed, these activities become much more complicated and labor intensive. Lastly, we have found that child care providers and parents are much more cooperative and willing to provide information once they have been assured that public health officials are not likely to close their facility. Removal of this threat makes the whole process much more collaborative.

Communicate the Findings

The last step to an outbreak investigation is to communicate the findings to those who have a need to know. A well-designed protocol should present a plan for communicating findings. At a minimum, a report documenting activities and results should be drafted for department files. The protocol should specify whether copies will be provided to the child care facility, licensing agency, or other governmental bodies. Parents should be considered in the flow of information. Unless there are extremely extenuating circumstances, the flow of information to parents should normally be through the director of the child care facility. However, confidentiality statutes may prohibit the release of medical information to persons other than parents or legal guardians. Therefore, it may be necessary to get permission to release information to the providers. In such instances it can be very helpful to have prior policies and procedures for this situation already in place.

Depending on the seriousness of the situation, the media may take an interest in the investigation. Here again, a protocol can help identify communications pathways. If media attention becomes likely, it is a good idea to notify the child care facility ahead of time. While confidentiality statutes in many areas may prohibit release of information about a facility, parents may notify the media, and a bit of coordination and planning ahead of time may prevent major problems and embarrassment later on.

Lastly, a post-outbreak review of activities should be conducted. The purpose of this review is to determine what worked, what did not work, and how the process can be improved. The results of this review should be used to revise protocols and procedures.

SUMMARY

Although no two outbreaks are exactly alike, they all share a number of common aspects, and planning and preparation can make significant differences in the quality of investigations. The establishment and revision as needed of written protocols will help refine the investigative process and avoid many of the problems that arise when working in an emotional climate such as a child care facility in the midst of an outbreak of serious illness. This chapter provides a framework for protocol development. We would add that our society is such that out-of-home child care is a vital commodity that is often in short supply. The vast majority of child care providers take great pride in their work and are committed to the health and well-being of their charges. A collaborative approach to both surveillance and outbreak investigations in this setting is much more likely to be successful in both immediate and long-term goals than one based on authority and confrontation.

REFERENCES

1. Sherman, I.L., Langmuir, A.D. (1952). Usefulness of communicable disease reports. *Public Health Rep* 67, 1249–57.
2. Addiss, D.G., Sacks, J.J., Kresnow, M.J., et al. (1994). The compliance of licensed US child care centers with National Health and Safety Performance Standards. *Am J Public Health* 84, 1161–64.
3. Bartlett, A.V., Englender, S.J., Jarvis, B.A., et al. (1991). Controlled trial of *Giardia lamblia*: control strategies in day care centers. *Am J Public Health* 81, 1001–6.
4. Tauxe, R.V., Johnson, K.E., Boase, J.C., et al. (1986). Control of day care shigellosis: a trial of convalescent day care in isolation. *Am J Public Health* 76, 627–30.
5. Mohle-Boetani, J.C., Stapleton, M., Finger, R., et al. (1995). Communitywide shigellosis: control of an outbreak and risk factors in child day-care centers. *Am J Public Health* 85, 812–16.

APPENDIX 16–1. INTRODUCTORY SCRIPT FOR DISEASE INVESTIGATIONS CONDUCTED BY TELEPHONE INTERVIEWS

1. Verify whom you are speaking with, introduce yourself, and explain the purpose of your call.
   Hello, is this the _____ residence? Am I speaking with Mrs _____? My name is _____ and I am with the County Health Department. I'm calling about your daughter's recent Giardia infection. Do you have a few minutes to talk with me about it?

2. Start by asking about illness (e.g., onset, symptoms, etc.). (Interest and knowledge at this stage help validate the nature of your call in addition to confirming information from reporting sources—don't hesitate to ask about discrepancies).
   Mr_____ our records indicate that your daughter became ill on the 10th yet you said she became ill on the 5th? I know it's tough to recall dates several weeks ago, but can you help us determine which is correct?

3. Determine number of household members.
   Mrs _____, counting yourself how many people live in your household?

4. Get names, ages, and occupations (including child care).
   Would you mind giving me the names and ages of these four people?

Do you work outside the home?

How about your husband Jim? Does he work outside the home?

Now you say Billy is 4 and Suzie is 18 months old. Are they in any sort of child care—baby sitter, or preschool, or other child care program?

5. Clarify child care and set groundwork for communication with child care facility.

Mrs _____, you say Billy and Suzie aren't in day care, yet you and Jim both work. Who looks after the children while you two are at work? Does Ms _____ come to your home or do you take your children to hers? I see. Does she care for any children other than your own? Does she know Suzie was ill? Do you know if any of the other children have been ill recently? Would you mind if we gave Ms _____ a call? We may be able to help her keep the other children from becoming sick.

APPENDIX 16–2. EXAMPLES OF CONTROL METHODS

- Notify families of the situation at the child care facility.
- Recommend keeping symptomatic children at home.
- Initiate a program to cohort exposed, asymptomatic and convalescent children.
- Recommend that staff limit the number of children they work with and that they work with only a specific group of children.
- Improve hand washing in both staff and children. Supervise hand washing in children and give training on hand washing to staff.
- Clean and disinfect surfaces, toys, or other potential sources for disease transmission.
- Limit treats and snacks for children to those that are commercially prepared and individually wrapped.
- Eliminate potential sources for spread of disease such as wading pools, water tables, dress-up clothes, and communal floor mats.
- Eliminate communal play areas where all age groups congregate during early morning and late hours.
- Be cautious if the child care facility unilaterally implements control measures such as using only bottled water. The public may expect the health department to rescind these measures when there was no valid reason to start them in the first place.

17

FIELD INVESTIGATIONS OF OCCUPATIONAL DISEASE AND INJURY

William E. Halperin

Earlier chapters of this book have concentrated mainly on field investigations of acute infectious disease problems. For the most part, the operational and epidemiologic tools and methods that have been described are relatively simple, straightforward, and complementary: the request for help, the local social and political scene, and the "players" involved generally seem logical, understandable, predictable, and cooperative. Moreover, the field investigator will usually know or have a good idea of the clinical, laboratory, and epidemiologic characteristics of the disease under study.

Imagine an industrial setting where you may never have set foot before, where you have few or no technical skills and little understanding of the manufacturing process, where there are often many social "agendas" playing off each other and yourself, and where your investigation may subsequently be faulted as biased because of real or perceived allegiances. Furthermore, very often in this scenario you will not know what is the responsible agent; whether it is an agent used in production, a contaminant, or a product; where it came from; how workers were exposed; or other critical clinical and epidemiologic aspects of the condition. Lastly, your performance of operational and epidemiologic functions may be significantly compromised because their conflicting forces can limit studies, muddy interpretation, and jeopardize valid conclusions.

Welcome, then, to the world of occupational disease and injury—a highly challenging and difficult area requiring not only great operational and technical skills but in many ways, a different mindset for the field epidemiologist.

PREPARATIONS FOR THE INVESTIGATIONS

The Request for Assistance

The request for assistance may come from a variety of sources and entail several different kinds of investigations. State and local health officials may be notified of a possible problem by health care providers; by one or more workers who feel there is a health problem in the workplace; by management requesting an evaluation; or by a federal agency that needs support from local sources. Because of statutory and legal considerations, particularly at the federal level, agencies such as the Occupational Safety and Health Administration (OSHA) and the National Institute for Occupational Safety and Health (NIOSH) can and do perform investigations independently of other health agencies. Regardless of the source of the request and even your possible involvement in the field investigation, the field epidemiologist should have a good understanding of both the operational and epidemiologic imperatives for a successful investigation in the workplace.

The Right of Entry

You must know the legal basis for conducting a study in the workplace, otherwise known as the right of entry. Right of entry concerns one's ability to review records, to conduct interviews, to examine workers, to measure levels of exposure, and to perform all other aspects of a field investigation. A successful challenge to your right of entry will not only prevent completion of an investigation, but may also result in lost time and effort, as the legal challenge may only come after the groundwork and preparation for the site visit have been completed.

Right of entry is idiosyncratic to the auspices under which the investigation is being conducted. State health departments may or may not have specialized regulations for investigations of the worksite or may base their actions on general rights and responsibilities incurred in protecting the public's health. NIOSH's right of entry for responding to requests from workers or management is spelled out in federal regulations. An epidemiologist working for OSHA would also have a legal foundation for entry.

The auspices under which the investigation is conducted will determine whether workers have a right to be interviewed and examined in private, whether the information will be kept confidential, whether the workers will be compensated when away from their jobs, and whether there is a basis for preventing possible retribution for participation.

Epidemiologists who are not working under a governmental umbrella may find that they have no legal basis for investigation at the worksite and are dependent on a commitment of all parties to do what is necessary for the goal of prevention or on a negotiated agreement between management and labor.

Trade Secrets

Maintaining trade secrets is a serious consideration when conducting studies in the workplace. Trade secrets include such things as ingredients, processes, or other intellectual material developed by a company that provide it a legitimate advantage over commercial competitors not privy to that information. You have two quite different considerations concerning trade secrets. One consideration is to protect against purposefully or inadvertently divulging a legitimate trade secret. The best thing to do here is to ask the company to identify any trade secret information when and if it is provided to you. The second consideration is how to respond to an intransigent company that claims that everything up to and including the names of management officials are trade secrets. These issues are often better dealt with by those who specialize in the law, rather than in epidemiology. However, you should be forewarned so as not to enter into agreements that can not be undone.

Signing Contracts

It is not unusual to be asked to sign contractual documents before entering the workplace. Some documents will concern issues of liability regarding possible injury to you and your obligation to comply with health and safety requirements like wearing personal protective equipment such as hard hats and eye protectors. Others may concern the dissemination of results contingent upon review and approval. Earnest investigators have sometimes found themselves precluded from publishing information of public health value because of restrictions to which they agreed.

Comportment in the Field: Maintaining a Tripartite Relationship

Success in field epidemiology depends in part on technical skills and in part on social and interpersonal skills. You should not assume that the interests of the workers in the local workforce are consistent with those of local management, or that local interests are consistent with the interests of national management of either the union, if there is one, or the employer, if it is a national or international company. Similarly, interests of the medical department or the engineering department may be quite different from the legal department, which in turn may have different motivations from the insurers. All industries and unions are complex organizations that the epidemiologist, a newcomer to the scene, has very little chance of understanding.

One effective approach to a diverse set of partners in the workplace is to establish early on a tripartite group consisting of the investigative team, representatives of labor, and representatives of management. All of them should be openly informed about all aspects of the study from design through interpretation and conveyance of results to the affected workers. In addition, in more controversial situations, you may want to establish a professional advisory panel of experts in epidemiology, exposure assessment, or toxicology, for example, who can offer technical advice on the conduct of the study. Your overriding commitment must be the protection of the health of the workforce. While this sounds fairly reasonable, be forewarned that epidemiologic questions in the workplace often have huge economic consequences, and one side or the other may have disproportionate resources to offer (e.g., participation by expert consultant epidemiologists and the like), making it difficult to maintain either the perception or the reality of even-handedness between labor and management. Needless to say, evenhandedness in dealing with labor and management should not be equated to evenhandedness in protection of workers' health versus protection of commerce, because your role, as a health professional, is protection of health.

Be Realistic and Open about the Consequences of an Epidemiologic Investigation

The realistic and experienced epidemiologist understands that investigations often do not provide satisfying answers to the basic questions of whether there is a problem of occupational etiology in the workforce. This is particularly true of cluster investigations, but it is also true of preplanned large-scale cohort studies searching for an association between exposure and outcome. It is best to communicate the possibility of both success and failure to labor and management throughout the investigation so that expectations are not unreasonable when a final report is delivered. Labor and management can contribute by helping to provide or facilitate your realistic communication to the workforce throughout the investigation.

You should also not contribute to the misconception that management or labor leadership may have about the consequences of epidemiologic studies. While it is immutable that the goal of epidemiology is prevention, the consequences of learning the epidemiologic truth may result in adverse consequences for labor and/or management. In the short term, lawsuits may well be generated. There may be additional production costs such as reengineering of the manufacturing process or altering the architecture of the workplace. However, in the long term, there may be reduced morbidity and reduced operating expenses as the newer processes become safer and more efficient. Industrial processes that lose feedstock chemicals or the products of the manufacturing process into the work environment are wasting money for the employer as well as endangering the workers.

Participation of Company, Union, Newspaper, or Voluntary Organizations in Data Collection

Tight budgets for field research, limited availability of skilled personnel, and other limitations make it very attractive to accept help in conducting an investigation. The help may come in the form of collecting and copying company records or abstracting records for histories of exposure. Employers and unions may have epidemiologists who are willing to contribute their efforts by helping in the review of records, analysis of data, and formulation of reports. You need to exert strict control of the data and analysis in order to insure that bias and the appearance of bias are prevented. The introduction of bias can be subtle. For example, enthusiastic employees or volunteers using open-ended questions about exposure and disease may exert added effort to elicit responses consistent with their preconceived assessment of the likely association.

Notification of Results

Consider the issue of notification of employees about the results of epidemiologic studies early in the planning phase for the study. In this context there are two types of notification, personal and group. Individuals who participate in medical studies such as blood tests and pulmonary function tests should receive an individualized explanation of their results. How the results of epidemiologic analyses are handled depends upon the importance of these findings to the study subjects who then have personal decisions to make. On the other hand, you are also obliged to inform other cohort subjects of more ambiguous results, even if they were not voluntary participants in a study, but only members of a historical cohort that was the subject of an epidemiologic study in which there was no contact between the investigator and the cohort member. At a minimum, study results that have little if any practical impact on any conceivable decision by the cohort member could be communicated through town meetings, local newspapers, or company newsletters. An example would be communicating via the news media the completion of a cohort mortality study in which no excess risk of mortality was observed. At the other extreme, substantial effort should be made to contact and inform persons who could take effective preventive action, if they had access to the new information that your studies provide. For example, workers appropriately notified of an excess risk of bladder cancer, associated with a previously unrecognized bladder carcinogen, should be personally notified, because they may benefit from clinical intervention.

KINDS OF STUDIES IN THE WORKPLACE

There are four main circumstances in which an epidemiologist will be asked to conduct an investigation in a workplace. These are:

1. Investigation of one or more cases of previously recognized occupational disease or injury
2. Investigation of one, few, or many cases of disease or injury that are not well recognized as occupationally related
3. Determination of whether exposure is associated with an adverse health outcome
4. Evaluation of the effectiveness of an intervention

Investigation of Cases of Known Occupational Etiology

Case Study.   A nurse epidemiologist conducting surveillance in hospital emergency departments for cases of occupational agricultural disease and injury found several cases of carbon monoxide poisoning among farmers who used gas-powered high-pressure water sprayers for cleaning hog pens. Carbon monoxide poisoning is a well-recognized preventable occupational disease; however, its relationship to hog farming was not initially apparent. Investigation revealed that farmers kept their hogs indoors in cold weather and cleaned the barns of offal with gas-powered high-pressure water sprayers. Case finding led to the identification of other cases in hog farmers and later to the recognition of the carbon monoxide hazard of water sprayers when used indoors, particularly after flooding from heavy rains. An experiment in a typical home car garage in which a water sprayer was operated indoors showed that no degree of ventilation through windows and doors—even using fans—could prevent accumulation of dangerous levels of carbon monoxide.

Information on the hazards of indoor use of gas-powered water sprayers and other gas-powered equipment is now circulated periodically by NIOSH, the Consumer Product Safety Commission, and other groups. Also special public service announcements warning of these hazards are made after regional flooding.

The framework for investigation of conditions of known occupational etiology was established in the 1980s by David Rutstein, Professor Emeritus at Harvard Medical School, and colleagues at NIOSH. They developed the concept of the Sentinel Health Event (Occupational), SHE(O).[1] A SHE(O) is defined as an unnecessary disease, disability, or untimely death that is occupationally related and whose occurrence provides evidence that there has been a failure of prevention. These failures can be used to characterize the magnitude and trends of a problem such as industrial lead poisoning. They can also be used on a case-by-case basis as an impetus for defining what failures are responsible for a particular case and for developing interventions to remedy those particular failures. For example, an adult case of lead poisoning is a SHE(O) because the case represents a failure of prevention. The failure may have resulted from inadequate use of substitute materials, inadequate ventilation, inappropriate personal protective equipment (e.g., a respirator), or inappropriate medical management (e.g., use of chronic chelation to control poisoning). The role of an epidemiologist in investigations of sentinel health events is to assist in the recognition of such events; to participate in their evaluation, usually with the aid of an industrial hygienist; to arrange for appropriate interventions; and to summarize and disseminate appropriate information to prevent similar cases elsewhere. Examples of SHE(O) include lead encephalopathy in workers exposed to lead in radiator repair or battery reclamation; leukemia in workers exposed to benzene; and silicosis among workers in foundries. A SHE(O) list for occupational injuries, work-related musculoskeletal syndromes, and psychological outcomes has not yet been developed. The concept of sentinel health events is not limited to occupational exposures but characterizes much of what field epidemiologists and public health professionals do, namely, investigate individual cases and small clusters of other preventable conditions. This is in considerable contrast to performing analytic studies in much larger populations.

A pragmatic framework for investigation of one or more cases of a SHE(O) is an appreciation that in the workplace effective prevention is based upon the implementation of a *hierarchy of prevention*.[2] The essential three elements of the hierarchy are primary, secondary, and tertiary prevention. Primary prevention includes those techniques aimed at preventing the disease or injury process before there is a pathologic effect. Secondary prevention entails early detection of disease or injury before signs and/or symptoms appear, when it is presumably more easily treated. Tertiary prevention involves application of clinical care and rehabilitation. Assessing the hierarchy of prevention is important to the investigator, to determine if there has been a failure in prevention and to ascertain if you have successfully communicated to both the workers and employers the greater effectiveness of primary over secondary over tertiary prevention.

The cascade of techniques in the hierarchy of prevention for occupational disease includes the following examples: (*1*) Primary: premarket testing of feedstock chemicals; substitution of less for more toxic feedstock chemicals, engineering controls, such as enclosed systems; environmental monitoring to insure engineering effectiveness; and personal protective devices if engineering controls are not adequate. (2) Secondary: periodic biologic monitoring for absorption of toxins, periodic medical examination for early signs or symptoms of intoxication, and early medical diagnosis of disease. (3) Tertiary: appropriate therapy and rehabilitation. The more effective primary techniques for prevention are largely in the venue of the industrial hygiene and safety engineering staff.

Investigation of Cases of Unknown Etiology

Case Study. In 1988, union representatives at a chemical plant in upstate New York requested that NIOSH investigate a perceived excess of bladder cancer and cardiovascular disease among workers manufacturing chemicals for the rubber industry.[3] Case ascertainment was conducted via discussion with labor representatives and management. A rough estimate of the population potentially at risk was made by actual physical measurement of several sample personnel file drawers using a yardstick and an extrapolation to the total number of personnel file drawers. Initial assessment suggested that the number of known bladder tumors was more than would be expected based on this crude estimate of total numbers of current and former employees. A walkthrough of the plant by an industrial hygienist identified in the worksite the presence of and the real potential for worker exposure to a number of chemicals including ortho-toluidine—a suspect carcinogen—based upon published experimental animal studies. A retrospective cohort study was done in which all former and current employees were identified. Thirteen incident bladder tumors were diagnosed between 1979 and 1989 among 1749 current and former workers compared to an expected number of 3.6 tumors. This yielded an incidence ratio of 3.6. Seven of the cases occurred in workers who worked primarily in the chemical production department, giving a department-specific incidence ratio of 6.5. The initial estimate of excess risk on the initial site visit led to efforts to reduce exposure. In part, based on the more refined study that took several years to complete, ortho-toluidine has been recognized as a human carcinogen.

The scenario of investigation of cases of unknown etiology differs from the investigation of a SHE(O) where there is a well-established relationship between occupational exposure and disease. The motivation for investigation of a SHE(O) is identification of a failure of prevention. The motivation for investigation of conditions of unknown etiology is, in addition, the early identification of a heretofore unrecognized or unaccepted association between exposure and outcome. Clearly the difficulty here is distinguishing between a chance occurrence of an unrelated case of disease and the first signal of the occurrence of a new disease-exposure relationship.

There are many examples of investigations of small numbers of occupational cases that led to the discovery of a new disease-exposure relationship. These include the investigation of cases of angiosarcoma of the liver associated with vinyl chloride in plastics manufacturing, the association of oat cell carcinoma of the lung with bis-chlorl-methyl-ether exposure in chemical production, the association of azospermia with dibromo-chloro-propane, and many more.

As in all other realms of field epidemiology, the successful investigation requires not only technical expertise in methodology but judgment in differentiating the presence of a real causal association from happenstance. The United States is so large, composed of such a magnitude of workplaces, that, by happenstance, even rare events will cluster. There are attributes of cases and case clusters that suggest a cause-and-effect relationship with exposure rather than a random occurrence. Some of these attributes include pathologic or pathophysiologic aspects of the cases; multiple similar cases; unusual or distinctive pathology; many years of exposure in the case of carcinogens, suggesting an effect of a higher dose; many years since first exposure, suggesting sufficient latency or time since first exposure for carcinogens; a common unique exposure shared by the cases; a chemical relationship between a suspect intoxicant and a structurally similar known hazard; and, of course, biologic plausibility based on prior toxicologic studies in experimental animals. Clearly the more signposts of a real causal association, the less astute need be the epidemiologist.

In this instance, however, the scope of the investigation requires other expertise beyond that of the epidemiologist, necessitating the work of a team. Industrial hygienists are trained to understand industrial processes as well as measurements of exposure. If you attempt a field investigation without the benefit of an industrial hygienist, you run two major risks of failure. On the one hand, most industrial processes to some degree look and sound frightening, but in reality have been made reasonably safe through engineering controls, including ventilation, use of environmental monitoring, and use of personal protective equipment. Without the benefit of an industrial hygienist, you may easily overreact to innocuous exposures and processes. Similarly, without training or experience in exposure assessment or industrial processes, you are unlikely to recognize real hazards. While an industrial toxicologist would be a very effective third member of a field team, in reality, toxicologists are usually consultants rather than primary field investigators. A toxicologist plays an instrumental role in identifying possible hazards among the many chemicals that are either used; produced in normal operations; or inadvertently generated when, for instance, there are changes of temperature or pressure in the manufacturing process.

Does Exposure Cause Disease?

Case Study. Tetrachloro-dibenzo-dioxin (TCDD) has been described by toxicologists as the most potent manufactured toxin. It is a contaminant in the manufacturing of herbicides and other industrial processes. The concern about TCDD is based on exposure studies in experimental animals and mechanistic studies that have demonstrated a molecular basis for toxicity involving binding to subcellular receptors. Starting in the late 1970s, NIOSH investigators identified over 6000 workers, exposed to TCDD in the manufacture of herbicides, who were exposed at quantifiable levels decades before and at substantially higher levels than would be found from normal environmental exposure.[4] These workers were followed through time to see if their cancer mortality differed from what would be expected in the general population—which has low-level exposure. Some cancers of interest were specified a priori, based upon animal experimental studies or cluster investigations in humans. The study took about a decade to complete and has provided some of the best data on the human experience with high-level TCDD exposure. The study documented a significant increase in all cancers combined and a specific increase in a rare tumor, soft tissue sarcoma.

There are usually two typical situations in which the question is asked whether exposure can cause disease. In one situation, workers themselves or their employers have become aware of a potentially hazardous exposure. For example, a feedstock chemical may have been recently found to cause cancer in animal feeding studies. In the other situation, researchers have become aware of the potential toxicity of a chemical and are actively searching for an occupational group to study. In either situation, for an epidemiologic study to adequately answer the question of whether an exposure is related to a disease outcome, the study must overcome many obstacles, or you can be fairly well guaranteed of an inconclusive study— after a substantial amount of effort and time has been expended and expectations have been raised.

There are two ways, neither easy, of going about answering whether an exposure is related to a disease outcome. One way involves *risk assessment*. There are two essential ingredients here. First, the quantitative relationship between exposure and adverse effect must be known either from experimental studies, usually in laboratory animals, or much less frequently, from human data. Second, the exposure in the workplace must be characterized quantitatively. Based upon the level of exposure and the dose-response relationship, predictions of adverse effects can be attempted. Predictions of risk are very difficult for numerous reasons. Among the difficulties are inaccuracy in estimating exposure; extrapolation across species from experimental animal to humans; extrapolation beyond, usually below, the level of exposure even in human studies, to lower levels of actual exposure; and idiosyncrasies of susceptibility and differences in metabolism and pathological reaction among experimental animals and humans.

The alternative approach to answering the question of whether exposure in a workplace leads to disease is to *conduct a study*. Before raising expectations that a study will answer this question, you must consider whether a study will lead to an accurate or to a biased assessment. Numerous questions must be posed. Is the population large enough to avoid a falsely negative study? Has the population been exposed long enough to allow for expression of disease if it were going to occur? Were the exposures high enough to expect that cases would occur? There are even more pragmatic questions such as whether records of exposure exist, whether membership in the worker population over time is known, and whether there would be cooperation among management and workers in estimating exposure or ascertaining if disease or death has occurred.

Three study designs fit this situation. The first design is *cross-sectional*. This is the easiest design to carry out. The cross-sectional investigation studies workers who are currently at the workplace and do not need to be located. The workers can be questioned and examined, and exposures can be measured at the same time. There are major limitations to this approach. The current population may represent healthy survivors. Cases may be long gone along with other sick and well leavers. A cross-sectional study of survivors will falsely underestimate the adverse effect of exposure. Second, exposure measured now is relevant only if the interval, or latency, between exposure and outcome is short, as you would see with a short-acting poison. With carcinogens and other agents that require chronic exposure, the expected latency between exposure and outcome may be decades.

An alternate approach is a *cohort design* in which considerable effort is expended to acquire a complete worker roster over decades and to follow them through time to determine their disease or mortality incidence (see Chapter 7). There are two ways that a cohort can be followed through time. One is the historical, otherwise known as retrospective cohort study, and the other is the prospective cohort study. In the retrospective study, you identify a group or cohort of workers who were exposed to a potential hazardous agent many years in the past. Membership in the cohort is dependent upon their having a potential for exposure. The cohort is then followed through time to the present time or some other arbitrary recent date. Their mortality experience, for example, between 1940 and the present, is then compared with a nonexposed and otherwise comparable worker population or to the mortality experience of the general population.

Virtually all cohort studies of occupational disease are of the retrospective, or historical, type. However, in a pure prospective cohort study, membership of the cohort and determination of their current exposure is made in the present time, and the cohort is followed in time into the future to determine if their future disease experience is comparable to a nonexposed worker population or the general population. Cohort studies can be partially retrospective and followed into the future as well, and hence partially prospective. A further complexity is that exposure can have ceased in the past, continued through the present, or persist into the future.

There are overwhelming problems with the purely prospective approach in which exposure persists into the future. First, if there is sufficient cause for concern about the adverse effect of the exposure, precaution would argue for diminution of the exposure now. Second, even with a strong adverse effect, it usually takes a fairly sizable multiplant cohort to detect the adverse effect during decades of observation during which worrisome exposure persists. It may take an even longer period of observation for a smaller cohort from a single plant. There is an ethical problem of conducting a prospective cohort study when you suspect that the effect of current levels of exposure will be deleterious.

This discussion should emphasize that the role of the epidemiologist cannot be limited to statistical analysis alone, but must consider the toxicity of the agent of interest, the projected risk to the study population, if exposure persists; and the ethics of observation with or without intervention. Clearly an essential element of conducting occupational studies is estimation of the exposure for cohort members. The cohort design is preferable to the cross-sectional approach because the cohort contains cases and survivors whether they currently work at the plant site or not. In practice, the cohort approach is usually limited to retrospective studies of mortality rather than morbidity. Death certificates are readily available, whereas it is very difficult to locate, question, and examine all cohort members to determine rates of nonfatal disease, especially among those already deceased.

A third approach is the *case referent*, or *case-control*, design (see Chapter 7). The prerequisite here—since you are starting with cases rather than exposure—is for you to know specifically what disease is associated with the exposure. Often case-control studies can be performed by selecting all cases from a previously conducted cohort study and comparing them with a random sample of noncases— a so-called nesting approach. Finding all cases, rather than a potentially biased sample of cases, can take as much effort as identifying all cohort members and their death and disease status in a cohort design. However, considerable time can be saved by this method because you only have to estimate exposures in cases and a sample of the others. But this approach also requires that there be variation in exposure, otherwise you will find that cases and referents (controls) are equally exposed.

In the next scenario, you may be asked the more challenging open-ended question of whether the workplace is safe, rather than the more specific question of whether a known outcome is associated with a workplace exposure, or whether a specific exposure is associated with an adverse outcome. Answering this question is not a simple task. A knowledgeable industrial hygienist should be able to supply a generic list of potential exposures for generic occupations and industries. However, a thorough assessment of potential exposures will require a site visit by an industrial hygienist to assess, as examples, an industrial process, the feedstock chemicals used in the process, or the potential for the process to generate new chemical products. This can be a very sophisticated undertaking, as changes in manufacturing processes, such as changes in temperature and pressure, will produce different products than expected. The workplace should have a file of Material Safety Data Sheets (MSDS) required by OSHA for products that are in use. Your role in this situation, particularly if you are a physician, is primarily to see if there is a health concern that is motivating the inquiry. You are likely to be humbled if you are working with an insightful industrial hygienist, toxicologist, or ergonomist, because they may well find potential hazards that are otherwise not evident to the untrained eye. If you are requested to evaluate whether a workplace is healthful, attempt to have the question and your response also address issues of safety from injury as well.

When confronted with the question of whether exposure leads to disease, your major challenge is to recognize that it is the exception when this question can be answered in a specific workplace. Usually, a large-scale study is necessary to avoid a falsely negative study. Large studies are very expensive in time and effort. Even if the circumstances are adequate to launch an epidemiologic study, including exposure assessment, you must consider whether embarking on a demanding, multiyear investigation may inadvertently delay practical actions that could be taken much sooner to reduce exposure, the so-called paralysis through analysis.

Evaluation of an Intervention

Case Study.   Many states conduct surveillance of occupational lead poisoning by requiring that laboratories report cases with elevated levels of lead to the state health department. States vary in their use of the information: some analyze and disseminate the data, others offer consultation, and some states refer companies that do not accept consultation to OSHA, so that OSHA may conduct formal investigations into whether the workplace is in compliance with applicable regulations for worker protection.

In Michigan Rosenman used epidemiologic analyses to evaluate the effectiveness of referral by a state health department of workplaces with excessive blood lead levels to OSHA.[5] A comparison population consisted of companies using lead where blood lead levels were not in excess. Inspection by OSHA found more re-

mediable problems in companies with workers with elevated blood lead levels
than among companies where workers' blood lead levels were not in excess—
demonstrating the effectiveness of the referral program.

Field epidemiology goes beyond investigation of epidemics and can be applied to the evaluation of interventions as shown in the above example. There is
a continuum of techniques used for the prevention of occupational disease and
injury. These are described earlier in the section Hierarchy of Prevention. You
may be requested to evaluate the effectiveness of these interventions. For example, industry may invest substantial resources in campaigns to increase the
use of seat belts. A reasonable question might be whether the campaign approach
is effective in increasing seat-belt use. Epidemiologic approaches may be utilized ranging from establishing a surveillance program for seat-belt use before,
during, and after initiation of the educational intervention, to even conducting
a trial in which alternative interventions might be instituted in various plants of
a large company.

Other Considerations in Conducting Occupational Investigations

Wearing blinders

Think logically when you are studying the nature of an epidemic. An epidemic in the workplace may or may not be of occupational etiology. For example,
gastrointestinal symptoms may be related to a food product served in the cafete-
ria or in the community. The workplace may be a window through which a problem in the greater community can be observed. On the other hand, occupational
epidemics may not be restricted to the workplace. Community residents may be
affected either by toxins carried home by workers on their clothes or vehicles, or
by toxins emitted from the plant carried by air or water.

Consider outcomes other than cancer

The focus of occupational epidemiology for the latter half of the twentieth
century was in two areas: occupational cancer and pulmonary disease. Toward
the latter half of the century there was growth in interest in neurotoxicity, adverse
reproductive effects, and musculoskeletal disorders. The change in focus was
usually precipitated by the advent of a major epidemic and epidemiologic investigation. Future directions are somewhat unpredictable but will probably include
several long-standing problems that have been ignored regardless of their substantial toll on mortality (e.g., occupational injury) and morbidity (e.g., dermati-
tis). New areas of focus will undoubtedly reflect development of new technology

such as personal use of video display terminals and cellular telephones; new advances in biologic science, genomics that will provide opportunities to understand subcellular risk factors and mechanisms of disease; and greater interest in social and psychological factors, such as job stress and fatigue.

A special word on years of potential life lost (YPLL)

A YPLL is a year of potential life lost. Simply put, a death at 75 years rather than at an arbitrary expected age of 85 years results in (or costs) 10 years of life lost. A death at age 25 costs 60 years of life lost. Unfortunately, occupational epidemiologists have focused their interest mostly on relative risks as a measure of public health impact. For example, if one case of some disease or injury is expected and four occur, then the relative risk is 4. However, four deaths of disease A at age 75 cost a total of 40 YPLL and four deaths of disease B at age 25 cost a total of 240 YPLL. Occupational cancer that usually occurs in older age and occupational injury that usually occurs in younger age might have the same excess relative risk but will cause far different losses of life. A corollary to this is: given deaths from a common disease and deaths from a rare disease, many more YPLL will result from the common disease than the rare one, provided all deaths occur at the same age and the relative risks are the same for both groups.

Quantifying exposure

There is a saying in toxicology that "the dose makes the poison," meaning that the greater the dose, the more the toxic effect. Quantifying the relationship between dose and effect is essential to modern quantitative epidemiology and risk assessment. Demonstrating a greater adverse outcome with a higher dose adds to the weight of the evidence for causality. Therefore, in designing a study, you might logically limit the cohort to workers with the most years of exposure. This should increase the probability of your finding an adverse effect among the workers related to exposure and increase the efficiency of your study by permitting you to study fewer persons. The downside of this restriction is that the comparison group for the worker cohort is external to the worker population thus limiting the possibility of demonstrating a dose-related effect. A second problem in using a comparison population external to the worksite is the healthy worker effect. Studies of workers usually find them to be healthier than the general population, especially for cardiovascular disease. This healthy worker effect probably derives from the selection process workers go through to qualify for a job and from the social and economic benefits of employment.

Years of employment is a crude measure of exposure. More sophisticated measures include estimates of probability of exposure based on knowledge of the job. Even more sophisticated measures can include incorporation of environmental measurements that were made over time. Thus, workers can be characterized by levels of exposure-days, which, in turn, can be described as parts per million of exposure times days of exposure. Even more sophisticated measures may go beyond total dose and provide dose rates. Using progressively more sophisticated measures of exposure in an occupational study often provides more and more accurate views of the actual dose-response relationship. The cost of these dose characterizations, however, is substantial. You can limit the cost by using a fairly crude measure of dose, such as years of employment in the cohort analysis, then do a nested case-control study within the cohort (see above), using the most sophisticated measures possible to describe exposure of the cases and referents.

SOURCES OF INFORMATION

At the start of the investigation, you will benefit from two types of information: (1) information specific to the worksite and more general knowledge about the industry, occupation, exposure, or disease that has motivated the investigation. Every workplace that is under the jurisdiction of OSHA keeps a log, called the *OSHA 200*. Cases of injury and illness requiring more than first aid that occur in that particular workplace are supposed to be recorded in the log, which is kept for 5 years and is accessible at the worksite. This source is usually not a complete roster of cases of illness or disease, but it is a helpful starting point. The roster is a line-listing of cases, not a statistical analysis of the injury or illness experience of the workplace. The Bureau of Labor Statistics of the Department of Labor collects a national sample of *OSHA 200* logs and from this provides an Annual Survey which is a statistical analysis of illness and injury by industry. This information is helpful in comparing the experience of particular industries with the general experience of all industries and can also serve as a point of comparison for a particular workplace. The other sources of information about a worksite are the Material Safety Data Sheets, which should be available in the plant office for every commercial product that is being used at the plant site.

(2) The second type of knowledge is more general. While there is a myriad of sources and texts the following are starting points:

- Texts on industrial processes
  Burgess, William. *Recognition of Health Hazards in Industry. A review of materials and processes*. (1981) John Wiley and Sons, New York. ISBN 0-471-06339-8.

Cralley, Lester V., Cralley, Lewis J. (1982) *Industrial Hygiene Aspects of Plant Operations. Volume 1, Process flows; Volume 2, Unit operations and product fabrication.* Macmillan Publishing Co., New York. ISBN 0-02-949350-1.

DiNardi, Salvatore R. (Ed.) (1998). *The Occupational Environment—its evaluation and control.* American Industrial Hygiene Association, Fairfax, Virginia. ISBN 0-932627-82-X.

- Help from NIOSH

  The NIOSH telephone number is a toll-free technical information service that provides convenient public access to NIOSH and its information resources. 1-800-35-NIOSH (800-356-4674)

  The NIOSH website is: http://www.cdc.gov/niosh/homepage.html This website provides an excellent portal to information on chemicals and toxicity.

- Help from colleagues

  Duke University has pioneered an Occupational and Environmental Medicine List Service that now has over 2800 participants and provides a vibrant daily forum for professionals. Participants include clinicians, public health experts, and hygiene and safety professionals from 60 nations. Members seem ready and capable to offer information and technical expertise to professional colleagues on a broad range of subjects. See their website: http://occhealthnews.net

CONCLUSIONS

Field investigations in the workplace, like all other epidemiologic endeavors, share a reliance on basic methods of epidemiology used wisely as part of logical problem solving. While one would like to conclude that one needs only professional capability in epidemiology to work successfully in workplace investigations, that would be naive. Little in medical training and probably less in academic epidemiologic training prepares the investigator with a sufficient understanding of industrial processes, chemical toxicities, mechanisms of toxicity, industrial processes and their failures, personal protective devices and their deficiencies, and complex social and political organizations. At a minimum, to work in the occupational arena, one should form a team with an industrial hygienist. Expertise on interpretation of the social and economic complexities of the workplace is more difficult to find. You should avoid advice to stay neutral between the interests of labor and industry. Rather you should stay dedicated to the goal of prevention. In doing so you will find allies among both labor and industry and probably do an effective job in the epidemiologic investigation.

REFERENCES

1. Rutstein, D., Mullan, R., Frazier, T., et al. (1983). The sentinel health event (occupational): a framework for occupational health surveillance and education. *J Am Public Health Assoc* 73 1054–62.
2. Halperin, W.E. (1996). The role of surveillance in the hierarchy of prevention. *Am J Ind Med* 29, 321–23.
3. Ward, E., Carpenter, A., Markowitz, S., et al. (1991). Excess bladder cancer in workers exposed to ortho-toluidine and aniline. *J Nat Cancer Inst* 83, 501–6.
4. Fingerhut, M., Halperin, W., Marlow, D., et al. (1991). Mortality among U.S. workers employed in the production of chemicals contaminated with 2,3,7,8–tetrachlorodibenzo-p-dioxin (TCDD). *N Engl J Med* 324, 212–18.
5. Rosenman, K. (2001). Evaluation of the effectiveness of following up laboratory reports of elevated blood leads in adults. American Industrial Hygiene Association Journal 62:371–8.

18

FIELD INVESTIGATIONS FROM THE STATE AND LOCAL HEALTH DEPARTMENT PERSPECTIVE

Jeffrey P. Davis
Guthrie S. Birkhead

The underpinnings of state and local public health practice involve disease surveillance and epidemic field investigations, both of which can occur virtually anywhere and any time. The frequency and breadth of these activities throughout the United States far exceed what is done at the federal level. For example, in New York State several hundred outbreaks or "events" are reported each year that require some level of investigation, often by a local health unit. These range from relatively mundane and routine to highly charged and compelling. When new diseases or routes of transmission are discovered, this often grows out of an investigation beginning at the local level. You can never know, when the first call arrives, how big or important the investigation will become.

Working and networking diligently with colleagues and appropriately communicating ideas and information across jurisdictional lines and between scientific disciplines are key to the success of state and local field epidemiologic activities. However, you should be aware of certain critical factors that can provide new insights into the conduct of even the most routine investigations and related activities. The following framework for investigations in this field and discussion of issues in state and local surveillance are not intended to be comprehensive, but they should give you some insight into this area and help you focus on the realities of conducting these activities in the early 2000s. We have also selected some examples among the many consequential field investigations conducted by state and local field epidemiologists and their partners to illustrate the issues. Although we use the words state and federal throughout the chapter, they are completely interchangeable with provincial and national. Many of the issues discussed here apply, to a greater or lesser degree, to other countries and jurisdictions and their various constituents.

THE FRAMEWORK FOR FIELD EPIDEMIOLOGY

Statutes, Regulations, Codes and Ordinances

In the United States, the Constitution does not designate protection of health as one of the powers and responsibilities assigned to the federal government. These matters are left to the states. States thus have substantial powers and duties with regard to public health matters. Each state and some cities have a code of public health laws and regulations that charges the state or local government with the responsibility of protecting the public's health[1] (see Chapter 14).

In brief, the following factors relating to statutes, regulations, health codes, and ordinances are always determinants of public health practice at the state and local level: responsibility, authority, powers, the balance of public health actions with what is necessary and justifiable (from which arises the need for good data) to avoid abuse of powers, and the need to maintain the cooperation of all involved.

Laws and regulations provide state and local health authorities with specific powers to collect health-related data, to investigate health events or disease occurrences, and to take actions to protect health. These powers can sometimes be extraordinary, and they may overcome individual rights to privacy by giving health departments the ability to collect disease reports with personally identifying information. These laws and regulations can also abridge putative personal freedoms by providing health departments the power to quarantine or to close or restrict a place of business (e.g., a restaurant) that may be a source of disease.

If you are working under the power of these statutes and regulations, you must respect and protect confidentiality or risk losing cooperation of health care providers and the public—both essential to the success of your efforts. For example, the Minnesota Department of Health has a long history of reading a carefully worded statement to potential respondents during telephone interviews that states cooperation is voluntary and information will not be released in identified form (K. Moore, personal communication).

You should be frequently reminded that your primary goal in a field investigation at the state or local level is to facilitate and permit application of control measures. Research is only a secondary purpose within the context of the state or local legal framework. Nevertheless, consent from individuals to provide information about themselves is an important principle. Generally, consent is not needed for basic field investigations, although responses to questionnaires are voluntary. However, you may reach a critical point in your investigation where the line into research is crossed, thus requiring a formal consent. This situation will typically involve approval of an investigational review board.

In sum, always have a clear understanding of the legal framework in which you are collecting information and conducting investigations. In addition, you should be aware that the results of your investigation may be used to take legal action, making it important that the data are correctly collected, analyzed, and interpreted.

Fiscal and Personnel Infrastructure

The size of a health department, population served, funding opportunities, and eagerness of staff to seek resources all have a bearing on the scope of field investigations. Even in a country as rich as the United States, it is fair to say that many local and state health departments are strapped for resources (money, people, and technology) because of a chronic lack of support. In many local settings the "field investigator" is a public health nurse, sanitarian, or college graduate—all without specialized training—who often has a full-time job doing something else. Furthermore, there generally is substantial turnover of personnel at the state and local level, and it is difficult to recruit specialized staff (e.g., information systems specialists) owing in part to relatively low public sector pay scales. This creates a constant need for training. Currently Epidemic Intelligence Service (EIS) officers from CDC, former EIS officers, preventive medicine residents, and persons with masters degrees in public health or comparable training are key to maintaining and strengthening the epidemiologic workforce at the state and local levels.

Much field investigation capability at the state and, to lesser extent, the local level is funded by federal dollars.[2] So state and local agencies need to be able to "pounce" when funding becomes available. In recent years, categorical federal funds, focused on emerging infectious diseases and bioterrorism, have provided much needed support to many state and local health departments to enhance their investigative capabilities. Therefore, field epidemiologists need to take advantage of outbreaks or other events to help justify funding appropriate infrastructures at the state and local level. A recent example is the provision of funds from federal, state, and local governments to state and local health departments in the eastern United States for surveillance and vector control following the emergence in 1999 of the West Nile virus.

Effectiveness of Collaboration

A team effort is critical at state and local levels to conduct successful field investigations. The members of the team typically include epidemiologists, laboratory workers, sanitary engineers, environmental experts, information systems specialists, statisticians, media relations staff, attorneys or legal advisors, and additional support staff depending on the type of problem being investigated. In large or potentially important outbreaks, team members may include representatives from state and local health jurisdictions; other state/local agencies, such as those responsible for natural resources, the environment, conservation, or agriculture; and, as needed, police agencies and the Federal Bureau of Investigation.

You need to be comfortable working as part of the team and communicating with your counterparts to explain the strengths and weaknesses of the epidemiologic data. This often involves both learning the vernacular of different disciplines on the team and teaching the epidemiologic principles involved.

Networking and Information Sharing

Networking at the local level follows from the need for teamwork. Also, because many public health problems cross jurisdictional boundaries, good communication across city, county, regional, and state borders is necessary. Historically, state health departments have these responsibilities within states, and the CDC and other federal agencies (the Food and Drug Administration, the Department of Agriculture, and the Environmental Protection Agency) have these responsibilities at the national level. The CDC may become directly involved in state or local investigations at the invitation of the state epidemiologist and is often relied upon to provide technical and laboratory assistance even without direct investigative involvement. Because of complex networks, increasing sources of relevant information, and templates (e.g., standard questionnaires) that are readily available to field investigators, some information sharing and organizing tools are essential to enhance networking processes—particularly those that are Internet related. These include the *Epi Info*[3] computer software for outbreak investigation and the recently developed Epi-X system[4] developed by CDC to improve communication about currently active outbreak investigations (see Chapter 12). Electronic mail list-serves such as *Promed* provide a valuable communication forum on emerging public health threats.

Information Transfer and the Rapidity of Technologic Advances

Health-care systems

Economic trends and pressures within the health-care system, such as the emergence of managed care in the private and public sectors, have created the need for state and local field epidemiologists to find, understand, and use the resulting databases and information. Furthermore, computers, data transmission, and data storage technology coupled with standard software analytic packages have facilitated the increasing use of large databases (e.g., hospital discharge) by state and local epidemiologists. One use of these databases has been to evaluate the surveillance of a wide variety of diseases. For example, New York State was able to measure the completeness of meningococcal disease reporting by comparing traditional disease reports with computerized hospital discharge records.[5] Hospital charts were reviewed to confirm the diagnosis of meningococcal disease and to match surveillance records for 1991. Using methods for comparing reports of the same disease events from different, independent data systems (the Chadra–Sekar–Deming, or capture–recapture, method), the completeness of surveillance reporting of meningococcal disease in the state was found to be 93%.

There can be pitfalls, however, when you use large electronic databases. Coding issues, for example, can challenge you, depending on the underlying purpose for which the data were gathered. Merging and integrating data from different sources are difficult to do and require complementary database design and trained staff, who may not be available at the state or local level. Examples of both the potential promise and the pitfalls of electronic data for field epidemiologic investigations are described later in this chapter.

Other data sources and technologies

Standard field-tested instruments are of great value in fieldwork. Many state and large local health departments have developed a standard format for field questionnaires. Excellent examples are found in the *Epi Info*[3] package and the comprehensive and user-friendly Minnesota Standard Foodborne Disease Exposure Questionnaire that can be readily customized for use in the field (K. Smith, personal communication). A standardized questionnaire is also found in the *Foodborne Disease Handbook*.[6]

You should also be aware of a number of available resources regarding late-breaking health issues. Most state and many local health departments publish weekly, biweekly, or monthly reports that contain descriptions of important local health events. The CDC, in *The Morbidity and Mortality Weekly Report (MMWR)* and in the *MMWR Recommendations and Reports* series, publishes a wide variety of health-related information from local to international jurisdictions on late-breaking issues, secular trends, and recommendations related to prevention and control of many health concerns. The *MMWR* can be accessed at http: www. cdc.gov/mmwr. The *Emerging Infectious Disease* journal published by CDC and accessible at http: www.cdc.gov/eid is another source, an on-line journal for field epidemiologists who want to keep up with the latest investigations in the emerging infectious disease world. *Promed* is an electronic mail list-serve for exchange of information or posing questions, again in the emerging infectious disease area.

The *Epidemiology Monitor Newsletter* is a good source of information on available software, job openings, and other issues of interest.

The state or local public health laboratory is also a data source and an important partner. The rapid advances in DNA-based technology, such as pulsed-field gel electrophoresis (PFGE) and the emergence of networks to share data electronically (Pulsenet and Foodnet), have provided state health departments with much improved opportunities to prevent and control recently identified infections, keep up with new technologies, and communicate disease-related information. Concomitantly, these advances provide new challenges to respond adequately to field investigation and surveillance findings.

Politics: Local, State, Federal

Politics is omnipresent particularly at the state and local level, because most authorities responsible for public health (commissioners) report to political leaders. Nevertheless, objective data and information generated through rigorous field investigation can be used to educate and persuade, as needed, even in politically charged settings.

Examples of typical or common political issues for the field epidemiologist include territorial problems between large city and state health departments that can intensify when both health agencies will need to commit substantial resources to investigate an outbreak or other health event or when the timely sharing of information is integral. Generally, political considerations increase as the number of involved agencies and levels of government increase.

Naturally, there are varying views of the role of federal agencies by state and local level health officials, but efforts to generate positive partnerships are nearly always prudent and benefit the public's health. When federal resources are needed, the field epidemiologist may need to contend with pressure exerted by state or local policy makers characterized by "We do not need any help from anyone." When there is a good track record of cooperation and benefit from such assistance, it is important to emphasize prudently, if not extol, the virtues of such assistance. Conversely, when resources are limited, the pressure might be its corollary: "Why can't you do it? That's what the state is paying you to do!" Federal support in the form of assistance from federally assigned epidemiologists works best when there is continued participation and involvement by state or local field epidemiologists.

Whenever cooperation is needed, there are potential problems involving possession of data, authorship, responsibility, accountability, and other comparable issues. It is always valuable to discuss these issues early during an investigation or collaboration to obviate later concerns and to clarify roles that can ultimately enhance the conduct of the investigation.

Media

Working cooperatively with the media is valuable and important at the state and local level. Within states the types and markets of the media vary as do the catchment areas. Even so, the media are often instrumental in conveying important public health messages that can help you investigate successfully and implement control measures. The messages can be directive ("anyone who was sick, call this number" or "go to this location at such and such a time to get your immunization") or instructive, that is, the media can also give to the public information needed during an investigation. During a pressing investigation, the media may seek increased access to you and your team. At that time, it is useful to create a specific time interval each day for the media to have access to the appropriate spokesperson of the team. In brief, you will need to keep the media informed. Patiently working with the media to assure the clearest of messages is key (see Chapter 13).

ISSUES RELATED TO STATE AND LOCAL SURVEILLANCE

Public health surveillance, a critical activity for the field epidemiologist at all levels of government, is a core public health function as defined by the Institute of Medicine in its 1988 report, *The Future of Public Health*.[7] Historically, surveillance efforts in the United States had their beginnings in the late 1700s and early 1800s and became more codified and universal in the late 1800s and early 1900s. These efforts took the form of requirements for investigating and reporting of specific diseases where public health measures like quarantine could be applied (e.g., smallpox, cholera). This direct link between surveillance and disease control activities currently remains an important feature of state and local public health practice.

The authority to conduct surveillance and require disease reporting is found in state laws and regulations. Some large cities also have health codes promulgated by boards of health that mandate surveillance activities. Ideally, these same laws and regulations specify the purposes for surveillance. State and local laws permit certain actions to manage disease threats and to specify the confidentiality protections for surveillance data. A model state statute on privacy of surveillance data has been proposed by CDC to aid states in ensuring that the confidentiality of surveillance data are adequately protected.

A common misconception is that placing a disease or health event on a list of reportable conditions automatically means that it is under surveillance. True public health surveillance, as defined in Chapter 3, is not being practiced simply because a report is required from a health care provider. Resources must be available to set up surveillance systems, train staff and reporters, ensure timely analysis and dissemination of the data, and take appropriate action. Without each of these steps in place, a new reporting system will founder.

Physicians and other health care providers have historically not been effective disease reporters. Results of several statewide studies have demonstrated that a smaller proportion of communicable disease reports (only 6%–10%) originate from a physician's office compared to those (71%–77%) originating from clinical laboratories.[8,9] Lack of knowledge about reporting and lack of incentives or time to report are common reasons given by physicians for not reporting.[10,11] Some studies have examined ways to improve physician reporting. Active surveillance, such as regular telephone calls to solicit reports, may result in increased reporting, but this approach is expensive and may not have a lasting effect if not continued.[8] For these reasons, in the future, surveillance systems should try to harness data available in electronic form from laboratories, hospitals, and managed care plans wherever possible. However, you should not give up the traditional system of reporting by physicians, particularly for conditions that are not diagnosed by laboratory testing or may not result in hospitalization. The newer systems of reporting laboratory and health-care data can serve as an adjunct to the old system of reporting by individual physicians, but not as a replacement for it.

Maintaining the confidentiality of surveillance data is particularly important. While reporting is often a requirement of the system, surveillance and subsequent disease control efforts work best when those who report and the public cooperate. Breaches of confidentiality may damage the trust between these providers and the public health department. You should be aware that when analyzing data from small geographic or population areas, individuals may be identifiable by using small numbers in some table cells. This was a particular concern in the early phase of the AIDS epidemic. Most state health departments and CDC have now developed data release policies that limit small cell sizes in tabulated data.

Funding for surveillance at the state and local level has been irregular and uncoordinated at best. For example, much of the specific funding support for infectious diseases surveillance comes from the federal government.[2] Many of these federal surveillance dollars are attached to categorical disease control programs (e.g., tuberculosis, AIDS/HIV, vaccine preventable diseases). You should make every effort to coordinate and, if possible, integrate funding streams to develop core surveillance capacities in your health department. In the late 1990s and early 2000s, several federal grant programs acknowledged this need for integration and coordination, for example, bioterrorism preparedness and the National Electronic Disease Surveillance System (NEDSS).

ATTRIBUTES OF SUCCESSFUL STATE AND LOCAL FIELD EPIDEMIOLOGY PROGRAMS

At the risk of being prescriptive and encroaching on the definition of field epidemiologic capacity, we describe a variety of factors that can serve as goals and markers for a successful field epidemiology program.

Goals

The field epidemiologist and field epidemiology programs:

- Foster a rich array of collaborative opportunities to benefit the public's health
- Have support from political leadership, the medical community, and the general public
- Have access to adequate training
- Promote good working relationships with laboratories and other partners
- Have the ability to analyze and disseminate findings in timely fashion
- Have adequate staffing, resources, and a team approach

Markers for Success

The field epidemiologist:

- Has a considerable breadth of knowledge and is aware of cutting edge issues
- Is mindful of traditional and emerging non-traditional partners
- Uses all opportunities to extend his or her ability to answer important public health questions

EXAMPLES OF INVESTIGATIONS BY STATE AND LOCAL HEALTH DEPARTMENT FIELD EPIDEMIOLOGISTS

1. *State Responses to a Rapidly Emerging Disease: Wisconsin, Minnesota, and Iowa Responses to Toxic Shock Syndrome.*   In December 1979, the Wisconsin Division of Health (DOH) received a call describing three hospitalized women from Madison, all of whom had rapid onset of fever, hypotension, erythroderma, and delayed desquamation of the palms and soles. The year before a similar syndrome in children had been described by Todd and was named toxic shock syndrome (TSS).[12] Apart from Madison residence, the only readily apparent common factor among these patients was being a woman. Because of the ex-

treme rarity of this condition and the clustering of cases in women, an immediate field investigation began.

Record reviews rapidly generated four more cases in Madison hospitals; all had occurred within 6 months and were in females. Epidemiologic interviews revealed that six patients had been menstruating at onset of illness, and two had similar but milder illnesses during prior menstrual periods, suggesting the syndrome could recur. Because of the severity, rarity, and apparent newness of this syndrome, the DOH then informed all Wisconsin physicians of these patients, provided management recommendations, and established criteria for immediate statewide TSS surveillance.[13]

In Minnesota, also in December, five women with similar illnesses were hospitalized and subsequently were determined to have onsets during menstruation. These 12 cases from the two states and their apparent association of illness with menstruation was reported to CDC in January by the state epidemiologists of Wisconsin and Minnesota. These reports served as the stimulus for the creation of a nationwide program of surveillance for TSS by CDC.[14]

Retrospective assessment of menstrual and other possible risk factors for TSS was now needed, and the Wisconsin DOH conducted a case-control study in winter and early spring of 1980.[13] Thirty-five of 38 reported cases of TSS occurred during menstruation. Among menstruating women, 34 of 35 patients used tampons during every menstrual period compared to 80 of 105 controls ($p < .001$). TSS rates among women under 30 years old were 2.4- to 3.3-fold greater than among women 30 years old or older. Peak rates of nearly 15 cases per 100,000 menstruating women per year were noted among women 15–19 years old who were regular users of tampons. Lastly, analysis of tampon brand data in this study did not implicate a specific brand.[13]

By May 1980, 55 cases had been reported nationwide including 31 from Wisconsin; 52 (95%) cases occurred in women; and 38 (95%) of 40 with known histories had onset during menses.[15] By June 1980, the use of tampons as a risk factor for TSS was corroborated in a national case-control study conducted by CDC. This study also showed no significant differences in brand use.[14] In September 1980, CDC reported results of a second case-control study that corroborated earlier findings regarding menses and tampon use as TSS risk factors. The results showed that, although cases occurred in association with multiple brands of tampons, significantly more cases compared to age-matched controls reported using Rely brand tampons; and that the relative risk of developing TSS was greater with use of Rely brand tampons when compared to other brands.[16] In mid-September the manufacturer of Rely brand tampons voluntarily withdrew the product from the market.

Meanwhile, during August 1980 epidemiologists from the Minnesota, Wisconsin, and Iowa state health departments with university colleagues in each of the states initiated a multistate collaborative comprehensive study of menses-associated TSS risk factors.[17] The Tri-State TSS Study included the use of proprietary tampon fluid capacity (as a measure of absorbency) and the chemical composition associated with all brand styles of tampons that had been used in the marketplace up to early September. Eighty women with TSS and 160 age- and sex-matched neighborhood controls were selected. The odds ratio for developing menstrual TSS with any tampon use compared to no tampon use was 18.0 ($p <$ .001). When individual tampon brand use was compared to no tampon use, the brand-specific odds ratios ranged from 5.9 to 27.2, and odds ratios for individual brand style use compared to no tampon use ranged from 2.6 to 34.5. In multivariate analysis, tampon fluid capacity (absorbency) and Rely brand tampon use were the only variables that significantly increased the relative risk of TSS; the risk associated with Rely brand tampon use was greater than that predicted by absorbency alone.[17]

Each of the studies used highly comparable TSS case definitions. Despite divergent methods, the association of menstrual TSS with tampon use was established in six different case-control studies (four state-based studies conducted in five states and two CDC studies) by late 1980. The Tri-State TSS Study provides a superb example of an interstate–interagency collaborative field investigation that contributed seminal information for the prevention and control of TSS nationwide.

2. State and Local Collaboration to Investigate and Analyze Disease Outbreaks: The New York State Department of Health-led Investigation of Widespread Shellfish-Associated Outbreaks.

A good example of state and local collaborative relationships occurred throughout New York State attendant to widespread outbreaks of gastroenteritis in 1982.

By way of background, the New York State Department of Health has a communicable disease epidemiology unit that oversees statewide surveillance and outbreak investigation activities. The 57 counties of New York State and the City of New York each have a public health officer who, under state law, acts as an agent of the state health commissioner. Each county has one or more communicable disease control specialists who are often public health nurses or sanitarians, particularly in rural areas of the state. Each county collects disease reports, conducts surveillance, performs outbreak investigations, and applies appropriate public health control measures. Only a few counties have public health laboratory services.

In the summer of 1982, this communicable disease surveillance and control system in New York was challenged by the occurrence of widespread outbreaks of gastroenteritis thought to be due to consumption of contaminated shellfish.[18] As the number of outbreaks reported to the county health departments increased in early summer of 1982, the state epidemiologists suspected a possible link between the outbreaks. However, it appeared that the source of the outbreaks would be difficult to determine because local health departments might not be conducting investigations in a standardized fashion. To ensure comparability, the state established a system to collect standard epidemiologic data, laboratory samples, and environmental information to trace the source of implicated shellfish. Standard epidemiologic case definitions, data collection tools, and analytic protocols for case-control studies were developed and disseminated to county health departments. Procedures for the proper collection, storage, and shipping of stool, blood, and food samples were developed; and special specimen containers were distributed. Standard procedures were designed to obtain shipping tags and other information to trace the origin of implicated lots of shellfish. Telephone and on-site technical assistance was provided by state staff to ensure proper application of the various protocols.

Using a standard protocol, 21 county health departments in New York investigated and reported 103 outbreaks of gastroenteritis that were definitely or probably associated with shellfish consumption. More than 1000 ill persons were interviewed statewide. In most cases the clinical and epidemiologic characteristics of these outbreaks were typical of Norwalk viruslike illness. Laboratory diagnosis of Norwalk virus was made in five of seven outbreaks when laboratory specimens were available. Norwalk virus was identified in shellfish specimens from two outbreaks. Northeastern U.S. coastal waters were the source of the shellfish when the source could be determined. Heavy spring rains with runoff into shellfish beds in 1982 may have been responsible for the widespread outbreaks.

The availability of high-quality epidemiologic and laboratory data from these outbreaks permitted the state health department to confidently warn consumers about the risks of raw or undercooked shellfish consumption, to strengthen record keeping procedures for selling shellfish, and to block the sale of shellfish from implicated beds.

3. Mobilization of State/Local Field Epidemiologists to Investigate a Large-Scale Outbreak: Typhoid Fever among Conventioneers, New York 1989.

Large-scale communicable disease outbreaks constitute one of the true public health emergencies that a state or local health department may face. Epidemiologic forces must be marshaled quickly to get and analyze data from large numbers of persons at risk, to provide real-time information to release to the public, and to apply the correct control and prevention measures. Under conditions like these you may face some of the greatest challenges of your professional career.

An example of effective statewide mobilization occurred during the 1989 outbreak of typhoid fever among 10,000 conventioneers in New York.[19] This outbreak was detected when two persons with typhoid fever were reported to the state health department from different hospitals in Syracuse, New York, on the Friday evening after the Fourth of July. Typhoid fever is rarely reported in the

United States in persons without a history of recent international travel, and neither of the patients had traveled out of the state recently. However, both had attended a convention of fire fighters in the Catskill region of New York 3 weeks before the onsets of their illnesses. Initial information indicated that over 10,000 persons had attended that convention, and additional case reports among attendees were being reported to the health department within a day or two of the initial reports. Because typhoid fever is an unusual and potentially fatal illness that physicians may not easily recognize and is often spread to others by a carrier; and because transmission had very possibly been ongoing for 3 weeks, potentially exposing tens of thousands of visitors to this resort area, a full-scale field investigation was immediately started.

During the weekend following receipt of the initial reports, the state health department mobilized multiple teams to start immediate investigation of the outbreak. All county health departments in the state and epidemiologists in neighboring states were contacted by one team to report possibly related cases to the New York State Department of Health. Standard data collection tools were disseminated, and stool specimens were requested for laboratory analysis. A second team began several cohort studies by telephone, using lists of fire fighters who had attended the convention, as well as other convention groups that had met at the resort before or after the fire fighters group. The fire fighters convention had occurred 3 weeks previously, and all attendees had returned to their homes throughout New York and the northeastern United States. The analysis sought to determine the duration, the time of exposure, and the origin of the epidemic, as well as possible vehicles of infection. A third field team began investigating the resort area, administering questionnaires, and collecting blood and stool specimens from staff at the suspect hotel where the first reported typhoid cases had stayed. This team also helped conduct an environmental investigation of the hotel kitchen and potable water supply.

A total of 44 culture-confirmed and 24 probable primary typhoid fever cases were reported in the outbreak from New York, several neighboring states, and Canada, making it the largest outbreak of typhoid fever in the United States in a decade. While complete reporting of the cases took several weeks, the initial telephone survey was completed and analyzed within 24 hours, implicating Hotel A as the source of the outbreak. A second telephone survey of Hotel A guests identified a 48 hour time period as the likely period of transmission; no cases were found in persons staying at the hotel before or after this time period. The case-control study implicated orange juice as the likely vehicle (Odds Ratio = 5.6, 95% CI 1.1–54.7), and investigation of hotel employees revealed that the one and only ill employee had drunk orange juice. Another employee who prepared the orange juice had a positive stool culture for *Salmonella typhi*, the causative organism. This employee had no symptoms, was probably a typhoid carrier, and was presumed to have caused the outbreak.

Epidemiologists from the New York State Department of Health, several county health departments within New York, neighboring states, and CDC collaborated in the investigation of the outbreak, demonstrating that a large epidemiologic effort can be organized and conducted in a few days. The field studies provided critical information during the initial phase of the epidemic investigation: disease transmission was time limited, no other groups or time periods were implicated, the vehicle and source of the infection were identified quickly, and the culture-positive kitchen employee was removed from food preparation duties.

4. Modern Social and Technologic Advances in the Investigation of Disease Outbreaks: A Hepatitis A Outbreak in New York with a Distinctly Old-Fashioned Cause. Computers are now a familiar and tremendously useful tool of the epidemiologist. The laptop computer may become as ubiquitous a symbol of the field epidemiologist as the worn-out shoe leather of old. Computers have become indispensable for tabulation of questionnaire responses and for analysis of outbreak data (see Chapter 12). However, as the computerization of all aspects of society increases and computer records are kept for even the most mundane commercial transactions, the potential for use of data already stored and available in the field also increases.

A good example of the value of recent technological advances occurred during a large hepatitis A outbreak in the Rochester, New York, area in 1994 among patrons of a retail buyers club.[20] Retail buyers clubs are large, members-only department stores and supermarkets. These clubs verify membership at the point of sale and can maintain detailed records of each member's purchases and often use them to market items to specific members based on their buying history. These data may also be useful to confirm potential exposure (at least purchase, if not consumption) to food items suspected in a food-borne outbreak. Such databases also establish a cohort that can be used for calculating rates of disease or serve as a sampling frame for epidemiologic studies.

In the spring of 1994, routine surveillance follow-up by the Monroe County Health Department staff of persons with reported hepatitis A revealed that a number of the persons either were coworkers at Buying Club A in Rochester or had purchased food from the club. The county health department then reviewed all recently reported hepatitis A cases in the Monroe County area where Rochester is located. Between April 9 and May 31, 79 cases of hepatitis A had been reported in Monroe and surrounding counties. Nine of the cases occurred in employees of Buying Club A, and 55 occurred in persons who ate food purchased at the club. To confirm the possible association of illness with the club, laboratory-confirmed hepatitis A cases were compared to controls matched by telephone prefix and interviewed by telephone. Eleven of 17 case households reported buying food at the club compared to 7 of 34 control households (matched Odds Ratio = 8.5, 95%

CI 1.7–41.6). Cases by date of onset are shown in Figure 18–1 suggesting a common source of exposure.[20] To help identify food items as possible sources, a questionnaire was administered to the cohort of all employees. A history of eating any sugar-glazed item from the club bakery was associated with a relative risk of 4.4 (95% CI 1.2–15.9) for developing hepatitis A. No other food items were positively associated with illness.

Further investigation revealed that a food handler reported being ill with diarrhea, though jaundice was not noticed, approximately one month before the first club-associated cases began to occur (Figure 18–1). His duties during this time period included applying sugar glaze by hand to freshly baked items after cooking. Although the food worker professed to wearing plastic gloves for this task, other workers said that gloves were not always used. Furthermore, facilities for hand washing were not optimally designed and were reportedly used infrequently. Subsequently, the blood of the food handler was found to have antibodies to hepatitis A indicative of recent infection, leading to the conclusion that he was the source of the outbreak.

Although this investigation clearly implicated a logical source and mode of transmission of the hepatitis epidemic, the exact food item(s) and dates of purchase were not yet known. Since recall of food histories and other events fade with time— and because the incubation period of hepatitis A ranges from 15 to 50 days—it was decided not to administer a questionnaire to club members but, rather, to analyze computer purchasing records for this information. Record review showed that

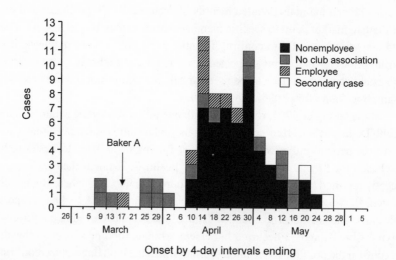

Figure 18–1. Cases of laboratory-confirmed acute hepatitis A by date of onset, greater Rochester area, New York, March 1–May 31, 1994. [*Source:* Weltman et al., 1996.[20] Used with permission.]

42 club members with hepatitis had purchased sugar-glazed products from the bakery during the period in question. The dates of purchase were compared to the dates that the implicated employee worked in the bakery. All but 3 of the 42 members with hepatitis A purchased glazed bakery products during one or both time periods (March 10–12 and March 21–24) that the employee was working and presumably infectious.[20] This information strengthened the conclusion that the outbreak was due to glazed products from the bakery prepared by this employee.

As computerized records of commercial transactions become more common, you should be aware of the potential uses of these data in outbreak investigations. Large buying clubs and other "mega-stores," in particular, may have very detailed data available on purchases by their members. This is fortunate, since these stores serve large numbers of people with the potential for widespread transmission of food-borne agents, if strict hygienic standards are not maintained. An interesting sidelight of the Monroe County investigation was the mechanism of transmission of hepatitis A by hand contamination in preparing sugar-glazed baked products. A similar mechanism of transmission was found during the classic food-borne outbreak investigation in West Branch, Michigan in 1968.[21,22] It seems that even though technology and computers are changing the world, some mechanisms of disease transmission never change.

5. The Potential Pitfalls of Using Administrative Data for Public Health Surveillance: A Pseudo-Outbreak of Cholera in New York State, 1991.

The decade of the 1990s saw a dramatic increase in use of electronic systems to capture health-care system data. Administrative data, such as health insurance billing claims, is one source of computerized information available for analysis and for control of health-care costs. Field epidemiologists have been encouraged to look at electronic systems of health data as a potential way to conduct public health surveillance. Such systems have the advantage of containing data on large numbers of persons, if not populationwide data. These data may be more or less readily available to you (usually some red tape is involved in gaining access) and can be analyzed by computer. However, you must exercise great care in using such data for public health purposes, including surveillance, as the following example illustrates.

In 1993, the communicable disease unit at the New York State Department of Health examined electronic health data for possible use as a supplement to existing reportable disease surveillance systems. Data were obtained from the fiscal intermediary for health insurance claims for 950,000 New York state and municipal employees, retirees, and their dependents for 1991. The analysis plan was to examine ICD-9 diagnostic codes from the insurance data for reportable communicable diseases and to compare these data with communicable disease cases reported to the state's communicable disease surveillance system. Table 18–1 shows the

Table 18–1.   Health Insurance Billing Claims and Public Health
Surveillance Reports for Selected Reportable Communicable
Diseases, New York, 1991

ICD CODE	DIAGNOSIS	INSURANCE CLAIMS*		SURVEILLANCE REPORTS[†]	
		PATIENTS	RATE	PATIENTS	RATE
001	Cholera	35	3.7	0	0.0
002	Typhoid	5	0.5	86	0.5
003	Salmonella	58	6.1	3474	19.3
004	Shigella	24	2.5	1058	5.9

*Health insurance billing claims for New York State and municipal employ-
ees, retirees, and their dependents. Rate per 100,000 insured persons.

[†]Public health surveillance reports for New York State excluding New York
City. Rate per 100,000 population. [*Source*: New York State Department
of Health.]

number of billing claims in the insurance database for 1991 for four reportable
communicable diseases: cholera, typhoid, salmonella, and shigella. The rate per
insured person for each disease was compared to the statewide disease rate calculated from the reportable disease surveillance data. Disease rates were lower, but
of the same order of magnitude, in the insurance data for salmonella and shigella,
and were the same for typhoid. However, the insurance data contained 35 patients
with a diagnosis of cholera with an ICD-9 code of 001, where none had been reported in the state that year through the traditional surveillance system.

To check the validity of the billing codes further, the insurance records were
examined to see if a stool culture was done, which is needed to confirm a diagnosis of any of these conditions. This was determined by looking for billing codes
for stool cultures in the insurance data. Of salmonella insurance claims, only 29%
reported a stool culture. The proportion was less for the other diseases (cholera:
3%, typhoid: 0%, shigella: 13%). These findings seriously challenged the validity of the diagnoses contained in the insurance database.

The cholera cases were of particular concern. No cases of cholera had been
reported in New York that year, but it is possible that the diagnosis had been missed
because physicians in the United States may not think of cholera in the differential diagnosis of watery diarrhea and may not order the appropriate laboratory tests.
However, this number of missed cases would constitute a public health emergency
and cast serious doubt on the traditional surveillance system. To gain further insight, detailed ICD-9 4-digit codes were examined. Of the 35 cholera patients, 25
(71%) were reported with an ICD-9 code of 001.1, indicating *V. cholerae*, el Tor
strain, a particularly virulent strain of cholera of major worldwide importance.
Particularly puzzling, moreover, was the fact that many of these records contained

a medical procedure billing code for "destruction by any method including laser, of benign facial lesions or premalignant lesions"—a procedure clearly unrelated to cholera. The investigators then realized that, while ICD-9 001.1 coded for cholera, ICD-9 110.0 coded for "dermatophytosis including infection by trychophyton, etc."—a condition that might fit better with the procedure code for treatment of benign facial lesions. They surmised that a simple numerical transposition of the ICD-9 disease code, as might occur in manual data entry, might have been responsible for the apparent pseudo-outbreak of cholera.

Computers and computerized databases are a boon to the field epidemiologist. However, using these databases may have pitfalls. It is incumbent on you, the field epidemiologist to learn as much about such databases as possible. Know where the data originate, how they are entered and handled, how they are checked and edited, and what coding systems are used before rushing to incorporate these data in surveillance or field investigation efforts. Such data must be completely characterized as to validity, sensitivity, specificity, and predictive value before pressed into use. In the case described here, a lot of unnecessary work by public health staff would have to be done to sort out the true diagnosis. Public health departments do not have the luxury of following up on too many blind alleys of this sort.

6. Epidemiology and Laboratory Collaboration to Detect Outbreaks: The Minnesota Department of Health E. coli O157:H7 subtyping system.

The public health laboratory is a key collaborator with the field epidemiologist in detecting and controlling communicable diseases at the state and local level. A good example of collaboration between epidemiologist and laboratory staff is the system established by the Minnesota Department of Health (MDH) to detect clusters of *Escherichia coli* O157:H7 subtypes, each of which may have a common source of transmission.[23] *E. coli* O157:H7 is a significant bacterial pathogen in the United States, causing outbreaks of severe, bloody diarrhea and, uncommonly, hemolytic uremic syndrome, a complication that can cause renal failure and death. *E. coli* O157:H7 is found in the intestinal tracts of cows and other animals, and outbreaks can occur by consumption of contaminated uncooked meat, particularly ground beef, and potable or recreational water contaminated by animal feces. Prevention and control of these infections depend on surveillance for early detection of potential outbreaks and investigation of possible sources of the bacteria.

Historically, surveillance for *E. coli* O157:H7 was based on clinical reports of clusters of patients with bloody diarrhea. However, *E. coli* are common in the human intestinal tract and may not be identified as pathogens in stool specimens. Now, since the emergence of the *E. coli* O157:H7 strain as an important pathogen, clinical laboratories have been encouraged to type *E. coli* isolates or submit isolates to appropriate laboratories for typing. Over time and in many areas of Minnesota, this has provided a baseline number of *E. coli* O157:H7 isolates for temporal, geographic, and demographic analysis. For example, Figure 18–2 shows the number of *E. coli* O157:H7 reports by week for the state of Minnesota in 1995.[23]

This method of surveillance can detect large disease outbreaks, but it is limited in its ability to detect smaller clusters. For example, examination of Figure 18–2 does not suggest any clustering patterns except an increase in cases in the summer that is similar to many enteric diseases. Recognizing these limitations, epidemiologists and laboratory personnel at the MDH applied a new laboratory technique, pulsed-field gel electrophoresis (PFGE), to improve the identification procedure in hopes of uncovering disease clusters. As can be seen in Figure 18–3, this "molecular fingerprinting" technique applied to the same *E. coli* O157:H7 isolates represented in Figure 18–2 shows multiple small clusters of subtypes that are likely related to a common source. Epidemiologists can then focus on each cluster as a discrete transmission event, determine the source, and implement control measures.

In Minnesota during 1994–95, 10 outbreaks and 35 clusters of *E. coli* O157:H7 disease were detected in large part due to the application of PFGE subtyping of isolates. The public health benefits of this epidemiologic and public health laboratory collaboration included identification of a number of outbreaks traced to consumption of contaminated meat and recreational water.

SUMMARY

Beyond the disciplined application of epidemiologic methods, the conduct of field epidemiologic investigations and surveillance activities by state and local health department staff and their partners occurs within a framework that involves: understanding state and local laws and codes; awareness of personnel and resource constraints; effective collaboration, networking, and information sharing; maximizing information transfer and appropriate incorporation of technologic advances;

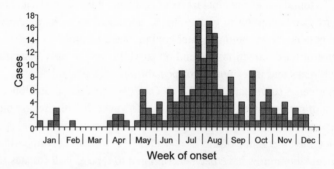

Figure 18–2. Cases of *E. coli* O157:H7 by date of onset, Minnesota, 1995. [*Source*: Bender et al., 1997.[23] Used with permission.]

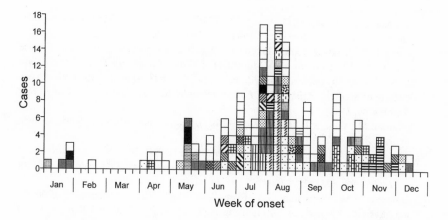

Note: Each white box represents a single, unrelated PFGE pattern, and each design represents multiple isolates of a unique PFGE pattern.

Figure 18–3. Cases of *E. coli* O157:H7 by date of onset, by pulsed-field gel electrophoresis (PFGE) type, Minnesota, 1995. [*Source*: Bender et al., 1997.[23] Used with permission.]

sensitivity to local, state, and federal political issues that are germane to field epidemiologists; and cooperative and productive working relationships using print and electronic media. Successful field epidemiologists and field epidemiology programs foster collaboration and adequate training, have broad medical and political support and adequate staffing, generate and disseminate findings and important information in a timely fashion, and use investigative opportunities to expand important public health knowledge. The legacy of investigations conducted by state and local health department field epidemiologists is truly broad, deep, rich, and rapidly expanding. This legacy will continue to serve as a premier foundation for you and all current and future field epidemiologists.

REFERENCES

1. Gostin, L.O. (2000). Public health law in a new century. Part II: public health powers and limits. *J Am Med Assoc* 283, 2979–84.
2. Osterholm, M.T., Birkhead, G.S., Meriwether, R.A. (1996). Impediments to public health surveillance in the 1990s: the lack of resources and the need for priorities. *J Public Health Manage Pract* 2, 11–15.
3. Dean, A.G., Arner, T.G., Sangam, S., et al. (2000). Epi Info 2000, a database and statistics program for public health professionals for use on Windows 95, 98, NT, and 2000 computers. Centers for Disease Control and Prevention, Atlanta.
4. Council of State and Territorial Epidemiologists. (2000). Support, development and implementation of the Epidemic Information Exchange (Epi-X). Position Statement EC-4. Available at http://www.cste.org/ps2000/2000-EC4.htm

5. Ackman, D.M., Birkhead, G., Flynn, M. (1996). Assessment of surveillance for meningococcal disease in New York, 1991. *Am J Epidemiol* 144, 78–82.
6. Morse, D.L., Birkhead, G.S., Guzewich, J.J. (2000). Investigating foodborne disease. In Y.H. Hui, J.R. Gorham, K.D. Murrell, et al. (Eds.), *Foodborne Disease Handbook: diseases caused by bacteria*, 2nd ed., vol. 1, pp. 587–643. Marcel Dekker, New York.
7. Institute of Medicine (1988). *The Future of Public Health.* National Academy Press, Washington, D.C.
8. Shramm, M., Vogt, R.L., Mamolen, J. (1991). Disease surveillance in Vermont: who reports? *Public Health Rep* 106, 95–97.
9. Harkess, J.R., Gildon, B.A., Archer, P.W., et al. (1988). Is passive surveillance always insensitive? An evaluation of shigellosis surveillance in Oklahoma. *Am J Public Health* 128, 878–81.
10. Konowitz, P.M., Petrossian, G.A., Rose, D.N. (1984). The underreporting of disease and physicians' knowledge of reporting requirement. *Public Health Rep* 99, 31–35.
11. Vogt, R.L., LaRue, D., Klaucke, D.N., et al. (1983). Comparison of an active and passive surveillance system of primary care providers for hepatitis, measles, rubella and salmonellosis in Vermont. *Am J Public Health* 73, 795–97.
12. Todd, J., Fishaut, M., Kapral, F., et al. (1978). Toxic-shock syndrome associated with phage-group-1 staphylococci. *Lancet* 2, 1116–18.
13. Davis, J.P., Chesney, P.J., Wand, P.J., et al. (1980). Toxic-shock syndrome: epidemiologic features, recurrence, risk factors, and prevention. *N Engl J Med* 303, 1429–35.
14. Shands, K.N., Schmid, G.P., Dan, B.D., et al. (1980). Toxic-shock syndrome in menstruating women: association with tampon use and *Staphylococcus aureus* and clinical features in 52 cases. *N Engl J Med* 303, 1436–42.
15. Centers for Disease Control (1980). Toxic-shock syndrome. *Morb Mortal Wkly Rep* 29, 229–30.
16. Schleck, W.F. III, Shands, K.N., Reingold, A.L., et al. (1982). Risk factors for development of toxic shock syndrome: association with a tampon brand. *J Am Med Assoc* 248, 835–39.
17. Osterholm, M.T., Davis, J.P., Gibson, R.W., et al. (1982). Tri-state Toxic-Shock Syndrome Study. I. Epidemiologic findings. *J Infect Dis* 145, 431–40.
18. Morse, D.L., Guzewich, J.J., Hanrahan, J.P., et al. (1986). Widespread outbreaks of clam- and oyster-associated gastroenteritis: role of Norwalk virus. *N Engl J Med* 314, 678–81.
19. Birkhead, G.S., Morse, D.L., Levine, W.C., et al. (1993). Typhoid fever at a resort hotel in New York: a large outbreak with an unusual vehicle. *J Infect Dis* 167, 1228–32.
20. Weltman, A.C., Bennett, N.M., Ackman, D.A., et al. (1996). An outbreak of hepatitis A associated with a bakery, New York, 1994: The 1968 "West Branch, Michigan" outbreak repeated. *Epidemiol Infect* 117, 333–41.
21. Schoenbaum, S.C., Baker, O., Jezek, Z. (1976). Common-source outbreak of hepatitis due to glazed and iced pastries. *Am J Epidemiol* 104, 74–80.
22. Roueche, B. (1982). The West Branch Study. In *The Medical Detectives*, pp. 233–52. Washington Square Press, New York.
23. Bender, J.B., Hedberg, C.W., Besser, J.M., et al. (1997). Surveillance for *Escherichia coli* O157:H7 infections in Minnesota by molecular subtyping. *N Engl J Med* 337, 388–94.

19

EPIDEMIOLOGIC INVESTIGATIONS IN INTERNATIONAL SETTINGS

Stanley O. Foster

We live in a global village. Natural disasters, outbreaks of infectious diseases, global epidemics, toxic exposures, terrorism, and civil wars have both local and global effects. Participating in investigations in areas with limited resources, that is, two-thirds of the world's population, provides unique opportunities for epidemiologists to learn about health problems in different ecologic, cultural, and resource settings; to utilize your skills in new ways; and to strengthen the epidemiologic capacities of national coworkers. The bottom line is health, as defined by the World Health Organization (WHO),[a] and strengthening the epidemiologic capacities of national colleagues.

Envision yourself assigned to investigate an epidemic of an unknown disease in an unfamiliar area of the world and in a country where both the language and the culture are different from anything you have previously experienced. Such an assignment encapsulates the challenge of field epidemiology in the international setting. Although the approach to international field investigations is similar to that described in Chapter 5, carrying out an investigation in unfamiliar settings has unique aspects.

International experience has frequently influenced the professional careers of epidemiologists. In a review of 226 international investigations carried out by

[a]"Health is a state of complete physical, mental, and social well-being, not just the absence of disease and infirmity."

CDC between 1946 and 1994, and a subsequent interview follow-up with a sample of the investigators, international experiences were identified as a seminal event in the development of the careers of most of the epidemiologists.[1]

BE PREPARED

If you have an interest in global health or are in a position that provides opportunities for global epidemiologic assistance, it is essential to be prepared, even though you never know what is coming. Twice in the author's career, Alexander D. Langmuir, the founder of the Epidemic Intelligence Service at CDC, called me and said, "If you are not on the plane by sundown, you are not going."

Being prepared to accept an international assignment often requires weeks (passport) or months (immunization). Those prepared get to go; those not prepared do not go. Preparation includes:

- an up-to-date valid passport, two photocopies of the identification page (in case the passport is stolen), and at least four extra pictures for visas;
- up-to-date immunizations for hepatitis A, hepatitis B, diphtheria, tetanus, poliomyelitis, and yellow fever (for tropical areas of Africa and South America). Rabies vaccine is recommended for veterinarians collecting specimens from animals and for joggers, and an international certificate verifying yellow fever immunization is required by international sanitary regulations;[b]
- a box of key items that you can easily forget in the last moment such as: a first-aid kit, flashlight with extra batteries, insect repellent, canteen, water purification tablets, and a solar operated calculator.

GETTING READY

Because many countries in the developing world have rudimentary disease reporting systems at best, most requests for epidemiologic assistance arise from adverse health events brought to the government's attention through the press or the political system. Outbreaks are generally of two types: (*1*) large outbreaks of a major epidemic disease (yellow fever, cholera, meningococcal meningitis) or (*2*) acute episodes of unexplained mortality, such as those caused by adulterated drugs or foods, toxic exposures, or rare hemorrhagic fevers. Detection is frequently de-

[b]A list of recommended vaccinations for adults can be found on the CDC website: http://www.cdc. gov/nip/recs/adult-schedule.pdf.

layed because of inadequate surveillance, poor communications, or the tendency of officials to overlook potential problems in the hope that the problems will eventually disappear. When the outbreaks do become public, there is often a sense of panic. For the public health official pressured to act, the arrival of technical assistance provides a visible sign of government response to the emergency. The request frequently carries with it the expectation of external resources to control the problem.

When a request for assistance is received, it is important to acknowledge receipt and provide a time frame in which a response will be forthcoming. Contact should be made with the World Health Organization (WHO), international and bilateral agencies working in the country, and the diplomatic mission to which you will be attached. These early contacts are useful in verifying the need for epidemiologic assistance; providing additional information on the outbreak; identifying other ongoing requests for assistance; and, most important, opening the channels of communication for in-country collaboration and support.

The typically short lead time between receipt of a request and departure (hours to days) requires that you prepare carefully. Place a high priority on arranging travel (some countries have only one flight in and out per week) and obtaining a visa or visas. The latter will require a current passport, passport-sized photos, and contact with the diplomatic mission accredited to grant visas. Clearances on the provision of technical assistance, preferably in writing, should be obtained from the requesting country, the funding agency, and your own supervisor. Advance information on the flight number and the arrival time should be communicated to an in-country contact with a request for airport assistance. Airport assistance will frequently reduce the hassle of immigration and customs and is especially important when the investigation requires carrying a computer (restricted in some countries); specimen collection materials such as needles, syringes; or laboratory equipment.

Your personal health merits attention. Written health guidelines for international travel are available from WHO and from many public health agencies. Sites relating to travelers' health available on the Internet can identify health hazards for individual countries. Experts on travelers' health can be found in larger health departments, major hospitals, and quarantine facilities. Travelers to malarious areas need to initiate appropriate chemoprophylaxis. If travel is to an area where *Plasmodium falciparum* is endemic and drug-resistant strains have been identified, a malaria expert should be contacted about current recommendations for chemoprophylaxis and back-up disease treatment. As medical facilities may be limited or of questionable quality in-country, you should assemble a basic medical kit for personal use that includes: a thermometer, antipyretics, antihistamines, antibiotic eye ointment, chapstick, oral rehydration salts (ORS) for treatment of dehydrating diarrheas, water purification tablets, antibiotics for severe diarrheal illness, and simple bandages.

Pack lightly. Men should include a jacket, and for women, native dress or a simple dress (long with long sleeves if custom expects it) for official visits. Take two sets of hand-washable comfortable clothes, good walking shoes, and sneakers. A small daypack and a carry-on roll-on bag are often sufficient and enable the traveler to avoid the hassle of waiting for baggage. Other important items to pack include a canteen, a flashlight with extra batteries, a Swiss Army–type knife (in checked baggage), hat, soap, towel, and plastic gloves (in case you are required to provide first aid), and an extra pair of glasses. While sunglasses are useful during travel, they are, in many cultures, a barrier to effective communication. Clear, not tinted, glasses are recommended during conversations.

As checked luggage may be delayed or lost en route, carry all essential items such as prescription medicines, one change of washable clothes, and toiletries *in your hand baggage.* If your luggage is lost, airlines will frequently provide money for an extra set of clothes. Replacements can often be obtained in the local market in a few hours.

Consider your money carefully. As credit cards and travelers' checks are not always accepted, cash may be needed. If it is possible that you will need to fund in-country travel, gasoline, or field staff, establish a mechanism for transfer of funds. For personal safety reasons, carrying large amounts of cash is not recommended. Wear a money belt. As investigations scheduled for a few weeks may on occasion last for several months, set aside one evening for family or close friends.

As international investigations frequently involve unknown or unfamiliar conditions, use the few available hours to read up on possible disease etiologies; collect a few key references; identify potential back-up technical expertise that will be available to respond if needed (e.g., epidemiologic, statistical, laboratory); and talk to individuals who have worked in the country. Depending on the nature of the request, consider the need for clerical supplies, a portable computer, and specimen collection and shipping materials. Keep a diary of events, persons met, and data in a bound notebook (loose pieces of paper can be a disaster). Be sure that any electrical equipment is compatible in voltage and plug type to what is available at your destination. Plugging a 110 volt computer into a 220 volt line will destroy the computer. It is important to back up your data on disks frequently; keep backup disks at a separate place. Computer crashes, theft, or accidents have compromised the results of many investigations. Solar calculators are an excellent investment, both for work in remote villages without electricity and as a token of appreciation for collaborating field staff.

Perhaps the most important part of the preparation is the collection of one or two books on the country and culture for reading in transit. Cultural differences are significant and important.[2,3] In certain societies, it is inappropriate to shake hands with members of the opposite sex. In others, showing the sole of your shoe is a major breach of etiquette. Mistakes will be made, but a few small steps demonstrating good faith and affirming your recognition and appreciation of the new culture will facilitate the development of effective working relationships. Knowledge of a country's history, geography, and greetings in the local language is a good place to start. Many cultures require that women's arms and legs be covered. While western dress is acceptable for women, wearing clothes similar to those of the women that you are working with is preferable and often more comfortable. Care should be taken not to wear the clothes of the elite.

E-mail and long distance telephones are both a blessing and a curse to the field epidemiologist. Both provide an opportunity to solicit information and advice that you and your national colleagues see as important. On the curse side is the tendency of some supervisors to micromanage the investigation from afar, frequently disrupting and paralyzing the collegiality of a field investigation. It is therefore important to establish ground rules with your supervisor in advance.

CHANGING DYNAMICS OF INTERNATIONAL EPIDEMIOLOGY

Over the last decade, there has been a significant shift in the role of the outside epidemiologist from that of "the outside expert" to a colleague with complementary skills. At least five changes have contributed to the strengthening of national epidemiologic competence: (1) advanced training in epidemiology at national and international academic institutions; (2) country-specific epidemiology training programs such as the Rockefeller Foundation's Schools without Walls and CDC's Field Epidemiology Training Programs; (3) global polio eradication, which has increased the understanding and practice of surveillance; (4) the global epidemic of HIV/AIDS with its broadening of epidemiology to include sentinel and behavioral surveillance; and (5) the increased access to knowledge, sharing of information, and training over the Internet.

THE FIRST DAY

The first day is important both in terms of whom you meet and the order you meet them. Critical to success is your attitude. Are you the knight in shining armor coming to solve an important problem or a colleague coming to work with national authorities to help them solve their problem?[4] The latter approach is the only appropriate one. In many cultures, it is necessary to establish rapport before proceeding with substantive discussions. Finding areas of common interest is an art that bears preparation and practice. During the protocol visits, a dependable national should be identified as responsible for the investigation. If you are not fluent in the language of the country, you will need an interpreter. Frequently, they are provided by the government. If you are responsible for recruiting an interpreter, be specific as to what you want—an individual willing to travel under difficult circumstances and to work long hours. Be sure to identify the source of funding and finalize the terms of employment in writing before departure to the field.

Before heading to the field, obtain maps, collect information on what is already known about the affected area, the health hazard, and the basic epidemiologic questions of who, what, when, and where. It is useful to determine how the outbreak came to public attention, the nature and timing of the response, and the reasons for the request. Be sure that you understand what is expected of you, and allocate top priorities to those tasks.

Logistics is a major challenge for the field epidemiologist. Request a vehicle with seat belts. Reliable transport, a driver, maps, gasoline, spare tire(s), a jack, and a lug wrench often require ingenuity and time to acquire. Do not take the driver's word that the vehicle is field ready; check out the transport yourself. Take the time to discuss with the driver your expectations regarding his driving, such as obeying the speed limit and not passing on hills. Ensuring compliance, especially during the first hour of travel, is good prevention. If the driver starts driving dangerously, ask the driver to stop. Calmly discuss again the rules of the road. The possibility of an accident in areas where blood supplies are not safe justifies expecting and enforcing safe driving practices. A reliable driver is worth his weight in gold. In most countries, it is dangerous to drive at night; so don't. If safe water and food are not available in the affected area, these, too, need to be procured in advance.

THE INVESTIGATION

Naturally, after days of preparation you will want to get on with the investigation and examine cases, however, the prelude to any field investigation is the introduction to the local authorities. These visits should be viewed not as protocol but as team recruitment. Local authorities will serve as guides, provide introductions at the community and household level, and facilitate community and family participation in the investigation. In addition, local authorities may have access to the only comfortable places to sleep and eat.

Once the existence of a health problem has been established, the next step in the investigation is the establishment of a case definition. This will require collecting a clinical history and a physical examination on several, preferably recently affected individuals. It is important to know that diseases often have a local name. For example, a search for yellow fever survivors for serologic tests in Ghana was totally unsuccessful until the investigators learned the local name—"horse-piss eye disease" (Newberry, D., personal communication). With that local definition, over 100 cases were found in an area where yellow skin, jaundice, or dark urine had failed to identify a single case. If timely laboratory support is not available, cases will usually be defined on clinical grounds. Where possible, use simple and workable definitions, such as those established by WHO. For example, the WHO case definition of poliomyelitis is acute onset of asymmetric flaccid paralysis without sensory change; that for neonatal tetanus includes breast-fed, cried normally during the first few days of life, stopped sucking, developed spasms, and died between days 3 and 21; and that for shigellosis is simply diarrhea with blood.

Once a case definition has been established, the next task is finding cases. Determining when and where cases occurred will frequently require the ingenuity and assistance of local political, religious, and traditional authorities. With a lay-adapted case definition and a list of geographic subunits (e.g., districts and villages), the challenge is to find the most efficient way to identify cases. This may utilize telephone contact among local authorities, police radio contact, or sending out traditional messengers on foot. On some occasions, it may be necessary to organize an active community-to-community search. Such surveys need to be well planned and involve several key steps: (1) recruitment and selection of personnel; (2) development and testing of the data collection instrument; (3) on-the-job training of the staff in field survey techniques; (4) utilization of field training to refine the survey instrument; and (5) mobilization of logistic support (see Chapter 11).

The conduct of the investigation will require an understanding of cultural norms and practices. For example, in some Muslim cultures, where men are not allowed to enter a house or talk to women, enumerators will have to be female. In developing the survey instrument and in carrying out interviews, knowledge of the local health belief model is useful. For individuals who traditionally attribute illness to a curse or to the supernatural, biologic causality does not make sense. You may often encounter events worthy of in-depth investigation and eventual publication. It is, however, important to give priority to the reasons for which your assistance was requested: the identification of etiology, the route of exposure, risk factors, and potential control strategies. Once an etiology is identified and control measures are agreed upon, control activities should become the primary focus of attention. Monitoring the quality and effectiveness of these control actions often requires new and creative approaches.

Fieldwork, even under ideal conditions, can be stressful. Absence from home, long hours, unfamiliar food, difficult climates, especially if accompanied by illness, often pose a health risk to the visiting epidemiologist. Consider your physical and mental well-being. A short half-day break may lead to a renewed sense of purpose and perspective. It is important to drink adequate "safe" fluids (kidney stones are an occupational hazard in dry climates). At times it will be difficult to stay calm when "things fall apart." Ability to laugh at yourself and a good sense of humor are essential.

COMMUNICATING AND REPORTING

An important aspect of the investigation is keeping those responsible informed. This includes the officials who requested the investigation, local health officials, political or traditional leaders cooperating in the investigation, and technical experts at the investigator's home institution. In areas where telephones do not exist or do not function, alternative means of communication need to be identified (e.g., police or short-wave radio). If communication is difficult, it is useful to set up a schedule for contact. Radio messages need to be discreetly worded to avoid misinterpretation by others with radio access. In some remote areas, couriers may be needed to transport messages via local transport or on foot.

Before leaving the country the investigative team has the responsibility to report the investigative findings and the recommended actions; first, to those responsible and, additionally, to others involved in the request or follow-up actions. It is important that your national counterpart have a prominent role in these debriefings. While hand-prepared audiovisuals such as transparencies are often useful in making the presentation, handouts or flip charts provide backup in case of power failure. Separate debriefings for those with different interests are often useful. This allows the debriefing messages to be targeted to meet special needs. Results of the investigation need to be clearly presented in a language understandable to the intended audience. Acknowledgments should be given to the individuals assisting in the investigation. Prepare and distribute a written draft report prior to departure. Promises of a report "next week" are seldom met, as one returns to family and long lists of urgent messages and e-mails. Delay in the availability of a report, frequently 2–3 months, compromises the implementation of recommendations.

As indicated in several chapters of this book, there is one key rule regarding the role of the visiting epidemiologist and the press: requests for information should be referred to the appropriate national authority. On rare occasions, when national authorities request a briefing with the media, the interviews should be carried out jointly.

PUBLICATION

When publication is appropriate, it needs to be sensibly handled. Authorship, including local collaborators, should be agreed to in advance. In large outbreaks, acknowledgment of the team with all contributors listed alphabetically merits consideration. In some field investigations the laboratory component deserves separate treatment in a companion article. All articles need clearance in writing from both the host country and the visiting epidemiologist's institution prior to publication.

MAINTAINING PERSPECTIVE

As a visiting epidemiologist, your salary may be 50–100 times that of your national colleagues. Living and working in such a situation require both wisdom and tact. Acceptance of hospitality from an impoverished village leader is difficult but necessary. As the leader's youngest children may go hungry when visitors are fed, a modest appetite is suggested. Maintaining team rapport often requires accepting accommodations that national team members can afford, rather than "fancy hotels." Small tokens of appreciation such as picture books of your city or country, commemorative stamps, postcards, or solar calculators are appropriate gifts. Except for drivers, monetary gifts are not recommended. Always carry a few family pictures both to keep in touch and to share.

On your return home, thank-you notes, technical publications, copies of photographs, provide appreciation and continuity to friendships that have developed.

SUMMARY

The opportunity to participate in epidemiologic investigations in cultures and countries other than your own is one of the challenges and rewards of epidemiology. During such investigations, you are a guest, whose responsibility is to work with national colleagues in solving their problems. This chapter describes practical steps for the field epidemiologist: getting ready, the first day in country, carrying out the field investigation, and communicating results.

REFERENCES

1. Foster, S.O., Gangarosa, E. (1996). Passing the epidemiologic torch from Farr to the world, the legacy of Alexander D. Langmuir. *Am J Epidemiol* 144 , S65–S73.
2. Brislin, R.W. (1982). *Cross-cultural Encounters*. Pergamon Press, New York.
3. Allegra, D.T., Nieburg, P., Grabe, M. (Eds.) (1984). Emergency *Refugee Health Care— a chronicle of experience in the Khymer assistance operation, 1979–1980.* Chapters 30–32, pp. 163–81. Centers for Disease Control, Atlanta.
4. Centers for Disease Control (1987). *Crossing Cultures? Some suggestions to smooth the way.* Centers for Disease Control, Atlanta.

20

BIOTERRORISM PREPAREDNESS AND RESPONSE: ISSUES FOR PUBLIC HEALTH

Scott R. Lillibridge
Kristy Murray-Lillibridge

Bioterrorism refers to the release or threat of release of biological agents or their toxins for the purpose of causing illness or death in civilian populations. In the fall of 2001, the United States experienced its first extensive, multi-state encounter with bioterrorism. Anthrax spores were found in letters mailed to members of the media, industry, and the federal government that resulted in illness and death within the population. Although this episode created great concern and fear in the general public, other possible scenarios—like that of an epidemic moving rapidly through a large population—would clearly cause greater fear and morbidity, as well as test the adequacy of our surveillance and management capacity, epidemiologic skills, laboratory detection, and other disease control measures.[1]

At the local and state level, public health departments have and will play a critical role in responding to bioterrorism through assessment and implementation of disease control measures such as quarantine and mass immunization. At the national level, the Centers for Disease Control and Prevention (CDC) and other federal agencies have played and will continue to play a leading role in preparing the public health community to detect and control such bioterrorist attacks.[2]

This chapter will briefly discuss some of the most important issues facing those who are responsible for preparing and responding to bioterrorism. Field epidemiologists are likely to be involved in assessing a threat or investigating a biological exposure or unexplained illness or death, so a broad knowledge of the action-oriented principles imperative for prevention and control of disease is essential to help protect the health of the community.

EARLY CONCERNS RELATED TO BIOTERRORISM

After World War II the United States Public Health Service began to address issues of bioterrorism preparedness by creating in 1951 an on-the-job training program for physicians and allied health professionals called the Epidemic Intelligence Service (EIS). Headquartered at the Communicable Disease Center (now the Centers for Disease Control and Prevention) in Atlanta, Georgia, this 2-year program taught the trainees how to perform disease surveillance and investigate epidemics in real-life situations to improve disease control nationwide.[3] As a broad strategy, the mission of this program was also to improve the capability of the United States to deal with the possibility of biological terrorism or warfare.[4] With the support and cooperation of the state and local health departments, more than 2500 epidemiologists have been trained over the past 50 years and many remain in active public health practice.[5]

After the fall of the Soviet Union in the early 1990s the public became aware of the large buildup of bio-offensive capacity by that country.[6] Moreover, as many as 17 nations have been suspected of having offensive biowarfare or bioterrorism capabilities involving the production of anthrax, smallpox, and other organisms.[7,8] Research by such nations, directed to facilitate the dissemination of such agents within populations and to enhance the virulence of biological agents, has the potential to challenge public health practice in the United States and threaten large populations with unexpected epidemics. In addition to these potential threats, the capabilities and motives of terrorist organizations operating outside of a nation–state framework are considerably less clear.

PUBLIC HEALTH GOALS FOR RESPONSE TO BIOTERRORISM

Public health officials have many unique roles and responsibilities following an act of bioterrorism.[9] However, their first objective is to detect and control the epidemic. Such disease control efforts will involve outbreak control measures described in other chapters in this book, along with some unique features that may be attendant with managing an outbreak related to bioterrorism. For example, implementing quarantine measures, mass medical prophylaxis, and/or immunization programs at the local level will require epidemiologists to determine quickly the population at risk and to identify tiers of risks, if the affected population is too large to manage immediately.[10] As part of effective planning, local communities need to review and update their legal authorities to cancel public gatherings and interdict travel, if such actions are required to control the epidemic.[11] If the victims require hospital services, shelter, food, and other support services, the local community could be overwhelmed without close cooperation between public health and emergency management authorities.

As in any emergency involving the health of the population, determination of the medical needs of victims will be needed to organize and guide the delivery of emergency medical services. Such information also includes baseline information on the capacities of health-care facilities in the local community and acute medical staffing needs, along with the pertinent support requirements such as patient food services, hospital beds, and ventilators. This information is critical if federal or state capacities are to be used efficiently to augment local medical resources. In addition to information on health-care facilities, health officials will need to assess rapidly the needs of displaced populations undergoing quarantine or some other form of infectious disease sequestration.

The emphasis of the emergency response is to detect and control the epidemic followed by expansion of the needed clinical services to treat or prevent the adverse health effects of the disease within the population.[12] This requires local public health authorities to work with the most senior levels of the state health officials and the emergency management community to ensure these objectives are met. The extent to which these state and local response activities link with federal response activities will determine the success of our national disease control efforts during such an emergency.

CANDIDATE BIOLOGICAL AGENTS FOR CONSIDERATION AND PREPAREDNESS

Certain biological agents have the unique capacity to harm large populations and have been produced by organizations involved in offensive biological warfare programs.[6,13] Such pathogens have been grouped into various categories for preparedness largely based on the vulnerability of the population.[2] In general, the pathogens with the greatest overall destructiveness (*1*) can be readily disseminated; (*2*) can be easily transmitted from person to person; (*3*) can cause high mortality; (*4*) can contribute to public panic or social disruption; and (*5*) may require specialized public health programmatic intervention. Such agents include: Variola major (smallpox), *Bacillus anthracis* (anthrax), *Yersinia pestis* (plague), *Clostridium botulinum* (botulism), *Francisella tularensis* (tularemia), and various hemorrhagic fever viruses (e.g., Ebola hemorrhagic fever). Other biological agents may pose a lesser threat to public health; these include those pathogens that could threaten the water or the food supply, as well as those agents that appear as new, emerging infectious diseases where the etiology and the control mechanisms are not immediately clear.

One bioterrorist act investigated by local and state health departments with CDC assistance was caused by salmonella-contaminated food.[14] Seven hundred and fifty-one cases of salmonellosis occurred among residents of The Dalles, Oregon, in the fall of 1984. Initial investigation clearly established salad bars in 10 restaurants as the source of the salmonella. However, intensive efforts failed to identify a food item as a single source of the salmonella. Later, with assistance from the public health laboratory, law enforcement officials were able to confirm a report that a religious commune had purposely contaminated the salad bars of the affected restaurants. This outbreak demonstrated valuable interplay between law enforcement and public health officials in solving a crime that involved biological agents. However, the bioterrorist dissemination of anthrax, largely through the mail in the fall of 2001 in the United States, captured the attention of the world and confirmed not only the capability of bioterrorists to deliver a lethal agent effectively but, in this instance, the vulnerability of the United States to the deliberate introduction of infectious diseases. These events have sensitized virtually every American to the reality of bioterrorism and served to highlight the importance of our public health infrastructure.

THE ROLE OF SURVEILLANCE

The broad subject of surveillance has been extensively covered in Chapter 3. Many of the same principles and practices outlined apply to surveillance in the realm of bioterrorism. The most important aspects of any surveillance system relate to their timeliness, sensitivity, and specificity; and these attributes are particularly important in bioterrorism assessment. How quickly the system recognizes a real epidemic and how well it differentiates a random event from a purposeful one is the true measure of the system. In addition, once an epidemic has been detected, public health officials will need to intensify surveillance activities for the purpose of monitoring progress of the control effort. The most important component of surveillance relates to early detection of diseases of concern for bioterrorism by alert clinical providers followed by prompt reporting of cases to local authorities.

DETECTION AT THE COMMUNITY LEVEL

An act of bioterrorism may initially look like any other outbreak of infectious disease within the community. In the absence of a warning, primary health care providers, hospital staff, and public health officials may become aware of increasing numbers of patients presenting for care with unexplained illnesses or death. By the time the outbreak is recognized by public health authorities, the disease can be well established in the population. Consequently, it is important that you begin to consider which factors might trigger the early recognition of an outbreak and whether it is naturally occurring or the result of bioterrorism. Much of the attention of the public health community involved with bioterrorism prepared- ness and response has been to promote the awareness of epidemiologic clues that would suggest an outbreak might be deliberate in origin.[2,13,15] The following sce- narios may be useful to help you recognize early a bioterrorism event. Recall that these situations share some similarities with the appearance of emerging infec- tious diseases or other naturally occurring outbreaks:

1. A single case of an unusual disease within the population whose appear- ance could not be explained by natural factors. Particularly good examples of this would be the sudden reappearance of smallpox, an eradicated dis- ease, and inhalation anthrax—as was seen in the fall of 2001—an ex- tremely rare disease in the United States.
2. Large numbers of persons with the same illness, syndrome, or cause of death whose onset is closely related in time, place, or personal character- istics, suggesting a common exposure.
3. A clustering of unexplained illnesses or death in a relatively discrete popu- lation that was not amenable to treatment or evaluation by standard clini- cal or laboratory diagnostic measures.
4. Higher morbidity and mortality of a disease than is normally present within the population.
5. The presence of disease with an unusual geographic or seasonal distribu- tion within a particular population.
6. Genetic sequencing similarities of agents from different geographic lo- cations that cannot be linked logically or by epidemiologic investigation.
7. An unusual, atypical, engineered, or antiquated strain of a particular virus or bacteria that has been isolated from an infected population.
8. Atypical transmission of a disease within the population.
9. Concurrent or presaging disease in the animal population.

OTHER CONSIDERATIONS

Many local communities have moved to enhance their surveillance activities for the purpose of improving "near real-time" detection of public health emergen- cies, particularly around special events such as conventions, meetings, and other mass gatherings. Some of these systems have implications for local bioterrorism preparedness. For example, during the political convention of 2000 in Los Angeles, emergency department surveillance activities were enhanced to detect specific syndromes or conditions that might suggest bioterrorism.[16] Other kinds of indicators of unexpected increases in morbidity include the number of ambulance runs, hospital bed capacity, and overall emergency department visits. Such systems represent expanded active surveillance during periods when the local population is considered at high risk for bioterrorism or from other public health hazards associated with crowding from special events.

Despite advances in public health practice, the first signal that the population has become victimized by bioterrorism might not come through formal infectious disease surveillance mechanisms, but through the awareness of community physicians or public health officials. Such cases of unexplained illness will require vigorous epidemiologic investigation to search for clues for causality. Case finding for unexplained deaths—in some contrast, depends heavily on how deaths are handled in the community under investigation and must be factored as part of any epidemiologic investigation. For example, in some instances only deaths occurring in hospitals may be reported to public health authorities. Other deaths may be reported only through law enforcement, the coroner, funeral homes, the media, or other nonpublic health entities. To get more information about the deceased, it may be necessary to interview survivors with similar illnesses and surrogates such as family, friends, or associates of the victims. Lastly, whatever system is used to enhance disease detection within the local community, it should lead to rapid expansion into a broader, more active, integrated surveillance activity that monitors the progress of disease control measures in the population.

THE THREAT

The most common bioterrorism-related situation confronting public health officials at the state and local level is when a person, location, or establishment is presented with a biological threat in the form of a package, letter, e-mail letter, or threatening telephone call.[18] Many local communities have developed standard protocols for dealing with these types of threats that include the cooperation of public health, local law enforcement, and emergency management services. Law enforcement will need to quickly determine the credibility of the threat and may need to consult with public health and medical content experts to assess the biological plausibility of a particular threat. *However, the key determinants necessary to assess the level of threat to public health are most related to whether biological agents have been confirmed and whether victims in the population have become ill.* In the absence of either of these two conditions, such a threat may predominantly rest with law enforcement officials.

THE RESPONSE

It is certainly within the realm of possibility that an epidemiologist may be one of the first in the field to investigate an epidemic that is deliberate in origin. As with any outbreak investigation, you must quickly collect the usual time, place, and person data; orient them; and pose tenable hypotheses that will explain the cause, mode of transmission, time and place of exposure, and the number of potentially exposed persons. If you *suspect* bioterrorism because the clinical, laboratory, or epidemiologic information suggests that an outbreak was deliberate, notify appropriate law enforcement authorities immediately. Otherwise, you and your team should proceed with the investigation and respond to the outbreak as appropriate for the public health community.

Once law enforcement authorities have been notified of the suspect bioterrorism event, it is reasonable to seek advice from experts in the fields of clinical and laboratory medicine, epidemiology, and other disciplines as needed. The purpose of subject matter experts is to broaden the differential of conditions and discuss possible confirmatory strategies. Further field investigation, especially interviews of patients, will be necessary as well as advanced laboratory capacities for detection and confirmation. In the case of unexplained deaths, the investigation should include the review of pertinent medical records, laboratory specimens, and tissue review by pathologists, particularly those skilled in the use of advanced molecular diagnostic techniques whereby tissues can be examined for genetic products associated with various bacteria, toxins, or viruses.

After the possibility of bioterrorism is communicated to local, state, and federal authorities, public health officials will become part of a larger response. Provisions for specialized and more detailed laboratory testing of a forensic nature along with a plan to protect the population from further exposure will all be essential. A combined local, state, and federal response will unfold. Public health officials will need to leverage resources toward epidemic control and the clinical needs of victims. Clear information will be needed continually on the extent of the outbreak within the community, the risk to the population, and exactly what is being done by those charged with responding to these emergencies. Recommendations to the public need to be clearly communicated by appropriate health authorities. Other chapters in this book have also highlighted the importance of developing a good communications strategy for public health emergencies.

It is reasonable to expect high-profile and fast-paced investigations in such an atmosphere, driven by the need to execute rapidly the necessary disease control measures. Besides the obvious need to implement an overall emergency plan, there are some critical field epidemiologic activities that public health officials may need to direct. They are as follows:

Conducting rapid surveys

As mentioned in several previous chapters, rapid surveys are absolutely essential in the early phases of an epidemic or natural disaster, most often to compare existing rates of disease with background or normal rates and to define high-risk populations. These surveys also help determine the geographic extent of the outbreak, the potential size of the affected population, and the mechanism by which the biological agents were disseminated.

Implementing standardized surveillance

Make sure that standard case definitions are adhered to, that case counts are representative, and that sources of data are comparable. This standardization becomes the measure of whether response efforts are failing or succeeding. Special attention to the mechanism of data collection, storage, and dissemination will be important in a response to bioterrorism as in any large-scale outbreak.

Coordinating laboratory specimens and testing

The presence of a competent, responsive, and well-trained laboratory staff is absolutely critical to the preparedness and support of a bioterrorism event. Proper laboratory investigations must be closely linked to the epidemiologic investigation and are key to the proper choice of therapeutic intervention or public health strategies that are chosen to control the epidemic. A plan for specimen routing is an essential component of local preparedness. Currently, state and local public health laboratories are linked to federal laboratories through the Laboratory Response Network for bioterrorism.[2] This network is coordinated through the Association of Public Health Laboratories (APHL). The network, which is supported by CDC, provides standardized training, consultation, and transportation of samples. In the future it is envisioned that electronic laboratory reporting will become an increasingly critical part of the national bioterrorism preparedness.

Organizing the flow of public health information

Rapid, regular, accurate, and nonambiguous communication with the public, the public health community, and medical professionals help allay fear, enhance cooperation, and improve surveillance. Public relations and information specialists provide invaluable advice and service under such critical circumstances, particularly if a change in public behavior is required to control the spread of disease (see Chapter 13).

IMPORTANT PUBLIC HEALTH AND GOVERNMENTAL LINKAGES FOR BIOTERRORISM RESPONSE

Local, state, or even national health agency responses to acts by bioterrorists will not occur in isolation from other emergency response sectors—all of whom are striving to meet the needs of the stricken population. Nor can they act without necessary contact with various law enforcement or other governmental agencies at different levels of responsibility. Yet public health responders need to be comfortable in conducting their activities within the context of a broader emergency response. As an example, a number of lessons were learned during the public health response to the 1999 West Nile virus investigation in New York City that highlight the importance of the interplay between public health and local emergency management.[18] During the initial days of the investigation it was unclear as to whether the cause was deliberate or merely the manifestation of a rare or emerging infectious disease. (This was also the case in October 2001 when the index case of inhalation anthrax bioterrorism was diagnosed in Florida.) Second, a number of vulnerabilities related to local, state, and federal epidemic response were noted following the emergence of the West Nile virus. Focus areas that needed expansion and improvement included the following:

- National investigative and laboratory coordination
- The need to link animal and human health concerns
- The development of "surge" emergency epidemiologic support
- The need for early, on-site involvement of subject matter consultants
- Augmented health information management during the emergency

The need for an effective local response and epidemic control plan, communication tree, and clear roles and responsibilities by responders is critical to successful management of the outbreak. Consider for a moment how many agencies, organizations, and government bodies have, and rightly claim, some degree of involvement following a bioterrorism attack. Such a list might include, at the local level: city and county health departments; police or sheriff's departments; the mayor's office, the Civil Defense Agency, and the Red Cross; at the state level: the health department, the state police, the human resources department; the environmental and natural resources agencies; and the governor's office; and at the national level: the Office of Homeland Security, the Department of Health and Human Services, CDC, National Institutes of Health, Food and Drug Administration, Department of Defense, Federal Bureau of Investigation, Federal Emergency Management Agency, and National Guard. All of these organizations will need to work together to respond to such crises.

In the public health arena, specific cross-sector planning must include consideration for the need to enforce quarantine, conduct mass vaccination, dispense mass pharmaceutical treatment or prophylaxis, ensure security for staff, and conduct expanded case finding and enhanced surveillance. Despite involvement in the response by a wide range of agencies and organizations, the most direct responsibility for the health of the population will likely rest with local public health officials and the medical community.

CONCLUSIONS

The recent emergence of bioterrorism has already tested this country's public health infrastructure—albeit, so far, to a somewhat limited extent. These events have clearly established (*1*) the critical role of a coordinated, timely public health response and (*2*) the need for new tools for emergency response and linkage to emergency management.[5,19] Public health officials play a key role in mobilizing resources for epidemic control. The ability to control the epidemic and to respond to medical needs at the local level is paramount to saving lives and protecting our population. An awareness of the indicators of a possible bioterrorism event, proper communication, and basic epidemiologic investigation skills are critical to control disease and to set priorities for the relief community.[20]

Early recognition of and public health response to bioterrorism should include improved clinical awareness of diseases of concern, electronic linkage of hospitals and public health facilities to facilitate reporting, and methods to detect aerosolized agents from airborne samples. However, the continued investment in improving critical public health infrastructure and emergency public health capacities provides the broadest base for national readiness for bioterrorism.

REFERENCES

1. Lillibridge, S.R., Trueman, S.W. (1998) Public health issues in disasters. 1169–1173 In Wallace, R.B. (Ed.) *Public Health and Preventive Medicine*, 14th ed., Appleton & Lange, Stamford, CT.
2. Centers for Disease Control and Prevention (2000) Biological and chemical terrorism: strategic plan for preparedness and response—recommendations of the CDC strategic planning workgroup. *Morb Mortal Wkly Rep* 49 (RR4), 1–14.
3. Langmuir, A.D., Andrews, J.M. (1952) Biological warfare defense—2: The Epidemic Intelligence Service for the Communicable Disease Center. *Am J Public Health* 42, 235–38.
4. Thacker, S.B., Goodman, R.A., Dicker, R.C. (1990) Training and service in public

health practice, 1951–1990—CDC's Epidemic Intelligence Service. *Public Health Rep* 105, 599–604.

5. McDade, J.E. (1999) Addressing the potential threat of bioterrorism—value added to an improved public health infrastructure. *Emerg Infect Dis* 5, 591–92.

6. Alibek, K., Handelman, S. (1999) *Biohazard: the chilling true story of the largest covert biological weapons program in the world—told from the inside by the man who ran it.* Random House, New York.

7. Cole, L.A. (1996) The specter of biological weapons. *Sci Am* 275, 60–65.

8. Davis, J.C. (1999) Nuclear blindness: an overview of the biological weapons programs of the former Soviet Union and Iraq. *Emerg Infect Dis* 5, 509–12.

9. Khan, A.S., Morse, S., Lillibridge, S. (2000) Public-health preparedness for biological terrorism in the USA. *Lancet* 356, 1179–82.

10. Centers for Disease Control and Prevention (2000) Use of anthrax vaccine in the United States: recommendations of the Advisory Committee on Immunization Practices (ACIP). *Morb Mortal Wkly Rep* 49 (RR-15), 1–8.

11. Gostin, L.O. (2000) Public health law in the new century: Part 1: Law as a tool to advance the community's health. *J Am Med Assoc* 283, 2837–41.

12. Hamburg, M.A. (2000) Bioterrorism: a challenge to public health and medicine. *J Public Health Prac* 6, 38–44.

13. Franz, D.R., Jahrling, P.B., Friedlander, A.M. (1997) Clinical recognition and management of patients exposed to biological warfare agents. *J Am Med Assoc* 278, 399–411.

14. Torork, T.J., Tauxe, R.V., Wise, R.P., et al. (1997) A large community outbreak of salmonellosis caused by intentional contamination of restaurant salad bars. *J Am Med Assoc* 278, 389–95.

15. Noah, D.L., Sobel, A.L., Ostroff, S.M. (1998) Biological warfare training: infectious disease outbreak differentiation criteria. *Mil Med* 163: 198–201.

16. Bancroft, E.A., Treadwell, T., Glynn, K., et al (2001) Real-time, web-based syndromic surveillance during the Democratic National Convention—Los Angeles, 2000. Presented at 50th Annual Epidemic Intelligence Service (EIS) Conference, Atlanta.

17. Centers for Disease Control and Prevention (1999) Bioterrorism alleging use of anthrax and interim guidelines for management—United States, 1998. *Morb Mortal Wkly Rep* 48, 69–74.

18. West Nile Virus Outbreak. Lessons for Public Health Preparedness. United States General Accounting Office, Health, Education and Human Services GAO/HEHS-00-180. September 11, 2000. [Download pdf file: http://www.gab.gov:8765]

19. Centers for Disease Control and Prevention (1998) Preventing emerging infectious diseases: strategies for the 21st century. Overview of the updated CDC plan. *Morb Mortal Wkly Rep* 47 (RR 15), 1–14.

20. Pavlin, J.A. (1999) Epidemiology of bioterrorism. *Emerg Infect Dis* 5, 528–30.

21

FIELD INVESTIGATIONS
OF NATURAL DISASTERS

Eric K. Noji
Michael B. Gregg

No matter where you live and work, as a practicing field epidemiologist you may be called upon to assess the health needs of your community during and/or following a natural disaster. Floods, hurricanes, earthquakes, and other occurrences are, unfortunately, relatively common events that can exact a heavy toll of death and suffering. During the past 30 years they have claimed about four million lives worldwide, have adversely affected the lives of at least a billion more people, and have resulted in property damage exceeding $100 billion.[1] The world was hit by a record number of natural disasters in the year 2000, and a rising population will only aggravate the situation. The number of natural catastrophes reached a new absolute high, with more than 850 recorded worldwide, 100 more than in the previous record year of 1999 and 200 more than the average for the 1990s. A devastating fire in the United States destroyed thousands of square kilometers of forest mainly in the western United States and in New Mexico. Thousands of people had to be evacuated.[2]

The future appears to be even more frightening. Increasing population density in floodplains and in earthquake- and hurricane-prone areas points to the probability of future catastrophic natural disasters with millions of casualties.[1,2] Many natural disasters of large magnitude occur in remote areas, far from population centers and hospitals. The roads frequently become impassable, bridges collapse, and inclement weather adds to the difficulties. The more remote the area, the longer it takes for help to arrive, and the more the community will have to rely on its own resources, at least for the first several hours, if not days.

THE HISTORICAL DEVELOPMENT OF FIELD EPIDEMIOLOGY IN DISASTERS AND EMERGENCIES

The practical application of epidemiology to disaster management really began during the massive international relief operations mounted during the civil war in Nigeria in the late 1960s.[3] Epidemiologists developed survey tools (such as the quakstick, a simple field device for estimating nutritional status by measuring height and upper arm circumference) and methods that rapidly assessed the nutritional status of large displaced populations so relief could be targeted to those with the greatest need. Subsequently, surveillance became critical in monitoring how the nutritional status of the population was affected by the quantity and types of foods delivered. Rapid assessment proved invaluable in evaluating food distribution practices in the face of rapidly changing conditions of health and relief. Now, nutritional surveillance has become a routine part of relief work in famine areas and in refugee populations.

During the 1970s, the need for disaster epidemiology became even more apparent in many relief operations.[4] Managers and planners with no public health expertise and no reliable or relevant information were forced to direct major relief efforts. In the absence of good information, their response was often dictated by the donors of relief and medical assistance or was based on "conventional wisdom," unverified reports, or myths thought to be appropriate by donor agencies. As a result, disaster scenes were often cluttered by unnecessary, outdated, or unlabeled drugs; vaccines that were ineffective, not needed, or improperly used; medical and surgical teams without proper training, experience, or logistical support; and relief programs that did not address immediate or real needs of the affected population. However, in the 1980s and 1990s relief agencies progressively accepted the role of epidemiology in disaster responses, their reliance on ad hoc crisis management has lessened substantially, and rates of disaster-related morbidity and mortality have fallen.

PROBLEMS YOU WILL FACE IN THE FIELD

General Considerations

Before we discuss the challenges you will face in the field, you may want to consult Appendix 21–1 for descriptions of the medical and public health effects of major natural disasters.

The overall objectives of post-disaster epidemiologic investigations are to assess the needs of disaster-affected populations, match available resources to needs, prevent further adverse health effects, evaluate relief program effectiveness, and permit better contingency planning.[4] Just after a disaster, when no information is available about the medical needs of the population, you may have to provide advice about probable health effects, establish priorities for action, and convince the powers that be to get accurate information to make intelligent decisions about relief efforts. More specifically, you may also be responsible for performing one or more of the following studies:

- Starting a surveillance system
- Evaluating the effectiveness of clinical management
- Determining risk factors
- Assessing the disaster's public health impact
- Describing the natural history of the disaster and its long-term effects

The success of your efforts after a disaster will be measured directly by (1) how rapidly you collect and analyze data to identify appropriate prevention strategies; and (2) how effectively decision makers implement these measures. Therefore, successful investigations require, among other activities, continuous coordination between the epidemiologist, who gathers data and identifies issues or strategies, and the decision makers, who must understand the data and strategies presented by you and implement the required policies and interventions.[3]

Conducting post-disaster assessments and establishing surveillance systems are fairly straightforward and logical, but you must rely heavily on your skills in management, communication, public relations, and epidemiology to succeed (see Chapters 4 and 7). However, to accomplish these tasks entails facing some technical and operational problems—like many referred to in earlier chapters—but often much more profound because of the nature of the disaster itself (see Table 21–1).[5]

Logistics

Logistic constraints will influence the collection, analysis, interpretation, and dissemination of surveillance data. For example, disasters can sever telecommunications systems; impede normal transportation routes; or disrupt or destroy the public health infrastructure such as hospitals, health departments, and their personnel.[6] Such disruptions may require hiring untrained personnel as fieldworkers, possibly affecting the quality of the data collected. You can hire outside or expatriate workers to do the work, but their unfamiliarity with local languages and

Table 21–1. Methodologic Issues in
Post-disaster Assessment and Surveillance

Compromise between timeliness and accuracy
Competing priorities for information
Logistical constraints
Absence of baseline information
Denominator data unavailable
Underreporting of health events
Lack of representativeness
Resource costs of collecting and analyzing data
Lack of standard reporting mechanisms

---

customs might compromise data quality or impair the delivery of preventive services. If possible, at least one member of the assessment team should be familiar with local language, customs, and conditions (e.g., cultural norms, practices, and usual medical care received) (see Chapter 19).

Determination of Rates

Baseline population and health information may be absent or unavailable. The size of the population at risk may be difficult to obtain, and, as has been emphasized in earlier chapters, you must have denominator data to calculate rates and make valid comparisons.[7] Comparing absolute numbers of a health event in two groups may be misleading if the underlying populations at risk differ in size or other characteristics. In the United States, census data are readily available in electronic form, but in the developing world data may be difficult to get in timely fashion. However, because the impact of the disaster within a particular geographic area is frequently not uniform, you may need more refined and localized estimates of the population at risk. You may also need baseline information to determine whether the post-disaster health problems represent true increases rather than simply improved case ascertainment.

For example, after Hurricane Andrew struck south Florida in 1992, surveillance data gathered at emergency medical facilities were difficult to interpret because the expected proportion of visits to a clinic for a particular reason, such as diarrhea, was unknown before the disaster. You may also need information on health or disability status before the disaster to identify groups that are particularly vulnerable and to estimate the magnitude of the disaster. In evacuation camps following floods, for example, rapid migration of people often means you will not know key information on the displaced community such as age, gender, or baseline communicable disease and nutritional status. These uncertainties hamper targeting relief efforts appropriately and make early collection of this information through rapid assessment a priority.[8]

THE RAPID EPIDEMIOLOGIC ASSESSMENT

Timeliness

The critical component of any disaster response is the early determination of urgent needs and relief priorities. Such a disaster assessment provides relief managers with objective information about the effects of the disaster on the population, generated from rapidly conducted field investigations.[9,10] Initially, timeliness and accuracy are more important than more scientifically sound methods of collection and analysis. Unfortunately, simultaneously satisfying these needs usually requires trade-offs or compromises such as using less than ideal sampling methods (see Chapter 11). Such situations have prompted practical adages such as "being roughly right is generally more useful than being precisely wrong" and "quick and dirty techniques." So try to gather a small amount of relevant information quickly (usually 2 to 4 days after a sudden-impact disaster such as a hurricane or earthquake). You may need to have a multidisciplinary team with you (e.g., a statistician, sanitary engineer, nutritionist, and primary health nurse), and you will probably rely on visual inspection, interviews with key local emergency personnel and community leaders, and simple surveys.[11] But get out into the field as quickly as possible after the disaster's impact.

Objectives

Specifically, you should try to determine the following:

- Overall magnitude of the impact of the disaster (geographic extent, number of affected, and estimated duration)
- Impact on health (e.g., number of casualties, mortality, morbidity)
- Number of damaged houses, homeless persons
- Integrity of health services delivery systems (e.g., nonfunctioning hospitals, clinics)
- Specific health-care needs of survivors (surgical, primary health care, reproductive health)
- Disruption of other service sectors (e.g., community "lifelines" such as electrical power, water, gas, sanitation) that can potentially affect public health
- Extent (and effectiveness) of response to the disaster by local authorities

Methods

Surveys

The techniques used to collect this information (primarily sample and systematic surveys and simple reporting systems) are usually methodologically straightforward. The most valuable data are generally simple to collect and analyze. You will not need elaborate sampling techniques in the acute phase following a sudden-impact natural disaster; but you will need to create a practical balance between ensuring that survey procedures are simple, yet effective, and achieving the highest degree of validity and reliability possible under the circumstances. Use standard clinical case definitions like, fever, cough with fever, watery or bloody diarrhea, and fever with rash. And put the definitions in writing so others can use them.

Since this information will be used to plan and implement immediate responses, the earliest assessments should address the most basic questions for which decision makers need answers. Later on, surveys can more carefully examine availability and quality of medical care, the need for specific interventions (surgery), nutrition, immunization status, and epidemic control.[12]

Sometimes after rapid-onset disasters, time constraints and disruption require you to conduct rapid assessment surveys using nonprobability sampling methods. However, you may get biased results because they are often based on purposive, convenience, or haphazard selection samples. Recall, too, that focusing on the most affected areas rather than on the entire disaster area can introduce sampling bias.

Recently, however, a modified cluster-sampling method was designed to perform a rapid assessment after hurricanes.[13] In the first survey conducted 3 days after Hurricane Andrew struck, clusters were systematically selected from a heavily damaged area by using a grid that had been overlaid on aerial photographs. Survey teams interviewed seven occupied households in consecutive order in each selected cluster. Results were available within 24 hours of beginning the survey. Surveys of the same heavily damaged area and of a less severely affected area were conducted 7 and 10 days later, respectively. The survey team found few households with injured residents, but a large proportion of households were without telephones or electricity. This directed relief workers to focus their limited resources on providing primary health care and preventive services to pediatric, gynecologic, and elderly populations. Otherwise, efforts would have been diverted to establish unnecessary high-tech surgical and mass-casualty trauma services.[14]

Although cluster-survey techniques hold promise for providing information rapidly after a disaster, in certain other settings these techniques may be less applicable. For example, epidemiologists who used a cluster-survey technique after the January 1994 earthquake in Northridge, California, found that the technique needed some modification. Unlike the damage from hurricanes, which is generally uniform over a large geographic area and when cluster-sampling can be useful, earthquake-related damage varies considerably over different terrain, where some areas experience little destruction and others heavy destruction. Therefore, cluster-sampling after an earthquake may cause you to miss seriously affected areas and, thus, to underestimate overall damages.

Other Issues

Other considerations include problems related to the political environment and problems caused by rapidly changing social conditions and demographics. To solve these problems, you must be flexible, innovative, and able to adapt to new situations. You must collect reasonably objective data rapidly under adverse environmental conditions during the immediate emergency period.[15] Table 21–2 outlines time and resource requirements and data-gathering techniques for different levels of assessment methods. Critical information about the immediate effects of disasters on people (e.g., locations where people are trapped, methods of victim extrication, the quality of on-site medical care rendered); the extent of damage to buildings, personal property, and community "lifelines"; economic activities; unsubstantiated rumors; and available natural resources—all must be gathered within the first few hours to days. Otherwise, evidence is rapidly lost during the rescue, clean-up, demolition, and recovery process. Such information has been described by experienced disaster investigators as "perishable," since it is usually irretrievably lost unless collected early.

SURVEILLANCE AFTER DISASTERS

General Considerations

The definition, kinds, functions, purposes, methods, and applications of public health surveillance have been described in detail in Chapter 3. Virtually all these attributes apply in disaster situations to a greater or lesser degree. We will highlight the more pertinent aspects of surveillance as they relate to disaster relief.

In disaster situations surveillance aims to collect, analyze, and respond to data in a kind of a "cycle" that must turn many times: immediately, with rapid assessments of problems using rudimentary data collection techniques; then with short-term assessments involving the establishment of simple but more reliable sources of data; and later, using ongoing surveillance to identify continuing problems and to monitor the impact of medical and health interventions. Surveillance becomes a cyclical process, constantly monitoring and assessing simple health

Table 21–2. Characteristics of Data Collection Methods in Disaster Settings

| ASSESSMENT | REQUIREMENTS | | DATA-GATHERING TECHNIQUES | |
METHOD	TIME	RESOURCES	INDICATORS	ADVANTAGES
1. Pre-disaster "background" data	Ongoing	Trained staff	Reporting from health facilities and *practitioners*. Disease patterns and seasonality	Provides baseline data for detecting problems and assessing trends
2. Remote: airplanes, helicopter, satellite	Minutes/hours	Hardware	Direct observation, cameras. Destroyed buildings, roads, dams, flooding.	Quick; useful when ground transport out; useful to identify area affected
3. On-site "walkthrough" (ride through)	Hours/days	Transportation, maps	Direct observation, talks with local leaders *and health workers*. Deaths, homeless persons, numbers and types of diseases	Quick; visible; does not require technical (health) background
4. "Quick and dirty" surveys	2–3 days	Few trained staff	Rapid surveys. Deaths, no. hospitalized, nutritional status, (see also 3)	Rapid quantitative data; may prevent mismanagement; can provide data for surveillance
5. Rapid health screening system	Ongoing (as needed)	Health workers; equipment that depends on the data that are collected	Collect data from fraction of persons being *screened*. Nutritional status, demography, hematocrit, parasitemia.	Can be established quickly; collects data and provides services (vaccines, vit. A, triage) in migrating populations
6. Surveillance systems	Ongoing	Some trained staff; standard diagnoses; method of communicating data	Routine data collection *in standardized manner*. Mortality/morbidity by diagnosis and age	Timely; expandable; can detect trends
7. Survey	Variable: hours/days	Experienced field epidemiologist statistician; reliable field staff	Random or representative *sample selection*. Varies according to purpose of survey	Large amount of specific data obtained in brief time

[*Source*: Adapted from Nieburg's model for data collection methods in disaster situations, in *Health Aspects and Relief Management After Natural Disasters. Center for Research on the Epidemiology of Disasters. Bruxelles, Belgium, 1980.*]

interventions. Sustained feedback about changing needs allows disaster response activities to be modified based on hard evidence.

In disaster settings you will face major hurdles that will test your ability to perform good surveillance. Some of them are: (*1*) data must be collected rapidly under highly adverse conditions; (*2*) multiple sources of information must be integrated in a cohesive fashion; (*3*) circumstances and forces may impede the flow from one step in the surveillance cycle to the next; and (*4*) the cycle from information to action must be completed rapidly, accurately, and repeatedly.

Surveillance systems in disaster settings should have a high degree of sensitivity, that is, they should have the ability to detect cases or events. This will help ensure that the health outcomes of interest are counted, and it will also provide early, although perhaps nonspecific, warnings of unusual occurrences. Disruption of communications and transportation systems can easily impede reporting and decrease the sensitivity of the system. Also, events that occur outside the domain of the health-care system may go undetected. For example, deaths in evacuation or tent camps may be underestimated or even go unnoticed because deaths may only be counted in hospitals and other medical facilities.

In August 1992, in Louisiana, for example, the state Office of Public Health (OPH) set up an active emergency surveillance system for getting information on injuries and illnesses associated with Hurricane Andrew. Officials contacted hospital emergency departments, coroners' offices, and public utilities in the 19 parishes (counties) that were in the path of the hurricane. The OPH created a case definition for hurricane-related fatal or nonfatal injury or illness and developed a questionnaire to obtain demographic information and data on the nature and cause of the injury or illness. OPH personnel made periodic telephone calls to stimulate reporting of hurricane-related events. Of the 42 hospital emergency departments contacted, 21 participated; 5 of 19 coroners' offices and 1 of 2 public utilities also participated in the system. Of the 17 fatal outcomes reported, 8 occurred before the hurricane reached landfall; the majority (86%) of the 383 nonfatal events were injuries, most commonly cuts and lacerations.

This system showed the feasibility of collecting morbidity and mortality data from existing emergency medical facilities. The Louisiana experience also underscores several difficulties in operating such a system. Data on morbidity and mortality are available through many sources—hospital emergency departments, police, rescue, fire departments, the Red Cross, medical examiners, and coroners' offices—but these sources frequently use different methods of defining, ascertaining, and reporting cases and causes of injury or illness. All of which emphasizes the need to establish standard, simple guidelines for those who contribute to your surveillance system. Underreporting may result from complex case definitions; overreporting from increasing reporting areas or increased awareness or interest. And remember, no reports does not mean no disease.

Active Surveillance

A sudden-impact disaster can severely damage existing medical care facilities, requiring you and others to start a surveillance system immediately. In such circumstances, relief teams have used temporary shelters such as school gymnasiums or makeshift medical facilities as sources of key health information. After Hurricane Andrew the medical system suffered severe damage. Many acute-care facilities and community health centers were closed, and many physicians' offices were destroyed in the impact area. State and federal public health officials, the American Red Cross, and the military established temporary medical facilities to care for the affected population. During the 4 weeks after the hurricane struck, officials established active surveillance at 15 civilian free-care centers, at 8 emergency departments in and surrounding the impact area, and at 28 military free-care sites.[16] Data from this system showed that injuries were an important cause of morbidity among civilians and military personnel, but that most injuries were minor and due to clean-up activities. The system was particularly useful in responding to rumors about the occurrence of communicable disease outbreaks (and in avoiding widespread administration of typhoid and cholera vaccines) and in determining that large numbers of volunteer health care providers such as surgeons and medical specialists were not needed.

Although this active surveillance effort achieved its objectives, there were several real problems. First, various relief agencies needed to coordinate their efforts. Data from the civilian and military systems had to be analyzed separately because different case definitions and data-collection methods were used. Second, there was no baseline information available to determine whether health events were occurring with a frequency greater than expected. Third, rates of illness and injury could not be determined for civilians because the size of the population at risk was unknown.

Sentinel Surveillance

Sentinel surveillance in disaster situations may be useful to monitor health events when: (1) there is no preexisting surveillance system; (2) the existing surveillance system has been disrupted; (3) information about the event cannot be readily obtained by using existing systems; or (4) time and resource constraints prohibit collecting information through population-based surveys. However, sentinel surveillance systems can provide a limited amount of information in a timely fashion.[17]

In the immediate aftermath of the eruption of Mount St. Helens in Washington State, on May 18, 1980, surveillance activities for respiratory and other illnesses related to ash-fall were established in the 18 main hospitals located in the path of the ash-fall east of the volcano.[18] In July 1990, a major earthquake struck a widespread area in Luzon Island in the Philippines. Because of widespread destruction of medical facilities and disruption of communications, sentinel surveillance for diarrhea and measles was established in each of the areas affected by the earthquake.

In both instances the sentinel systems provided extremely important information very rapidly: the extent of serious respiratory distress from ash-fall in Washington and, remarkably, no increases in diarrhea or measles in Luzon. Health information like this, so rapidly and accurately obtained, helped dispel rumors and reassure the public.

In sum, the advantages of sentinel surveillance are its timeliness, flexibility, and acceptability. But establishing sentinel surveillance requires overcoming the same challenges posed by other methods of surveillance. Recruiting and training participants and standardizing data-collection procedures consume time and resources. Rare events can easily be missed simply because those who report see only a fraction of the affected population. Finally, the representativeness of the sentinel system can be difficult to estimate. Nonetheless, sentinel surveillance can be a practical method to gather information from a variety of sources such as: shelters; field tent clinics; disaster-assistance centers; and other nontraditional sources such as police, fire departments, civil defense organizations, humanitarian aid agencies, medical examiners, religious officials, pharmacies, and schools.

INVESTIGATIONS OF RUMORS

Rumors frequently circulate in disaster settings, and you may, by necessity, be involved in proving or disproving their truth. Rumors arise from a variety of circumstances, such as poor communication between the affected population and civil/political authorities, loss of control and uncertainty among those usually in charge, or fears of epidemics from misconceptions about infectious diseases and decaying corpses. Sources of rumors may come from: (1) health workers' misdiagnoses of common, nonthreatening diseases; (2) the media and individual anecdotes and testimonials; (3) politicians and others who want command and control, and (4) civil authorities and relief agencies who report different body counts and the like.

To investigate a rumor, try to confirm it by answering the following questions: Who reported the event? What is the basis for the rumor? Has the event been confirmed using reliable methods (e.g., laboratory confirmation or corroboration by multiple observers)? Have officials consulted other independent sources to confirm the existence of the event? One designated spokesperson (local, state, provincial, or national health official) should report the findings of the relief teams to the public, media, government agencies, and all others who need to know.

Through regular, often daily, updates and briefings, this spokesperson should be the "point person" for all information that is to be disseminated[19] (see Chapter 13).

SPECIAL CONSIDERATIONS

The Laboratory

Although outbreaks of communicable diseases are uncommon following natural disasters, particularly in the United States, these diseases have caused substantial morbidity and mortality in certain international and wartime settings.[20–21] In camps for refugees and displaced populations, diarrheal diseases, malaria, measles, and acute respiratory illness are among the leading causes of death.[22] Therefore, you should seriously consider using the laboratory to help verify the clinical data. The laboratory will confirm the clinical diagnosis and help direct prevention efforts and clinical management.

Recall, you do not have to culture every suspect patient; only a few of the most typical cases will usually do. Also, you do not have to wait for laboratory confirmation before you quarantine, isolate, or immunize. You can almost always act upon good clinical and epidemiologic data.[23]

Standardized Reporting

It is very important that field epidemiologists develop standardized reporting methods. Unfortunately, standardized and widely accepted case definitions for disaster-related deaths or injuries do not exist,[24,25] although attempts are being made to rectify this situation both nationally and internationally. One such effort is the Sphere Project, a non-governmental, Red Cross/Red Crescent initiative to enhance the accountability of the humanitarian and disaster response system, primarily by identifying basic minimum requirements, skills, and knowledge base for effective disaster response.[26]

Communicating the Surveillance Data

What you learn from the surveillance system must be disseminated as a hard copy document through appropriate channels as quickly as possible. Define in advance on paper your methods, purposes, and target audience. If possible, make contact with your most important constituents before you start your communication system. Do not confuse your daily reports to the media with this more formal, scientific, surveillance report. However, this surveillance report can be given to the press if need be. Consider the following as your possible audience: those who provided the data (the feedback), key representatives of the affected population, other health officials, cooperating agencies, the political establishment, the policy makers, and the media. And last, but not least, make the reports simple to read and understand. Write for the least sophisticated of your audience. Use charts and graphs liberally to help the reader visualize the findings. Few, if any, field epidemiologists have been faulted for creating clear, nontechnical scientific reports. Above all, remember who you are trying to inform, educate, and convince.[27]

Coordination

In disasters, the epidemiologist and the government decision makers must be coordinated. You will not be successful in a post-disaster setting if you operate on your own, since you must rely on governmental relief authorities for access to transportation, communication, security, and often the very ability to gain entry to a disaster site. Furthermore, developing and operating a surveillance system in a disaster setting could be perceived by government officials and other decision makers as diverting resources from other important relief programs and services that have been established, such as building shelters and latrines, providing clinical medical services, and bringing in food and water. Decision makers such as politicians, particularly those who are not familiar with public health or surveillance, may view such diversions as unacceptable unless you develop a system that can demonstrate to those who control the pursestrings that the benefits from collecting such information outweigh the costs. In other words, your presence in the field must be viewed as a very inexpensive, cost-effective measure with high "pay off" in comparison with the high costs of shipping tons of food, vehicles, and equipment to a disaster site.

SUMMARY

In disaster relief and other forms of humanitarian assistance, important and often irreversible decisions must be made rapidly. The need for reliable early data to assist decision making is crucial. An organized approach to data collection in disasters can greatly improve decision making by presenting those in charge with a variety of options to choose from. Collecting more information will not automatically improve disaster response. Much of the information currently generated by governments, relief agencies, international agencies, voluntary relief organizations, and other groups is of questionable validity; and a lot of it is improperly collected, analyzed, and used. The effectiveness of information management following a disaster can be measured by: (1) how rapidly you collect and analyze the data; (2) how well you identify prevention strategies; and (3) how well the decision makers execute the appropriate policies and strategies. Field epidemiology, especially including public health surveillance, represents the most effective decision-making tool to prepare for and respond to the disruption and destruction that natural disasters bring.

APPENDIX 21–1. SUMMARY OF THE MEDICAL AND PUBLIC HEALTH EFFECTS OF MAJOR NATURAL DISASTERS

FLOODS

Floods are the most common natural disaster. They affect more people worldwide and cause greater mortality than any other type of natural disaster. They occur in almost every country, but 70% of all flood deaths occur in India and Bangladesh. In the United States, floods cause more deaths than any other natural disaster, with most fatalities resulting from flash floods. Fast flowing water carrying debris such as boulders and fallen trees accounts for most flood-related injuries and deaths—the main cause of death being drowning, followed by various combinations of trauma, drowning, and hypothermia. Although the health impact of many floods has not been studied at all or only rudimentarily, the few that have been well studied suggest that among flood survivors, the proportion requiring emergency medical care is reported to vary between 0.2% and 2%. Most injuries requiring medical attention are minor and include lacerations, skin rashes, and ulcers. For some floods, substantial numbers of casualties caused by fire have been documented, because fast-flowing water can break oil or gasoline storage tanks.

Floods may disrupt water purification and sewage disposal systems, cause toxic waste sites to overflow, or dislodge chemicals stored above ground. There may be the potential for water-borne disease transmission of such agents as *Escherichia coli*, *Shigella*, *Salmonella*, and hepatitis A virus. In endemic areas, the risk of transmission of mosquito-borne diseases such as malaria, yellow fever, and the encephalitides may be increased because of enhanced vector-breeding conditions. Upper respiratory tract diseases can increase and be rapidly spread in overcrowded temporary shelters for flood victims. Despite the potential for communicable diseases to follow floods, mass immunization programs are almost always counterproductive: they divert limited personnel and resources from other critical relief tasks, and they may create a false sense of security. Unfortunately, after floods, the public often demands typhoid vaccine and tetanus toxoid, although no epidemics of typhoid after floods have ever been documented in the United States. The vaccine can produce mild to moderate systemic reactions, takes several weeks to develop immunity, and even then produces only limited protection. Likewise, mass tetanus vaccination programs are not indicated. Management of flood-associated wounds—like any wounds—

requires a tetanus immunization history and immunization only if indicated. As with all disasters the proper approach to communicable disease prevention and control is to set up a public health surveillance system to monitor disease occurrence.

TROPICAL CYCLONES (HURRICANES OR TYPHOONS)

The greatest natural disaster in U.S. history occurred on September 8, 1900, when a hurricane struck Galveston, Texas, and killed more than 6000 people. Cyclones, hurricanes, and typhoons have killed hundreds of thousands and injured millions of people during the last 20 years. In 1970, deaths resulting from a single tropical cyclone striking Bangladesh were estimated to exceed 250,000. As population growth continues along vulnerable coastal areas, deaths and injuries resulting from tropical cyclones will increase. Although hurricane winds do great damage, wind is not the biggest killer in a hurricane. Hurricanes are classic examples of disasters that trigger secondary effects such as tornadoes and flooding that, together with storm surges, can cause extraordinarily high rates of morbidity and mortality. This was seen following the 1991 cyclone and sea surge in Bangladesh in which 140,000 people drowned and during Hurricane Mitch in Central America in 1998 with thousands of drowning deaths. Nine of 10 hurricane fatalities are drownings associated with storm surges. The major rescue problem is locating persons stranded by rising waters and evacuating them to higher land. Other causes of deaths and injuries include burial beneath houses collapsed by wind or water, penetrating trauma from broken glass or wood, blunt trauma from floating objects or debris, or entrapment by mud slides that may accompany hurricane-associated floods. Many of the most severe injuries occur to persons who are in mobile homes during the storm or who are injured or electrocuted during the post-disaster cleanup. Most persons who seek medical care after hurricanes do not require sophisticated surgical or intensive care services and can be treated as outpatients by primary care physicians. The great majority suffer from lacerations caused by flying glass or other debris; a few have closed fractures; and others, mostly penetrating injuries. As with flood-related wounds, emergency medical care providers should be aware that such wounds may contain highly contaminated material such as soil or fecal matter.

People are often severely crowded in storm shelters. As with flood disasters, this crowding increases the probability of disease transmission via aerosol or fecal–oral routes, particularly when sanitary facilities are insufficient. Trauma after a cyclone is not usually a major public health problem when compared with the need for water, food, clothing, sanitation, and other hygienic measures. Sending fully equipped mobile hospitals and specialized surgical teams that usually arrive much too late at the disaster site is an ineffective response to a cyclone disaster.

Nonmedical relief (such as epidemiologists, sanitary engineers, shelter, food, and agricultural supplies) is probably more effective in reducing mortality and morbidity. However, field hospitals and emergency medical teams from outside the disaster-affected area may, indeed, be useful to provide ongoing primary health-care services to the community when all other health-care facilities have been destroyed or severely damaged.

TORNADOES

Tornadoes are among the most violent of all natural atmospheric phenomena. Although almost 700 tornadoes occur in the United States each year, only about 3% result in severe injuries requiring hospitalization. Of 14,600 tornadoes between 1952 and 1973 for which data exist, only 497 caused fatalities, and 26 of these events accounted for almost half of the fatalities. The destruction caused by tornadoes results from the combined action of their strong rotary winds and the partial vacuum in the center of the vortex. For example, when a tornado passes over a building, the winds twist and rip at the outside. Simultaneously, the abrupt pressure reduction in the tornado's eye causes explosive pressures inside the building. Walls collapse or topple outward, windows explode, and the debris from this destruction can be driven as high-velocity missiles through the air. Buildings of nonreinforced masonry, wood frame buildings, and those with large window areas are likely to suffer the most. The leading cause of death is craniocerebral trauma, followed by crushing wounds of the chest and trunk. Lacerations and fractures are the most frequent nonfatal injuries. Also frequent are penetrating trauma with retained foreign bodies and other soft tissue injuries. A high percentage of wounds among tornado casualties are heavily contaminated. In many instances foreign materials such as glass, wood splinters, tar, dirt, grass, and manure are deeply embedded in areas of soft tissue injury. Sepsis is common in both minor and major injuries; sepsis affects one-half to two-thirds of patients with minor wounds.

VOLCANIC ERUPTIONS

The U.S. Geological Survey has identified approximately 35 volcanoes in the western United States and Alaska that are likely to erupt in the future. Most of these are in remote rural areas and are not likely to result in human disaster. A few, like Mt. Hood, Mt. Shasta, Mt. Rainier, and the volcano underlying Mammoth Lakes in California, are located near population centers. Most volcanic deaths are caused by immediate suffocation and, to a lesser extent, by burns or blunt trauma. Eruptions have immediate life-threatening health effects through suffocation from inhalation of massive quantities of airborne ash, scalding from blasts of superheated steam, and surges of lethal gas. Pyroclastic flows and surges are particularly lethal. These are currents of extremely hot gases and particles that flow down the slopes of a volcano at tens to hundreds of meters per second and cover hundreds of square kilometers. Because of their suddenness and speed, pyroclastic flows and surges are difficult to escape. Sudden release of these gases can be catastrophic: carbon dioxide released from Lake Monoun and Lake Nyos in Cameroon in 1984 and 1986, respectively, claimed 1800 lives. Other toxic effects of these gas releases include pulmonary edema, irritant conjunctivitis, joint pain, muscle weakness, and cutaneous bullae. Mud flows, or lahars, account for at least 10% of volcano-related deaths. These are flowing masses of volcanic debris mixed with water. The mud is sometimes scalding hot, causing severe burns. A volcanic eruption may also generate tremendous quantities of ash-fall. Buildings have been reported to collapse from the weight of ash accumulating on roofs, resulting in severe trauma to the occupants. The ash can also be irritating to the eyes (causing corneal abrasions), mucous membranes, and the respiratory system. Upper airway irritation, cough, and bronchospasm, as well as exacerbation of chronic lung diseases, are common findings in symptomatic patients. With extremely high concentrations, volcanic ash may cause severe tracheal injury, pulmonary edema, and bronchial obstruction leading to death from acute pulmonary injury or from suffocation.

After the eruption of Mount St. Helens in 1980, 23 immediate deaths were reported. Postmortem examinations revealed that 18 of these deaths resulted from asphyxia. Finally, a delayed onset of ash-induced mucus hypersecretion or obstructive airway disease may occur. Hospitals in the vicinity of both active and dormant volcanoes should be prepared to deal with a sudden influx of victims with severe burns and lung damage from inhalation of hot ash, as well as multiple varieties of trauma.

EARTHQUAKES

An earthquake of great magnitude is one of the most destructive events in nature. During the past 20 years, earthquakes have caused more than a million deaths and injuries worldwide. Hospitals and other health-care facilities are particularly vulnerable to the damaging effects of an earthquake. The primary cause of death and injury from earthquakes is the collapse of buildings. Deaths may come from severe crushing injuries to the head or chest, external or internal hemorrhage, or drowning from earthquake-induced tidal waves (tsunamis). Rapid death occurs within minutes or hours and may come from asphyxia from dust inhalation or chest compression, hypovolemic shock, or exposure. Heavy dust, produced by crumbling buildings immediately following an earthquake, may cause asphyxiation or upper airway obstruction. Asbestos and other particulate matter in the dust are both subacute and chronic respiratory hazards for trapped victims, as well as for rescue and cleanup personnel. Burns and smoke inhalation from fires are also major hazards after an earthquake.

Paralleling the speed required for effective search and extrication is the speed needed for emergency medical services—for speed is of the essence. The greatest demand occurs within the first 24 hours. Injured people usually seek medical attention at emergency departments only during the first 3 to 5 days; afterward the case mix patterns return almost to normal. Moreover, a surprisingly large number of patients require acute care for nonsurgical problems such as acute heart attacks, exacerbation of chronic diseases such as diabetes or hypertension, anxiety and other mental health problems, and near drowning because of flooding from broken dams.

Finally, an earthquake may precipitate a major technologic disaster by damaging or destroying nuclear power stations, hospitals with dangerous biologic products, hydrocarbon storage areas, and hazardous chemical plants. As with most natural disasters, the risk of secondary epidemics is minimal, and only mass immunization campaigns based on results of public health surveillance are appropriate following earthquakes.

REFERENCES

1. Walker, P., Walter, J. (Eds.) (2000). *World Disasters Report 2000: focus on public health*, pp. 159–87. International Federation of Red Cross and Red Crescent Societies, Geneva.
2. Munich Re. (2000) *Natural Catastrophes 2000*. Munich Re, Munich.
3. Western, K. (1972). *The epidemiology of natural and man-made disasters: the present state of the art* [dissertation]. University of London, London.
4. Noji, E.K., Toole, M.J. (1997). Public health and disasters: the historical development of public health responses to disasters. *Disasters* 21, 369–79.
5. Noji, E.K. (1992). Disaster epidemiology: challenges for public health action. *J Public Health Policy* 13, 332–40.
6. Binder, S., Sanderson, L.M. (1987). The role of the epidemiologist in natural disasters. *Ann Emerg Med* 16,1081–84.
7. Telford, J. (1997). *Counting and identification of beneficiary populations in emergency operations: Registration and its alternatives*. Good Practice Review No 5, Relief and Rehabilitation Network (RRN). pp. 1–45. Overseas Development Institute, London.
8. Lechat, M.F. (1990). Updates: the epidemiology of health effects of disasters. *Epidemiol Rev* 12, 192–97.
9. Lillibridge, S.A., Noji, E.K., Burkle, F.M. (1993). Disaster assessment: the emergency health evaluation of a disaster site. *Ann Emerg Med* 22, 1715–20.

10. Guha-Sapir, D., Lechat, M.F. (1986). Information systems and needs assessment in natural disasters: an approach for better disaster relief management. *Disasters* 10, 232–37.

11. Guha-Sapir, D. (1991). Rapid assessment of health needs in mass emergencies: review of current concepts and methods. *World Health Stat Q* 44, 171–81.

12. World Health Organization (1999). *Rapid Health Assessment Protocols*, pp. 1–34. WHO, Geneva.

13. Malilay, J., Flanders, W.D., Brogan, D. (1996). A modified cluster—sampling method for post-disaster rapid assessment of needs. *Bull World Health Organ* 74, 399–405.

14. Hlady, W.G., Quenemoen, L.E., Armenia-Cope, R.R., et al. (1994). Use of a modified cluster sampling method to perform rapid needs assessment after Hurricane Andrew. *Ann Emerg Med* 23, 719–25.

15. Noji, E.K. (Ed.) (1997). *The Public Health Consequences of Disasters*. Oxford University Press, New York.

16. Lee, L.E., Fonseca, V., Brett, K.M., et al. (1992). Active morbidity surveillance after Hurricane Andrew—Florida. *J Am Med Assoc* 270, 591–94.

17. Pan American Health Organization (2000). *Natural Disasters: protecting the public's health*, pp. 1–9. Scientific Publication No. 575, Washington D.C. PAHO.

18. Bernstein, R.S., Baxter, P.J., Falk, H., et al. (1986). Immediate public health concerns and actions in volcanic eruptions: lessons from the Mount St. Helens eruptions, May 18–October 18, 1980. *Am J Public Health* 76 (Suppl), 25–37.

19. Churchill, R.E. (1997). Effective media relations. In E.K. Noji (Ed.) *The Public Health Consequences of Disasters*, pp. 122–32. Oxford University Press, New York.

20. Perrin, P. (1996). *Handbook on War and Public Health*. International Committee of the Red Cross, Geneva.

21. Seaman, J. (1984). Epidemiology of natural disasters. *Contrib Epidemiol Biostat* 5, 1–177.

22. Medecins Sans Frontieres (MSF) (1997). *Refugee Health: an approach to emergency situations*. Macmillan, London.

23. Centers for Disease Control (1992). Famine-affected, refugee, and displaced populations: recommendations for public health issues. *Morb Mortal Wkly Rep* 41 (No.RR-13), 1–76.

24. Combs, D.L., Quenemoen, L.E., Parrish, R.G., et al. (1999). Assessing disaster-attributed mortality: development application of a definition classification matrix. *Int J Epidemiol* 28, 1124–29.

25. Noji, E.K. (1993). Analysis of medical needs in disasters caused by tropical cyclones: the need for a uniform injury reporting scheme. *J Trop Med Hygiene* 96, 370–76.

26. Roy, J., Kreysler, J. (2000). Minimum standards in health services. In *The Sphere Project: humanitarian charter and minimum standards in disaster response*, pp. 219–269. Oxfam Publishing, Oxford.

27. Western, K.A. (1982). *Epidemiologic Surveillance after Natural Disasters*, pp. 1–59. Pan American Health Organization, Washington, D.C.

22

LABORATORY SUPPORT FOR THE EPIDEMIOLOGIST IN THE FIELD

Janet K. A. Nicholson
Elaine W. Gunter

This chapter provides general guidelines on what specimens are appropriate to collect when investigating an infectious disease problem or when studying a potential toxic chemical exposure and what types of tests should be done to confirm an exposure or infection. The lists of specimens to collect and tests to perform are not exhaustive and may not include newer investigative or research tools such as genome probing. For the microbial agents, no effort was made to include all possible agents, only the more common ones that you are likely to encounter. Because most field investigations will involve specimen collection , *it is absolutely essential to contact the appropriate laboratory personnel prior to specimen collection and preferably before you enter the field* (see Chapter 5).

Although these guidelines are intended for epidemiologists doing field investigations, they also apply to specimens collected in other settings, as indicated in the sections below. Many of the local support laboratories can perform the tests described below—particularly those relating to infectious diseases. However, the laboratory services of the Centers for Disease Control and Prevention (CDC) will always serve as a necessary backup. And remember, make early contact with your support laboratory, and seek out the local, state, or provincial laboratory as appropriate.

This chapter is divided into three parts: the first deals with specimen collection for the detection of toxic chemicals; the second covers the identification of infectious pathogens; and the last addresses general issues related to shipping specimens.

COLLECTION OF SPECIMENS FOR POTENTIAL CHEMICAL TOXICANTS

General Instructions

In cases of suspected chemical toxicant exposure, it is extremely important to work in conjunction with your analytic support laboratory or, if needed, the Division of Laboratory Sciences (DLS) in the National Center for Environmental Health (NCEH) of CDC. DLS will provide laboratory support for environmental health studies and emergency response in these situations, and, as with other epidemiologic investigation, these studies must be planned and submitted for all appropriate processing as early as possible. For all analyses to be performed by DLS, it is imperative to contact the laboratory personnel prior to specimen collection, because a detailed specimen collection protocol must be prepared and included as an appendix to any study protocol.

The section below describes only general instructions on how to collect specimens. An example of the necessary detail and care required to collect certain kinds of specimens is also given to emphasize the critical nature of the methods used (see Appendix 22–1). In the rare event that you might be part of a team responding to chemical or biological terrorism events, see Appendix 22–2. It outlines simplified instructions for first responders who will be collecting specimens for identification of suspected chemical agents. All specimens will be sent to CDC's Rapid Response and Technology Laboratory (RRAT Lab), where they will be initially triaged for Class III or IV biological agents (the most dangerous and easiest to spread agents in the laboratory setting). They will then be irradiated before being transferred to the DLS, NCEH for chemical agent identification and quantitation.

If, on the other hand, you are contemplating collection and transport of specimens for chemical toxicant examination at CDC, it is imperative that you make contact with the NCEH DLS laboratory prior to collection. This is absolutely essential because of the highly specialized collection and analysis required for these toxicants. In some cases DLS is the only place where certain assays are performed. DLS has or will create detailed protocols for you. If there is an emergency, DLS is on call and will send materials and instructions as soon as possible—and, if necessary, provide personnel to assist in field specimen collection.

In chemical exposures, many toxicants or their metabolites may be rapidly cleared from easily accessible specimens, such as blood, either through excretion or sequestration in tissues. One must know the proper specimen matrix to collect to reflect either recent acute exposure, or body burden through chronic exposure. To meet this need, DLS maintains dedicated specimen collection supplies that have been pretested for any background contamination and abbreviated collection instructions (by specimen type) that can be rapidly shipped by air or prepared to accompany the investigator. The information that follows and the urine collection procedure in Appendix 22–1 are examples of these instructions.

A good rule of thumb in the case of an emergency where acute exposure(s) may have occurred is to obtain biological specimens (blood, serum, and urine) as soon as possible, even if it means using materials not pretested by the support laboratory or CDC. In these cases, follow the basic guidelines to control extraneous contamination, and cool the specimens as soon as possible. To allow evaluation of possible extraneous contamination from the collection materials, randomly select at least three of each item used (e.g., three randomly selected empty test tubes), seal them in a clean container, and store and ship them with the specimens. However, it is still important to obtain the state support laboratory or CDC-supplied collection materials as soon as possible for all subsequent sampling.

For both regularly scheduled studies and emergency response, laboratory results are only as good as the specimens collected, regardless of how sophisticated the analytic method may be. The small amounts of clinical specimens that are often collected and the low toxicant concentrations in the specimens may require methods with sensitivities as low as parts per quintillion (10^{-18}). Extraneous substances from the ambient air or a person's skin or clothing, or interfering substances in collection supplies will be concentrated and measured along with the specimens. Specimens must be kept at low temperatures to prevent degradation. For these reasons, detailed specimen collection protocols are found below.

Materials Required

Materials available locally

The following materials must be supplied or available locally by prior arrangement with a support laboratory:

- Centrifuge capable of spinning tubes as large as 16 mm in diameter by 100 mm long for separation of serum. After the blood in the red-topped tubes has been allowed to clot at room temperature for at least 30 and no more than 60 minutes, centrifuge the tubes for 15 minutes at 2400–2800 RPM (i.e., RPMs necessary to attain a force of $1000 \times G$)
- Refrigerator (4–8°C) and freezer (≤ –20°C, preferably *not* frost-free)
- Dry ice, 20–30 lb on hand (10–12 lb per shipping container)

Materials supplied from DLS

- Materials: All other materials needed are contained in the supplies provided by DLS. A collection protocol will be provided, since specimen collection requirements may vary for each study.

  All of these materials (collection tubes, pipets, aluminum foil, etc.) will have been screened or specially washed to minimize extraneous contamination. *Use only the materials supplied* for specimens if they are to be sent to CDC, and do not open the supplies until they need to be used. Return any unused intact and nonexpendable supplies to CDC.

- Instructions: Detailed instructions for collecting each specimen type should be included as well as the protocol for packing and shipping specimens. These instructions have been abbreviated to the extent possible to accommodate emergency situations.

Three general considerations must be kept in mind at all times:

- Specimen collection and processing conditions should be aimed at minimizing contamination from extraneous sources, such as hands, body parts, clothes, and ambient air.
- Specimens should be refrigerated or frozen, *as instructed*, as rapidly as possible after collection. If the field situation prevents access to specimen processing for 6–8 hours, the laboratory staff will provide stability information about the specimens. A cooler and reusable cold-packs will be provided for this purpose during specimen collection and transport for processing.
- Bar-coded labels with ASTRO numbers (CDC's unique specimen identifiers required for "cradle-to-grave" specimen tracking) will be provided by the laboratory to label all tubes collected, vials processed, and related paperwork. ASTRO specimen tracking software will be provided to the field epidemiologist on a laptop computer so that any required subject demographic information can be combined with the specimen list when the samples are returned to CDC. A specimen transmittal list must be prepared to accompany the specimens.

Specimen collection teams should be provided copies of these instructions and trained in their use prior to the time of anticipated need.

Guidelines for Collection of Clinical Specimens

Table 22–1 is provided to assist collection teams in determining which specimens should be collected in various situations based on the type of toxicant exposure and the types of specimens collected, by priority. For example, if problems are

Table 22–1. Blood or Urine to Collect for Suspected Environmental Toxicants

SUSPECTED TOXICANT	SPECIMEN PREFERRED (IN DECREASING ORDER OF PRIORITY)	ADULTS AND CHILDREN (10 YEARS OLD AND OLDER)	BABIES AND CHILDREN (LESS THAN 10 YEARS OLD)
Organic	Serum	two 10 mL tubes, no antigoagulant	one 5.0 mL tube, no anticoagulant
	Urine†	20 mL	10–20 mL†
	Whole blood (heparin)	one 7 mL tube	one 7 mL‡
Inorganic	Urine^d	20 mL	10–20 mL
	Whole blood (EDTA)	one 2 mL tube	one 2 mL tube
	Serum¶	one 7 mL trace metals–free tube	one 7 mL trace metals–free tube
Unknown	Serum	two 10 mL tubes, no anticoagulant	one 5.0 mL tube, no anticoagulant
	Urine*	20 mL	10–20 mL
	Whole blood (EDTA)	one 2 mL tube	one 2 mL tube
	Whole blood (heparin)	one 7 mL tube	one 7 mL tube‡

*Urine is preferred specimen to be collected if a cholinesterase inhibitor is suspected, such as organophosphate pesticide.

†For babies and children too young to be toilet trained, disposable urine collection bags or special collection tampons placed in the diaper may be used.

‡Preferred specimen if toxicant is suspected volatile organic compound. If time permits, the preferred tube here is a 7 or 10 mL gray-top (sodium oxalate/sodium fluoride anticoagulant) prepared by DLS.

dSpecimen pretreatment required ONLY for a separate aliquot for urine mercury if toxic mercury exposure is suspected. DLS will provide collection containers with a small amount of Triton X-100 surfactant and sulfamic acid to stabilize this specimen. Urine specimens for all other metals (e.g., As, Ni, Sn, Sb, Pb, Cd, Cr) or heavy radionuclides (e.g., U, Th, or Pu) will be stabilized with Ultrex nitric acid upon receipt at DLS.

¶For essential trace metals such as Se, Fe, Zn, Cu, Mg, Mn only, in case of overload.

encountered while collecting specimens from a 6-year-old boy by venipuncture for a suspected inorganic toxicant such as lead, cadmium, or mercury, the EDTA-anti-coagulated whole blood tube should be obtained before collection of blood for serum is attempted.

Contact the support laboratory or DLS, NCEH (770-488-4305 or 770-488-7932) and establish the date and time to ship the specimens.

Examples of possible environmental toxicants are:

• *Organic*: dioxins, furans, coplanar and non-coplanar polychlorinated bisphenol compounds (PCBs), persistent pesticides, volatile organic compounds (VOCs), cotinine and other markers of tobacco exposure, nonpersistent pesticides, organophosphate pesticides, polyaromatic hydrocarbons (PAHs), phthalates, paranitrophenol.

- *Inorganic*: heavy metals such as lead, arsenic, nickel, mercury, chromium, beryllium, or tin; essential trace metals such as selenium, iron, zinc, copper, calcium, magnesium, manganese (in overload cases); radionuclides such as uranium, thorium, plutonium, radioactive iodine.

For autopsy material such as liver, adipose, kidney, and lung tissues; and for fluids such as whole blood, urine, and stomach contents, place freshly cut tissues or fluids in sterile plastic screw-capped containers provided by DLS. Do not use formalized tissues.

The authors wish to thank the following persons who contributed to the preparation of this chapter: Carolyn M. Black, Ph.D., Scientific Resources Program; David L. Trees, Ph.D., Division of AIDS, STD, and TB Laboratory Research; John T. Roehrig, Ph.D. and May C. Chu, Ph.D., Division of Vector-Borne Infectious Diseases; Cheryl A. Bopp, M.S., Division of Bacterial and Mycotic Diseases; Harvey T. Holmes, Ph.D., Division of Healthcare Quality Promotion; Pierre E. Rollin, M.D., Division of Viral and Rickettsial Diseases; and Mark L. Eberhard, Ph.D., Division of Parasitic Diseases; all from the National Center for Infectious Diseases, and Eric J. Sampson, Ph.D.; James L. Pirkle, M.D., Ph.D.; John Liddle, Ph.D.; Daniel Huff, M.T.(ASCP); Charles Dodson, M.T.(ASCP); all from the Division of Laboratory Sciences, the National Center for Environmental Health.

APPENDIX 22–1. URINE COLLECTION PROCEDURE FOR SPECIMENS FOR METALS AND PESTICIDES ANALYSIS

URINE COLLECTION (FIRST MORNING VOID SPECIMEN IF POSSIBLE)

Urine collection cups will be provided for each participant. Instruct each person to do the following for urine collection to obtain a "clean catch" sample:

- Hands should be washed with soap and water.
- Do not remove the cap from cup until ready to void. Exposure to air should be minimized.
- Collect at least 30 mL urine in the cup as a midstream collection.
  - Do not touch the inside of the cup or cap at any time.
  - Recap the specimen and deliver to investigator.
  - Place a label for *URINE CONTAINER* on cup.
  - For a child younger than 3 years of age, pediatric urine collection bags may need to be used. Follow the directions accompanying the bags for use.

A total of 3 aliquots is needed. Prepare them in the order given below. If the sample is insufficient for all aliquots, do as many as possible with the amounts required for each test.

1. *Urine Pesticides*: Gently swirl the capped container to resuspend any dissolved solids. Pour 20–30 mL urine into the provided 2 or 4 oz plastic specimen container. (At DLS, one 1.0 mL aliquot of this specimen will be used for a urine creatinine measurement to correct the concentration of the metals or pesticides for specimen volume differences.) If a pediatric collection bag was used, tilt the bag slightly so the corner of the bag can be clipped with clean stainless steel scissors. Carefully pour the urine into the containers through this small hole.
2. *Urine Metals*: Transfer 4 mL urine to a 5 mL plastic cryotube.
3. *Urine Mercury*: Add urine to 4.5 mL line on tube with red dot. This tube contains a small amount of a surfactant and a mild acid to preserve the mercury and must be mixed well by inversion after being securely capped to dissolve this preservative.

All aliquot tubes should be labeled with the appropriate barcoded label with the participant ID number and aliquot type. Ship to DLS on dry ice.

SHIPPING LIST

A transmittal log is provided to record samples that are collected. Mark the appropriate spaces indicating which aliquots were collected, date collected, and any problems that were encountered in collection, storage, or shipping.

SHIPPING PROCEDURE

1. Pack the shipping box with the boxes of urine samples. Place each box in the Ziplock bags before packing. Fill the shipper with dry ice, cover with the styrofoam lid, and tape down the cardboard outer flaps. Place a dry ice label on the outside of the container and write in the amount of dry ice in the shipper.
2. Ship to the following address:
   Specimen Receipt Coordinator
   Division of Laboratory Sciences
   Centers for Disease Control and Prevention
   Building 17 Loading Dock

4770 Buford Highway NE
Atlanta, GA 30341-3724

3. Call (770) 488-4305 on the day the shipment is made or if any questions arise.

APPENDIX 22–2. SUMMARY INSTRUCTIONS FOR SPECIMEN COLLECTION IN CASES OF SUSPECTED CHEMICAL TERRORISM EVENTS

SPECIMEN COLLECTION

(*Do not use personal identifiers on samples; adhere to forensic evidence chain of custody protocols.*)

- Urine: at least 20 mL; use screw-capped plastic container.
- Serum: the yield from two 10 mL *no-anticoagulant* [U.S. color code red-top] tubes (*do not use SST tubes*) in plastic screw-capped vials.
- Whole blood: one 5 mL or 7 mL NaOxalate/NaF anticoagulated—gray-top tube (or one 5 mL or 7 mL heparinized/[*U.S. color code green-top*] tube) unopened, *plus* an empty tube to check as a blank.

COLLECTION OF SPECIMENS FOR MICROBIAL IDENTIFICATION

General Instructions

It is essential that the field epidemiologist contact the specific support laboratory prior to collecting specimens, because each testing laboratory has its own protocols. If you plan to send your specimens to CDC, you should know that the National Center of Infectious Diseases (NCID) does not have a single point of contact for specimen collection and testing. NCID published a document entitled, "Reference and Disease Surveillance," in February 1993, that specifies the kinds of specimens that will be processed for state health departments, the kinds of tests that will be performed, and considerable detail regarding the collection and shipment of specimens to CDC. NCID provides laboratory services to state health departments under special, clearly defined circumstances. NCID does not normally accept specimens submitted to it from county health departments, hospitals, or private physicians, as these specimens should initially be sent to the state health department laboratory. If the state laboratory subsequently deems it necessary to call upon the laboratories of NCID for support and if the specimens satisfy the CDC requirements, then the NCID laboratories will accept the specimens. Under some circumstances, individual NCID laboratories will accept specimens directly;

however, these are special circumstances, and these arrangements must be made in advance with the specific laboratory.

When an epidemiologist encounters an illness likely to be of infectious etiology, there is no substitute for good clinical judgment. Inappropriate, insufficient, or inappropriately collected specimens may result in misidentification or the inability to identify the causative agent. In this regard, many of the suggested laboratory tests provide information to support a diagnosis, not make it.

Universal precautions statement

Since medical history and examination cannot reliably identify all persons infected with HIV or other blood-borne pathogens, "universal blood and body fluid precautions" should be used when obtaining and handling specimens of blood and certain other body fluids from *all persons* (*Morbidity and Mortality Weekly Report* 37:377, 1988). Other body fluids include amniotic, pericardial, peritoneal, pleural, synovial, and cerebrospinal fluids (CSF), and semen and vaginal secretions. In addition, any body fluid containing visible blood and body tissues should be handled as though it may be infectious.

Gloves should be worn whenever handling blood or the specified body fluids and when performing phlebotomy. Barrier precautions should be used whenever appropriate to prevent skin and mucous membrane exposure during specimen acquisition and handling. Gowns should be worn if splashing or spattering of fluids is likely. If splashing of the mouth and face are possible, masks and protective eyewear are indicated. Specimens are to be transported in leakproof containers.

Take care to prevent injuries when using needles, scalpels, and other sharp instruments or devices and when disposing of used instrument sharps. Do not recap or remove needles from disposable syringes by hand; and do not bend, break, or otherwise manipulate used needles by hand. Dispose of needles and sharp equipment in puncture-resistant containers designed for this purpose.

Specimen collection

Tables 22–2–9 provide information on the type of specimen needed and the assays used for identification of the microbial agent. Some considerations for collection and shipment of specimens are found below.

Serum specimens for serology should be separated from whole blood using aseptic technique. Contaminated serum specimens are unsuited for almost all purposes. Paired serum specimens are preferred and in many cases required. The first specimen should be obtained as soon after the onset of illness as possible and refrigerated. The second specimen should be collected 2–4 weeks later. The optimal interval for collecting the serum specimens will vary with different infectious diseases. Paired serum specimens, though desirable, are difficult to obtain and are not required for serologic tests of mycotic or parasitic diseases or for syphilis.

Table 22–2. Bacterial Diseases—General*

AGENT OR DISEASE	SPECIMEN(S) TO COLLECT	METHOD OF CONFIRMATION OR IDENTIFICATION	COMMENTS
Brucellosis	Blood, bone, marrow, or site of localization	Culture	Prolonged incubation (4–5 days) may be necessary
	Sera	Tube agglutination or EIA	2-mercaptoethanol agglutination test distinguishes IgG from IgM antibodies and may be diagnostic for chronic brucellosis. *B. canis* infection requires specific serologic test
Cat scratch disease	Skin biopsy Lymph node Blood Pus	Culture, FA	
Chlamydia pneumonia	Nasopharyngeal swab	Culture, PCR	Maintain cultures at 4°C, or –70°C if transport time >24 hr
Diphtheria	Throat swab	Culture	Put swab directly into Pai slant
H. influenzae	Blood CSF Sterile site specimen	Culture	Antigen tests sensitive but culture strongly preferable
Legionellosis	Sera Lung tissue Resp. secretions Water Urine	FA FA, culture-confirm by SAT Culture Antigen detection (RIA)	Positive IFA not conclusive, culture strongly preferable

(continued)

Table 22–2. (*Continued*)

AGENT OR DISEASE	SPECIMEN(S) TO COLLECT	METHOD OF CONFIRMATION OR IDENTIFICATION	COMMENTS
Leptospirosis	Blood	Culture	Leptospiremia occurs during first week of illness. Leptospiruria occurs after the second week of illness. Growth occurs after several days to several weeks
	Urine	Culture	
	Sera	MAT	
Listeriosis	CSF		Serology neither sensitive nor specific
	Blood		
	Site of infection	Culture, PCR	
	Placenta		
	Food		
Lyme disease and other borrellioses	Sera	FA, EIA	Serotyping and subtyping indicated for epidemiologic investigation; not for confirmation or identification
	Blood, skin biopsy	Culture, PCR	Clinical case definition necessary
	CSF	Culture, EIA, PCR	Culture requires special medium
	Synovial fluid	EIA, PCR	Indicated for patients with neurologic involvement
Mycoplasma pneumoniae	Throat swab, sputum	Culture	
	Sera	CF, EIA, indirect hemagglutination, IIF	

Organism	Specimen	Test	Comments
Neisseria meningitidis	CSF Blood Throat Sera	Culture, serotype, latex agglutination	Serotyping and subtyping indicated for epidemiologic investigation; not for confirmation or identification
Trachoma (*C. trachomatis*)	Conjunctival swab	NAAT	Maintain at −70°C in sucrose phosphate transport medium without penicillin
Tularemia	Blood, lymph node, sputum, lesional material Lymph node, lesional material Sera	Culture, serology, FA, IHC Direct fluorescent antibody test Microagglutination	Culture requires chocolate agar Laboratory hazard
Group A streptococcus	Culture	Throat swab	
Group B streptococcus	Placenta, blood	Culture, subtyping	
Plague	Blood, lymph node, lymph aspirate, sputum, lesional material Lesional material, lymph node Sera	Culture, IHC FA Passive hemagglutination or EIA	Culture recovery on general lab media
Psittacosis (*C. psittaci*)	Sera	CF	

*See Appendix 22–3 for definitions of acronyms.

Table 22-3. Bacterial Diseases—Sexually Transmitted*

AGENT OR DISEASE	SPECIMEN(S) TO COLLECT	METHOD OF CONFIRMATION OR IDENTIFICATION	COMMENTS
Chancroid	Swab from lesion	Gram strain, culture: colonial morphology and texture (catalase, porphyrin, oxidase [tetra], nitrate reductase, alkaline phosphatase	Organism dies rapidly. Transport swabs in deep rabbit blood agar and Isovitalex swabs or freeze at −70°C in defibrinated rabbit's blood
Lymphogranuloma venereum (LGV) (*C. trachomatis*)	Bubo aspirate Lymph node biopsy Sera	Culture, NAAT NAAT CF, MIF	Culture: maintain at 4°C or −70°C if transport time >24 hr Negative CF or MIF test rules out LGV
Genital non-LGV (*C. trachomatis*)	Endocervical swab Urine	Culture, NAAT NAAT	Culture: maintain at −70°C in sucrose-phosphate transport medium without penicillin
Gonorrhea	Heterosexual men: U(T)† Women: C, R, T† Homosexual men: U, R, T† Urine	Culture: acid production from carbohydrates, enzyme substrate tests. Serologic tests: FA coagglutination DNA probe, NAAT	Suspend growth from pure culture in 75% glycerol in TSB. Store at −70°C, transport on dry ice (frozen strains may be stored at −20° for 1–2 weeks)
Syphilis	Sera	Nontreponemal/treponemal tests, DNA and Reiter absorption, WB	Treponemal tests available on postmortem bloods
Congenital	Sera	FTA-ABS, IgM (19S) IgM EIA	Mother's and baby's serum and history requested
Neurosyphilis	CSF Autopsy, biopsy, lesional material	FTA-ABS CSF, VDRL (CSF), WB DFA-TP	Paraffin blocks, slides, or fixed material acceptable; must state fixative

*See Appendix 22–3 for definitions of acryonyms.
†U = urethra, R = rectum, T = throat, C = cervix.

Table 22-4. Bacterial Diseases—Food-Borne

AGENT OR DISEASE	SPECIMEN(S) TO COLLECT	METHOD OF CONFIRMATION OR IDENTIFICATION	COMMENTS
Bacillus cereus	Stool Food	Culture Assay for toxin	Need at least 10^5 organisms per gram of incriminated food
Campylobacter jejuni	Stool Food	Culture	Serotyping done in special circumstances
Botulism (*Clostridium botulinum*)	Stool NG aspirate Food Serum	Culture, mouse assay for toxin Culture, mouse assay for toxin Mouse assay for toxin	Call Foodborne and Diarrheal Diseases Branch ASAP if you suspect botulism
Clostridium perfringens	Stool Food	Culture Assay for toxin	Need 10^5 organisms per gram of incriminated food Serotyping is done in special cases
E. coli	Stool Food Serum	Culture, serotyping, assays for toxin production and for invasiveness Assay for lipopolysaccharide (LPS) antibody	Specialized testing is needed to determine if *E. coli* belongs to one of the four groups recognized as enteric pathogens
Salmonellosis	Stool Food	Culture, serotyping	Antibiograms are useful epidemiologic markers. Molecular subtyping (e.g., PFGE) is done in special circumstances

(continued)

Table 22-4. (*Continued*)

AGENT OR DISEASE	SPECIMEN(S) TO COLLECT	METHOD OF CONFIRMATION OR IDENTIFICATION	COMMENTS
Shigellosis	Stool Food	Culture, serotyping	Antibiograms are useful epidemiologic markers. Molecular subtyping is done in special circumstances
Staphylococcus aureus	Stool Food Vomitus Nasal swabs	Culture, phase typing Assay for toxin	Need 10^5 organisms per gram of incriminated food or Detection of toxin in implicated food (not done at CDC)
Vibrio cholerae O1 and O139	Stool Food Sera	Culture, serotype, assay for toxin production Vibriocidal and antitoxic antibodies	Cholera is the disease caused by toxigenic *V. cholerae* O1 and O139 Call the Foodborne and Diarrheal Diseases Branch ASAP if you suspect cholera
Vibrio cholerae non-O1	Stool Food	Culture, serotype Assay for toxin production	Serotyping is done in special cases
Vibrio parahemolyticus	Stool Food	Culture Serotyping Hemolysin testing	Human isolates produce a thermostable direct hemolysin or thermo-stable direct-related hemolysin or both
Yersinia enterocolitica	Stool Food Sera	Culture, serotyping	Serotyping done in special circumstances

Table 22–5. Viral Diseases—General*

AGENT OR DISEASE	SPECIMEN(S) TO COLLECT	METHOD OF CONFIRMATION OR IDENTIFICATION	COMMENTS
Adenovirus	Throat swab, stool, eye swab	Culture, EIA	
	Sera	HI, CF, NT, EIA, IIF	
AIDS (retroviruses)	Blood, body fluids	Culture	
	Sera	EIA, WB	
Cytomegalovirus (CMV)	Urine, throat swab	Culture	Serologic tests of limited diagnostic value
	Sera	EIA, CF, indirect hemaglutination	
Coronaviruses	Throat swab	Culture	Serologic tests of limited diagnostic value
	Sera	CF, HI, NT, EIA	
Coxsackie	CSF, stool, rectal swab	Culture swab, throat swab	Serologic tests of limited diagnostic value
	Sera	NT, EIA	
Epstein–Barr	Blood, throat swab	Culture	
	Sera	OCH, IIF	
Echoviruses	CSF, stool, rectal swab	Culture	Serologic tests of limited diagnostic value
	Sera	EIA	
Hepatitis A	Blood	EIA	
	Sera	EIA, RIA	
Hepatitis B	Blood	EIA	
	Sera	EIA, RIA	
Hepatitis (Delta)	Blood	EIA	
	Sera	EIA	
Hepatitis C (non-A, non-B) (NANB)	Sera	EIA, RIA	

(continued)

Table 22–5. (*Continued*)

AGENT OR DISEASE	SPECIMEN(S) TO COLLECT	METHOD OF CONFIRMATION OR IDENTIFICATION	COMMENTS
Enterically-transmitted Hepatitis E	Sera	EIA, FA	
Herpes simplex	Vesicular fluid, brain biopsy	Culture, EIA, DFA	
	Sera	EIA, CF, indirect hemagglutination	Serologic tests of limited diagnostic value
Influenza	Throat swab	Culture, EIA	
	Sera	CF, HI, EIA	
Lassa fever	Blood	Culture	Isolation of agent in lab requires biosafety level 4 containment
	Sera	IIF, NT	
Lymphocytic choriomeningitis	Brain	Culture	
	Sera	CF, IIF, NT	
Measles	Throat swab	Culture, EIA	Serology preferred for diagnosis
	Sera	EIA, HI, CF, NT	
Mumps	Throat swab	Culture, EIA	
	Sera	HI, CF, NT, EIA	
Norwalk virus	Stool	EIA, immune electron microscopy	
	Sera	EIA	
Parainfluenza	Throat swab	Culture, EIA	
	Sera	CF, HI, EIA, IIF	
Parvovirus	Blood	EIA	
	Sera	EIA, RIA	

Organism	Specimen	Test	Comment
Picornaviruses	Stool, rectal swab, throat swab Sera	Culture NT, EIA	
Polioviruses 1–3	Stool, rectal swab, throat swab, CNS tissue Sera	Culture NT, CF	
Rabies	Brain, skin biopsy Sera	Culture, DFA RFFIT, IFA	
Respiratory syncytial virus	Throat swab Sera	Culture, EIA CF, EIA, NT	
Rotavirus	Stool Sera	EIA, culture, electron microscopy, gel electrophoresis EIA, NT	
Rubella	Throat swab Sera	Culture, EIA EIA, HI, Latex Agglutination, IIF	Serology preferred for diagnosis
Vaccinia	Vesicular fluid, scabs, brain Sera	Culture, Electron microscopy EIA, HI, NT	
Varicella-zoster	Vesicular fluid Sera	Culture, electron microscopy IIF, CF	

*See Appendix 22–3 for definitions of acronyms.

Table 22–6. Viral Diseases—Vector-Borne*

AGENT OR DISEASE	SPECIMEN(S) TO COLLECT	METHOD OF CONFIRMATION OR IDENTIFICATION	COMMENTS
California encephalitis	Sera	EIA, HI, CF, NT	
	Brain	Virus isolation	Except where noted freeze specimens for virus isolation at –65°C (dry ice)
	CSF	Virus isolation, EIA	
	Mosquitoes	Virus isolation, EIA	
Colorado tick fever	Whole blood clot	Virus isolation	Do not freeze samples for CTF virus isolation.
	Sera	IIF, EIA, CF, NT	
	Ticks	Virus isolation, EIA	
Dengue 1–4	Sera	Virus isolation, HI, CF, NT, EIA, PCR	
	Liver, lung, lymph nodes	Virus isolation, antigen detection	Freeze tissues at –70°C and fix in formalin
Eastern equine encephalitis	Sera	Virus isolation, HI, CF, NT, EIA, IIF	
	Brain	Virus isolation	
	CSF	Virus isolation, EIA	
	Mosquitoes	Virus isolation, EIA	
	Horse sera	HI, CF, NT, EIA	
St. Louis encephalitis	Sera	HI, CF, NT, EIA, IIF	
	Urine	EIA, virus isolation	
	Brain	virus isolation, EIA, IIF	
	CSF	virus isolation, EIA	
	Mosquitoes	virus isolation, EIA	

Agent or Disease	Specimen(s) to Collect	Method of Confirmation or Identification	Comments
Venezuelan equine encephalitis	Sera	Virus isolation, HI, CF, NT, EIA, IIF	Isolation requires biosafety level 3 containment
	Brain	Virus isolation, IIF, EIA	
	CSF	Virus isolation, EIA	
	Mosquitoes	Virus isolation, EIA	
	Horse sera	Virus isolation, HI, CF, NT, EIA	
Western equine encephalitis	Sera	HI, CF, NT, EIA, IIF	
	Brain	Virus isolation, IIF, EIA	
	CSF	Virus isolation, EIA	
	Mosquitoes	Virus isolation, EIA	
	Horse sera	Virus isolation, HI, CF, NT, EIA	
West Nile virus	Sera	HI, CF, NT, IFA	Isolation requires biosafety level 3 containment
	Brain, brain stem, spinal cord	Virus isolation, EIA, IFA	
	CSF	Virus isolation, EIA	
	Mosquitoes	Virus isolation, EIA	
Yellow fever	Sera	Virus isolation, EIA, PCR, CF, HI, NT, IIF	Isolation requires biosafety level 3 containment with HEPA filtered exhaust air flow
	Liver	Virus isolation, histopathology, EIA	Yellow fever immunization required
	Mosquitoes	Virus isolation, EIA	

*See Appendix 22–3 for definitions of acronyms.

Table 22–7. Rickettsial Diseases*

AGENT OR DISEASE	SPECIMEN(S) TO COLLECT	METHOD OF CONFIRMATION OR IDENTIFICATION	COMMENTS
Q fever	Sera Lung, blood	CF, IIF Culture	Isolation of organisms in lab requires biosafety level 3 containment
Rocky Mountain spotted fever	Sera Brain, spleen, blood	IIF Culture, FA	Isolation of organisms in lab requires biosafety level 3 containment
Murine typhus	Sera Blood	IIF Culture	
Ehrlichiosis	Blood, spleen Sera	Culture IIF	

*See Appendix 22–3 for definitions of acronyms.

Table 22–8. Mycotic Infections*

AGENT OR DISEASE	SPECIMEN(S) TO COLLECT	METHOD OF CONFIRMATION OR IDENTIFICATION	COMMENTS
Aspergillosis	Sera Tissue, site of infection	ID Histology, direct examination, culture	
Candidiasis	Sera Tissue	ID, LA, EIA Histology, culture	
Cryptococcosis	Sera Tissue, site of infection CSF	TA, LA Histology, FA, direct exam, culture	
Histoplasmosis	Sera Tissue, site of infection Urine	ID, CF Direct exam, culture, ID (exoantigen), histology, FA Antigenuria	
Nocardiasis	Sera Tissue, site of infection	ID Direct exam, culture	
Sporotrichosis	Sera Tissue, site of infection	TA, LA Histology, FA, direct exam, culture	

*See Appendix 22–3 for definitions of acronyms.

Table 22-9. Parasitic Infections*

AGENT OR DISEASE	SPECIMEN(S) TO COLLECT	METHOD OF CONFIRMATION OR IDENTIFICATION	COMMENTS
Amebiasis	Sera	IHA	
	Tissue	Direct examination	
	Formalin- and PVA-preserved stool	Trichrome stain	
	Water from suspect source		
Cryptosporidiosis	Formalin-preserved stool	Direct examination of concentrated stool stain by modified Kinyoun (acid-fast) stain or DFA	
	Tissue	Histopathology	
	Sera		
Cyclospora	Formalin-preserved stool	Direct exam of concentrated stool by Kinyouns modified acid-fast stain or hot safranin stain	
	Potassium dichromate–preserved stool	PCR	
	Suspect food sample	PCR	
Giardiasis	Formalin-preserved stool	Direct examination of concentrated stool or DFA	
	PVA-preserved stool	Trichrome stain	
Leishmaniasis	Sera	CF or IFA	
	Tissue	Direct exam of H&E or Giemsa stained tissue or impression smears	
	Tissue impression smears	Culture	
	Whole blood		

(continued)

(continued)

Table 22–9. (*Continued*)

AGENT OR DISEASE	SPECIMEN(s) TO COLLECT	METHOD OF CONFIRMATION OR IDENTIFICATION	COMMENTS
Malaria	Blood smear Sera	Direct exam of Giemsa stained smear IFA	
Schistosomiasis	Formalin-preserved stool Fresh urine (examine within 45 minutes or preserve with formalin) Sera	Exam of concentrated stool for eggs Examination of centrifuged urine sediment EIA	Tissue diagnosis occasionally necessary for diagnosis; rectal biopsy more common Serologic tests helpful in acute or ectopic schistosomiasis
Toxoplasmosis	Sera Tissue	IFA or ELISA Direct exam	IgM antibodies against toxoplasma indicate recent exposure but may be detectable by EIA for 6 months to a year after infection
Trichinellosis	Sera Tissue sample of suspect meat	EIA Direct exam of biopsied tissue	In addition to pork, other meats such as bear, cougar, moose, walrus, and horse meat have been implicated as the source of infection

However, when neonates are being tested for congenital syphilis, serum specimens are required from the newborn and the mother. Serologic tests for neurosyphilis require serum and CSF specimens.

When whole blood is sent for isolation of certain viral, bacterial, and parasitic agents, the blood should be kept cold, but not frozen, prior to shipment and shipped in wet ice, not dry ice. Water ice should not be used for packing when taken directly from the ice maker or ice trays. Rather, the wet ice should be held in a container until some liquid water collects, indicating the ice is starting to thaw. The liquid may be poured off and the specimen packed with the remaining solid ice with less fear of ruining the specimen by freezing en route. Provision should be made to prevent leakage of the water as the wet ice melts and to keep this water from the specimen (a good sealed container will suffice). Be sure that the specimen is so arranged that it will not be broken by the solid ice in which it is packed. Whole blood submitted for rickettsial isolation must be packed in dry ice and shipped frozen. Because some microbial specimens require different handling procedures, be sure to check with the diagnostic laboratory prior to shipping.

Slides with tissue sections, blood films, and smears of clinical material should be dry, free of immersion oil, properly labeled, and carefully packed in a slide mailing container. If it is unstained, it should be fixed prior to shipping to minimize the chance of sending live organisms. If a cardboard slide mailer is the only mailer available, it should be placed in another shipping container to ensure that the slides are not broken in transit.

Cultures of etiologic agents should be cultivated and shipped in a medium that will protect and ensure the viability of the microorganism during transit. This medium is used to minimize growth of both the organism and unwanted contaminants during transport.

Optimum containers for different groups of etiologic agents vary depending upon the agent and the distance involved in shipment. In all instances, the primary container should be of a durable material that, when properly packaged, is leakproof and can withstand the temperature and pressure variations likely to occur in the air and on the ground during shipment.

When in doubt about what to collect, when to collect, and how to handle specimens, consult your support laboratory or the NCID laboratory contact. If time is of the essence and that person(s) cannot be reached, refer to a standard microbiology text for this information.

SPECIMEN SHIPPING PROTOCOL

This protocol applies for specimens to be tested for chemical or microbial exposures. Shipping regulations have changed over the years, so it is prudent to refer to current regulations prior to shipping specimens. For assistance in determining how to ship specimens contact your support laboratory or the CDC Office of Health and Safety website: (http://www.cdc.gov/od/ohs/biosfty/biosfty.htm).

Temperature Requirements

The following types of specimens must be shipped frozen in containers with dry ice:

- Serum/plasma (when directed by protocol)
- Urine
- Frozen food
- Tissue
- Red blood cell hemolysates (if prepared by special protocol)

The following types of specimens must be sent refrigerated, in containers with reusable cold-packs or, if necessary, double-bagged icepacks:

- Whole blood (e.g., the tubes collected for heavy metals such as Pb or the VOCs)
- Red blood cells (if separated for a special protocol)
- Food
- Serum/plasma (when directed by protocol)
- Urine (when directed by protocol)

The following types of specimens may be sent refrigerated or frozen:

- Water
- Soil[a]

List of Materials Needed

Available locally: 10–12 pounds of dry ice per shipping container (for frozen specimens). Shipping materials supplied by DLS for analysis of chemical toxins (for infectious specimens, refer to NCID laboratory for necessary materials):

- Styrofoam-insulated shipping container
- Cardboard storage boxes with dividers or foam inserts for anticoagulated blood collection tubes or processed specimens

[a]If soil is being sent from an international field site for chemical testing, DLS has a USDA-approved soil importation certificate. Contact the laboratory (770-488-7932 or 770-488-4305) for a copy and the required stickers for the soil container.

- Bubble wrap packing material (additional paper material such as paper towels or newspaper will be needed.)
- Clear or reinforced packaging tape
- Reusable cold-packs for refrigerated specimens: *These must be placed in a −20° Centigrade freezer for a minimum of 2 hours before use.*
- Air express courier shipping labels (with CDC's account number)

Procedures for Shipping Frozen Specimens to DLS or NCID Laboratory

- Assemble shipping container, packing materials, and dry ice. Work quickly so the frozen specimens will not be exposed to ambient temperatures for more than 5 to 10 minutes, if possible. It is imperative that the specimens be kept in a hard frozen state.
- Place the processed serum or urine samples into white cardboard boxes provided by the laboratory. Label the top of each box with the study name, and "Box 1 of 3," etc. Secure the box top with a large rubber band or packaging tape. Place a layer of dry ice on the bottom of the shipper, followed by a layer of newspaper or paper towels. Place the specimen boxes on top of the paper, followed by another layer of paper, and finally fill the container with additional dry ice on top for a total of 10–12 lb. In this manner, the specimens are protected from collision with each other and from direct contact with the dry ice. Use enough paper to pack the boxes so they will not move inside the shipping container, even as the dry ice sublimes and creates open space.
- The shipping container has an inner styrofoam lid and an outer cardboard lid. Secure the inner styrofoam lid, and place an envelope containing a copy of the completed transmittal list which contains the sample identifiers, dates of collection, and other pertinent information for the laboratory. Make sure the transmittal list reflects exactly in what order the specimens were placed in the boxes. Secure the outer cardboard top with strapping tape.
- Attach the mailing label provided and ship by air express courier such as Federal Express, UPS, or DHL so the specimens will be received by the support lab within 24 hours.
- Telephone the support lab or CDC laboratory (for specimens analyzed for chemical toxins, call 770-488-4305 or 770-488-7932; fax 770-488-4609) to alert them how specimens are being sent and when and where they will arrive. This is especially important if it is unavoidable that the specimens will be delivered on weekends or holidays.

Procedures for Shipping Refrigerated Specimens

- Assemble shipping container, cardboard storage boxes with foam inserts, frozen refrigerant packs, and packing materials.
- Place anticoagulated collection tubes in the foam inserts to keep them upright in the cardboard storage boxes during shipment. Place other processed specimens in the provided cardboard storage boxes.
- Place several frozen refrigerant packs at the bottom of the container, add a layer of paper, then the cardboard storage boxes. Add additional cold-packs on the side and on top of the boxes, if available. Pack the shipping container with additional paper to secure everything in place during shipment. The shipping container has an inner styrofoam lid and an outer cardboard lid. Secure the inner styrofoam lid, and place an envelope containing a copy of the completed transmittal list which contains the sample identifiers, dates of collection, and other pertinent information for the laboratory. Make sure the transmittal list reflects exactly in what order the specimens were placed in the boxes. Secure the outer cardboard top with strapping tape.
- Attach the mailing label provided and ship by air express courier such as Federal Express, UPS, or DHL so that the specimens will be received by the support lab or DLS, CDC within 24 hours.
- Telephone DLS (call 770-488-4305 or 770-488-7932; fax 770-488-4609) or appropriate NCID laboratory to alert them how specimens are being sent and when and where they will arrive. This is especially important if it is unavoidable that the specimens will be delivered on weekends or holidays.

APPENDIX 22-3. LIST OF ABBREVIATIONS

BF	Bentonite flocculation
CF	Complement fixation
CMV	Cytomegalovirus
CSF	Cerebrospinal fluid
DFA-TP	Direct fluorescent antibody for *T. pallidum*
DLS	Division of Laboratory Sciences
EIA	Enzyme immunoassay
ELISA	Enzyme-linked immunoabsorbent assay
FA	Fluorescent antibody test (direct or indirect)
FTA-ABS	Fluorescent treponemal antibody-absorption
H & E	Hematoxylin and eosin stain
HI	Hemagglutination inhibition
ID	Immunodiffusion

IEP	Immune electrophoresis
IIF	Indirect immune fluorescence
IHA	Indirect hemagglutination
IHC	Immunohistochemistry
LA	Latex agglutination
LGV	Lymphogranuloma venereum
MAT	Microscopic agglutination
MIF	Microimmunofluorescence test
NAAT	Nucleic acid amplification test
NCEH	National Center for Environmental Health
NCID	National Center for Infectious Diseases
NT	Neutralization test
OCH	Ox cell hemolysin
PAH	Polyaromatic hydrocarbons
PCB	Polychlorinated bisphenol compounds
PCR	Polymerase chain reaction
PHA	Passive hemagglutination
PVA	Polyvinyl alcohol
Resp.	Respiratory
RFFIT	Rapid fluorescent focus inhibition test
RIA	Radioimmunoassay
SAT	Slide agglutination test
TA	Tube agglutination
VDRL	Venereal disease research laboratory
VOC	Volatile organic compounds
WB	Western blot

APPENDIX
A WALK-THROUGH EXERCISE:
A FOOD-BORNE EPIDEMIC IN
OSWEGO COUNTY, NEW YORK

Michael B. Gregg

Chapter 5 describes in some detail how to investigate an epidemic. Although not "chipped in stone," the steps described in that chapter lead you logically through a broad series of actions and thought processes that virtually every field epidemiologist will take during an investigation. However, the beginner, the neophyte epidemiologist, may need a more detailed explanation of what to do, when to do it, and how to think. In other words, a "walk-through" kind of exercise might be of use to some of the readers of this book—particularly those who are local food inspectors responsible for investigating sicknesses associated with social functions and food establishments. This Appendix attempts to do just that.

The following story is true, and, although old in time, it represents a typical outbreak and subsequent investigation still performed by many local and state health departments to this day. Designed as the first exercise for introductory courses in epidemiology, the "Oswego problem," as it is known, has probably taught more budding epidemiologists than any other exercise of its kind in existence. It has been translated into many languages, is still used at CDC, and has weathered well the test of time as a true "classic."

Before we begin unraveling the story in Oswego County, New York, let us review the critical steps in a field investigation referred to in Chapter 5.

- Establish the existence of the epidemic
- Verify the diagnosis

- Define a case and count cases
- Describe the epidemic in terms of time, place, and person
- Determine who is at risk
- Develop a hypothesis
- Test the hypothesis
- Compare the hypothesis with the established facts
- Plan a more systematic study
- Prepare a written report
- Execute control and prevention measures

For our purposes here, we concentrate on all the steps that you will actually perform while you are in the field; therefore, we omit the steps of planning a study and writing a report.

Recall several important things:

- The order you do these steps will vary from epidemic to epidemic depending on many factors. You actually may do several steps at the same time. However different the circumstances may be, you will ultimately do them all to a greater or lesser degree.
- In this particular "walk-through" exercise, Dr. Rubin, the investigator in Oswego, was given, right at the beginning, some preliminary time, place, and person information that he necessarily had to take at face value. He did not collect the data, but, then, he would not have responded to the outbreak unless he thought that there was some reasonable chance a problem existed. This is true for all field investigations. You usually will have received "tip-of-the-iceberg" data, preliminary assessments, even rumors that will soon need verification and amplification.
- Some investigators might find it useful to think along two lines of activity: operational and epidemiologic. *Operationally*, as you investigate the epidemic, think of where you are "on that list," where you have been, and where you will be going next. Take the time to orient yourself to the tasks accomplished and those ahead of you. There is nothing more useful than a framework or a defined context to help you plan and execute your work. So take a deep breath now and then! *Epidemiologically*, think of the need for and the value of the hard facts of time, place, and person and how you will build the strongest possible case for your analyses, interpretations, and conclusions. Be sure of your data, for you may be challenged. So consider where you want to "do battle": on the quality of the data or on their analysis and interpretation.

In this walk-through, we describe the events much as they are written in the Oswego exercise and taken from Dr. Rubin's report, which is found in the records of the New York State Department of Health (CDC, unpublished data). Some minor changes have been made to enhance the flow and logic of the exercise. Periodically, we take stock of where we are in the investigative process by asking questions, looking at what we *know* and what we can *infer* or what we think the information is suggesting. It is quite important to keep these two processes very separate in your mind.

THE OUTBREAK

On April 19. 1940, the local health officer in Lycoming, Oswego County, New York, reported the occurrence of an outbreak of acute gastrointestinal (GI) illness to the District Health Officer in Syracuse. Dr. A. M. Rubin, epidemiologist-in-training, was assigned to conduct an investigation.

When Dr. Rubin arrived in the field that day he immediately went to the local health officer and was told that all persons known to be ill had attended a church supper on the previous evening and that most of them became ill the early morning of April 19. Eighty persons were known to have attended the supper and over 40 were ill. Family members who did not attend the supper did not become ill.

Would You Call This an Epidemic? Would You Call It an Outbreak?

Both terms, *epidemic* and *outbreak*, are usually defined as the occurrence of more cases of illness in a place (or population) and time than is normally expected. Here, 40 or more cases of GI illness spanning a 24 hour period, seemingly among a social group, are clearly more than one would expect.

The words "epidemic" and "outbreak" are used interchangeably by many epidemiologists, although some consider the term "outbreak" to refer to a more localized situation, and "epidemic" to a more widespread—and perhaps prolonged—occurrence. Try not to use the word "epidemic" when you are in the field; it can be very frightening to some and real fodder for the press.

What Do You Know Now?

- This is *an outbreak*, or epidemic, if you wish, because 40 plus cases of GI illness in such a short period of time is clearly unusual.
- *A probable time frame*: most identified illnesses occurred during one night.
- Most of the known ill had some kind of *GI illness*.
- The ill people *shared a common experience* the night before.
- GI illnesses, particularly those that start fairly soon after eating, often come from eating contaminated food.

- As of April 19, the day Dr. Rubin arrived, no family members who did not attend the supper had become ill.

What Can You Realistically Infer from This Information So Far?

- The 40 or more cases were probably the majority of church supper–related cases, yet there certainly could have been other cases not yet reported or found.
- Since there were no known cases among family members, this suggests a noncommunicable illness. However, remember, Dr. Rubin arrived less than 24 hours after the outbreak—for many communicable diseases, too short a time for secondary cases to appear.
- So, with an acute GI disease affecting some people who shared a common meal, in the absence of known disease elsewhere in the community, the logical inference is that these people were exposed to something at the supper—probably something they ate.

What Should You Do Now?

There are several possibilities, but, since your preliminary data suggest a possible food-borne epidemic, *one of the first things to do is to collect food, stool, and vomitus specimens*, if available, for laboratory testing. You do not know if these specimens will be needed, but time is critical in this kind of an outbreak, and it is better to have specimens you do not need than none at all, when you wish you had them.

Now, back to Oswego and the steps in the outline above: so far the facts and inferences strongly point to a food-borne outbreak among church members, but *you know very little about the disease* these people had, only that they had an acute GI problem. In no way have you made, much less confirmed, the diagnosis. And in order to develop a reasonable idea of what specific agent might have caused the epidemic, where it came from, and how it was transmitted—in short, its epidemiologic characteristics—you should try to get some idea of the clinical disease and what it resembles. If you are not clinically trained, you may very likely need a physician or health professional to help you in the differential diagnosis. But below is what Dr. Rubin reported:

> According to Dr. Rubin the onset of illness in all cases was acute, characterized chiefly by nausea, vomiting, diarrhea, and abdominal pain. None of the ill persons reported having an elevated temperature; all recovered within 24 to 30 hours. Approximately 20% of the ill persons visited physicians. No fecal specimens were obtained for bacteriologic examination. (Whether Dr. Rubin actually saw some cases, we do not know. If you had been he, before investigating any further, it would have been a good idea to visit several cases or, at least, to talk to the physicians who saw some cases.)

What Do You Know Now?

- Among those you know about, the illness was not severe or life threatening but very short-lived.
- The agent affected both the upper and lower GI tract without fever.
- The laboratory probably will not be of help; therefore you will have to rely heavily on the clinical picture and the epidemiologic findings for a presumptive diagnosis.

What Can You Infer?

- That all the cases have been reported to Dr. Rubin. (If you had serious doubts, you would throw the net wide and find as many cases as possible.) (See Chapters 3 and 5.)
- That all cases are related in some way and that their illnesses are probably due to the same agent.
- That no one died or was hospitalized. This may or may not be true, because you do not know how the local health officer conducted case finding. However, for our purposes, you can assume these are all the cases.
- The agent caused illness within a few hours after exposure. In other words, the agent probably has a relatively short *incubation period*—the time from exposure to the time of onset of illness.

What Should You Do Now?

This is where you will need someone clinically trained to help in the differential diagnosis. But before you look at the table below, there are a few things you should know that can be very useful. The major categories of agents that cause acute onset of GI diseases are:

- Infectious—caused by bacteria, viruses, or parasites
- Toxic/environmental—such as heavy metals, herbicides, household cleaning agents, or certain fish toxins
- Sociogenic—such as mass hysteria

When you try to "diagnose" an acute food poisoning outbreak, recall that nausea, vomiting, and diarrhea are normal body defense mechanisms designed to rid the body of harmful substances. So think of how and where in the GI tract the agent might affect the body. Ingestion of toxins predominantly affects the upper GI tract—the stomach, where their effect is usually within hours, causing nausea, vomiting, and, not infrequently, diarrhea. At the other extreme, bacteria, like salmonella and shigella, take more time—24 to 48 hours—to invade intestinal tissue (usually small and/or large bowel), to reproduce, and often to cause fever, cramps, diarrhea, and other symptoms. Fever is usually a sign that an agent or toxin has actually entered or invaded the body tissues—not just irritated the lining of the intestine. Many other agents exhibit considerable variations in their pathogenesis and presentation. Several of the more frequently encountered ones are listed in Table A–1.

What Are Some Important Things You Have Learned from This Table?

- Many agents have fairly similar presentations.
- Toxins predominately affect the upper GI tract.
- Staphylococcus produces a toxin that can have a very short incubation period.
- Finally, more clinical details on those who ate at the supper would help in the diagnosis.

What Should You Do Next?

With some general ideas about the time, place, and person of the epidemic; a good idea of who might be at risk; and a fairly reasonable hypothesis that the church supper could be responsible; you should get a list of the church supper participants, draw up a questionnaire, and ask the participants a series of questions primarily to focus on what unique exposures they may have had that made them ill. This is exactly what Dr. Rubin did.

What Information Do You Want To Know?

Minimally, for this investigation you would like to know (see Chapters 11 and 12):

- Identifying information: name, address, phone number, and respondent (self, parent, spouse)
- Demographic information: birth date or age, gender
- Clinical information: signs/symptoms, severity, time of onset, and duration of illness
- Epidemiologic information:
  - Did you attend the supper?
  - Did you eat food at the supper?
  - When did you eat?
  - What did you eat and drink?

Table A–1. Some Common Food-borne and Water-borne Agents that Cause Acute Gastroenteritis

AGENT	INCUBATION PERIOD	PATHOPHYSIOLOGY	SYMPTOMS	TYPICAL FOODS
Staphylococcus aureus	2–4 hours	Preformed enterotoxin	Sudden vomiting, cramps, diarrhea, no fever	Ham, meats, custards, cream fillings
Clostridium perfringens	6–24 hours, usually 10–12 hours	Enterotoxin formed in vivo	Abdominal pain, diarrhea, nausea, vomiting, fever usually absent	Meat, poultry
Salmonella (nontyphoid)	6–48 hours	Intestinal invasion of bacteria	Diarrhea, fever, chills	Poultry, eggs, meat
Shigella species	2–4 days	Intestinal invasion of bacteria	Diarrhea, often bloody, cramps, little or no fever	Foods contaminated by food handler, usually not food-borne
E. coli Escherichia coli (O157:H7 and others)	3–4 days	Cytotoxin	Diarrhea, abdominal cramps, little or no fever	Beef, raw milk, water
Norwalk-like viruses	24–48 hours	Unknown	Vomiting, cramps, headache, fever	Raw or undercooked shellfish, sandwiches, salads, water
Heavy metals (antimony, cadmium, copper, lead, tin, zinc)	Usually less than 1 hour	Chemical irritation	Vomiting	Foods and beverages prepared/stored/cooked in containers contaminated with offending metal.

From Dr. Rubin's investigation we learn:

The supper was held in the basement of the village church. Foods were contributed by numerous members of the congregation. The supper began at 6:00 p.m. and continued until 11:00 p.m. Food was spread out on a table and consumed over a period of several hours. Data were collected regarding onset of illness and food eaten or water drunk by each of the 75 persons interviewed.

Dr. Rubin put his data into what is called a *line-listing*—a presentation or a spread sheet of results of the questionnaires displayed in considerable detail. A line-listing is a grid containing information about persons who are under study. Each row shows data on a single case. Each column represents a variable such as identifying information, clinical data, and epidemiologic information, such as risk and exposure factors. Such a list can be very useful, particularly at the beginning of an investigation, to help you view the entire database as time progresses, to fill in gaps of information, to share the results with others on your team, and simply to "eyeball" for obvious errors, outliers, and trends. Table A–2 is Dr. Rubin's line-listing.

What Can You Glean from This Line-List?

Not a great deal; it is really a working document. Most of the ill attendees were adults, and many could not remember when they ate the meal; however, all remembered when they became ill, and all but two knew what they ate. This latter observation is truly remarkable. In many food-borne outbreaks there will almost always be persons who forget most or some of what they ate, particularly those who were not ill. Several things, however, may have come into play here: (*1*) the number of food items was small, making it easy to remember; (*2*) the questionnaire may not have had a space for the respondent to answer: "Don't know," thus forcing the repondent to give an answer, "yes" or "no"; (*3*) the outbreak was quite a vivid experience for everyone, thus sharpening their memory; and (*4*) since all the food was prepared by church members, they would have a better recollection of who prepared what foods and what they ate.

What Should You Do Next?

Now you have the necessary information to describe the epidemic in terms of time, place, and person—the essentials for developing hypotheses of why the epidemic occurred, who was at risk, and what was the definitive exposure. As was described in Chapters 5 and 6, one of the most useful ways to depict the *time aspect* of an epidemic is to draw an *epidemic curve*. By plotting cases of illness on the vertical (*y*) axis and a suitable time frame on the horizontal (*x*) axis you create a graph

Table A–2. Line-listing from an Investigation of an Outbreak of Gastroenteritis, Oswego, New York, 1940

ID	AGE	SEX	TIME OF MEAL	ILL	DATE OF ONSET	TIME OF ONSET	BAKED HAM	SPINACH	MASHED POTATOES	CABBAGE SALAD	JELLO	ROLLS	BROWN BREAD	MILK	COFFEE	WATER	CAKES	VAN. ICE CREAM	CHOC. ICE CREAM	FRUIT SALAD
1	11	M	UNK	N			N	N	N	N	N	N	N	N	N	N	N	N	Y	N
2	52	F	8:00PM	Y	4/19	12:30 AM	Y	Y	Y	N	N	Y	N	N	Y	N	N	Y	Y	N
3	65	M	6:30 PM	Y	4/19	12:30 AM	Y	Y	Y	Y	N	N	N	N	Y	N	Y	Y	N	N
4	59	F	6:30 PM	Y	4/19	12:30 AM	N	Y	N	N	N	N	N	N	Y	Y	N	Y	Y	N
5	13	F	UNK	N			N	N	N	N	N	N	N	N	N	Y	N	N	Y	N
6	63	F	7:30 PM	Y	4/18	10:30 PM	Y	Y	Y	Y	N	N	Y	N	Y	Y	N	Y	Y	N
7	70	M	7:30 PM	Y	4/18	10:30 PM	Y	Y	Y	N	N	Y	N	N	Y	Y	N	Y	N	N
8	40	F	7:30 PM	Y	4/19	2:00 AM	N	N	N	N	N	N	N	N	Y	N	Y	Y	Y	N
9	15	F	10:00 PM	Y	4/19	1:00 AM	Y	Y	Y	N	N	Y	Y	N	N	Y	N	Y	Y	N
10	33	F	7:00PM	Y	4/18	11:00 PM	Y	Y	Y	N	N	Y	N	N	N	Y	N	Y	Y	N
11	65	M	UNK	N			N	Y	Y	N	N	Y	Y	N	N	N	N	Y	Y	N
12	38	F	UNK	N			Y	Y	Y	Y	Y	Y	Y	N	Y	Y	N	N	Y	Y
13	62	F	UNK	N			Y	Y	N	N	N	N	N	N	N	N	N	Y	Y	N
14	10	M	7:30 PM	Y	4/19	2:00 AM	N	N	N	N	N	N	N	N	Y	N	Y	Y	Y	N
15	25	M	UNK	N			Y	Y	Y	Y	Y	Y	Y	N	Y	N	Y	Y	N	N
16	32	F	UNK	Y	4/19	10:30 AM	Y	Y	N	Y	N	N	N	N	Y	N	Y	Y	Y	N
17	62	F	UNK	Y	4/19	12:30 AM	N	N	N	Y	Y	Y	Y	N	N	Y	N	Y	N	N
18	36	M	UNK	Y	4/18	10:15 PM	Y	Y	N	Y	Y	Y	Y	N	N	Y	N	N	N	N
19	11	M	UNK	N			Y	Y	?	Y	Y	Y	N	N	N	Y	N	N	Y	N
20	33	F	UNK	Y	4/18	10:00 PM	Y	Y	Y	Y	Y	Y	N	N	Y	Y	Y	Y	Y	N

(continued)

Table A-2. (Continued)

ID	AGE	SEX	TIME OF MEAL	ILL	DATE OF ONSET	TIME OF ONSET	BAKED HAM	SPINACH	MASHED POTATOES	CABBAGE SALAD	JELLO	ROLLS	BROWN BREAD	MILK	COFFEE	WATER	CAKES	VAN. ICE CREAM	CHOC. ICE CREAM	FRUIT SALAD
21	13	F	10:00 PM	Y	4/19	1:00 AM	N	N	N	N	N	N	N	N	N	N	Y	Y	N	N
22	7	M	UNK	Y	4/18	11:00 PM	Y	Y	Y	Y	N	Y	Y	N	N	Y	Y	Y	Y	N
23	64	M	UNK	N			N	N	N	N	N	N	N	N	N	N	N	Y	N	N
24	3	M	UNK	Y	4/18	9:45 PM	N	Y	Y	Y	N	N	Y	N	Y	Y	Y	Y	Y	N
25	65	F	UNK	N			Y	Y	Y	Y	N	Y	Y	N	N	N	Y	Y	Y	N
26	59	F	UNK	Y	4/18	9:45 PM	N	N	N	Y	N	N	N	N	N	N	Y	Y	Y	N
27	15	F	10:00 PM	Y	4/19	1:00 AM	Y	Y	Y	N	Y	Y	Y	N	Y	N	Y	N	Y	N
28	62	M	UNK	N			N	Y	Y	N	Y	N	Y	N	Y	N	N	Y	N	Y
29	37	F	UNK	Y	4/18	11:00 PM	N	N	N	N	N	N	N	N	Y	N	N	Y	N	N
30	17	M	10:00 PM	N			Y	Y	Y	Y	Y	Y	Y	N	Y	Y	Y	N	Y	Y
31	35	M	UNK	Y	4/18	9:00 PM	Y	N	N	N	N	N	N	N	N	N	N	Y	N	N
32	15	M	10:00 PM	Y	4/19	1:00 AM	N	Y	Y	N	N	N	Y	N	Y	N	Y	N	Y	Y
33	50	F	10:00 PM	Y	4/19	1:00 AM	N	N	N	N	N	N	N	N	N	Y	Y	N	N	Y
34	40	M	UNK	N			Y	Y	Y	Y	N	Y	Y	N	Y	Y	Y	N	N	N
35	35	F	UNK	N			Y	Y	Y	Y	N	Y	Y	N	Y	Y	Y	N	Y	Y
36	35	F	UNK	Y	4/18	9:15 PM	Y	Y	Y	Y	Y	N	Y	N	Y	N	N	N	N	N
37	36	M	UNK	N			Y	N	N	N	N	N	Y	N	Y	N	Y	N	N	N
38	57	F	UNK	Y	4/18	11:30 PM	N	Y	N	Y	Y	N	N	N	Y	N	Y	N	Y	N
39	16	F	10:00 PM	Y	4/19	1:00 AM	Y	N	Y	N	N	N	Y	N	N	N	Y	Y	Y	N
40	68	M	UNK	Y	4/18	9:30 PM	Y	Y	N	N	N	N	N	N	Y	N	N	N	N	N
41	54	F	UNK	N			Y	Y	N	N	Y	Y	Y	N	Y	N	Y	Y	Y	Y
42	77	M	UNK	Y	4/19	2:30 AM	N	Y	N	Y	N	N	N	N	N	N	N	Y	N	N
43	72	F	UNK	Y	4/19V	2:00 AM	Y	Y	N	Y	Y	N	Y	N	Y	N	Y	Y	Y	N

No.	Age	Sex	Time	Ill	Onset Date	Onset Time
44	58	M	UNK	Y	4/18	9:30 PM
45	20	M	10:00 PM	N		
46	17	M	UNK	N		
47	62	F	UNK	Y	4/19	12:30 AM
48	20	F	7:00 PM	Y	4/19	1:00 AM
49	52	F	UNK	Y	4/18	10:30 PM
50	9	F	UNK	N		
51	50	M	UNK	N		
52	8	M	11:00 PM	Y	4/18	3:00 PM
53	35	F	UNK	N		
54	48	M	UNK	Y	4/18	12:00 MN
55	25	F	UNK	Y	4/18	11:00 PM
56	11	F	UNK	N		
57	74	M	UNK	Y	4/18	10:30 PM
58	12	F	10:00 PM	Y	4/19	1:00 AM
59	44	F	7:30 PM	Y	4/19	2:30 AM
60	53	F	7:30 PM	Y	4/18	11:30 PM
61	37	M	UNK	N		
62	24	F	UNK	N		
63	69	F	UNK	N		
64	7	M	UNK	Y	4/19	1:00 AM
65	17	F	10:00 PM	Y	4/19	12:30 AM
66	8	F	UNK	N		
67	11	M	7:30 PM	N		
68	17	M	7:30 PM	N		
69	36	F	UNK	Y	4/19	12:30 AM
70	21	M	7:30 PM	Y	4/19	1:00 AM
71	60	F	7:30 PM	Y	4/18	12:00 MN
72	18	F	UNK	N		
73	14	F	10:00 PM	Y	4/19	2:15 AM
74	52	M	UNK	Y	4/18	11:00 PM
75	45	F	UNK	Y		

that gives you an idea of the size of the epidemic, its relation to endemic cases, its time course, its pattern of spread, and where you are in the course of the epidemic— the upslope or the downslope of the curve. Figure A–1 shows the epidemic curve for the Oswego outbreak.

What Can You Learn from This Graph?

- Most cases form a tight cluster within a 6-hour interval, suggesting a single common exposure.
- There are two "outliers"—one very early and one late in the epidemic. Either one or both could represent background or endemic cases not related to the epidemic at all; or the early case could be the "source" of the epidemic; the late case could be a secondary case.
- You will want to investigate these cases later, but there are still much more important things to do.

Another aspect of *time* focuses on when the ill persons became sick in relation to when they ate or were exposed: the incubation period. Virtually all infectious diseases and many toxins have known or estimated incubation periods—a characteristic that can help you identify what agent caused the disease.

Dr. Rubin's questionnaire provides the data needed to determine the incubation periods of those ill persons (only 22 of the 46 ill persons) who remembered when they ate and when they became ill. See Figure A–2.

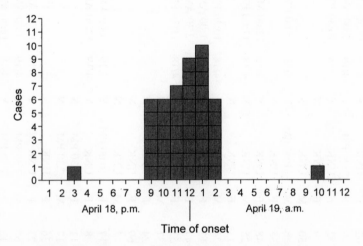

Figure A–1. Cases of gastrointestinal illness by time of onset of symptoms, Oswego County, New York, April 18–19, 1940. (CDC, Unpublished data).

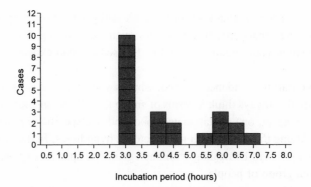

Figure A–2. Cases of gastrointestinal illness by incubation period in hours, Oswego County, New York, April 18–19, 1940. (CDC, Unpublished data).

What Can You Learn from Figure A–2?

- It is hard to generalize with such small numbers, but it looks as though there are two clusters of occurrence in time, one at 3 hours and one at about 6 to 6½ hours. Overall the median incubation period is 4 hours.
- Interestingly, the incubation period was shorter for those who ate later in the evening than those who ate earlier in the evening. This difference could be explained by a continuing production of enterotoxin by staphylococci in a food. It could also be explained by the fact that younger people ate later and perhaps ate more than the older folks who ate earlier. (This is an excellent example of a simple, creative analysis of basic demographic and epidemiologic data that can uncover fascinating and sometimes important aspects of a very common type of outbreak.)
- But most important, an incubation period of 4 hours fits well with incubation periods of agents such as staphylococcus, some fish toxins, and *Bacillus cereus*. Fish toxins can be ruled out, because fish was not served; *B. cereus* seems unlikely, because the foods usually associated with it (rice, custards, cereals) were not served either. So staphylococcal toxin seems the most likely agent, although it would be helpful to have more detailed clinical information.

Next, you will want to orient the data in terms of *place*. According to Dr. Rubin's report, all 75 repondents to the questionnaire ate at the supper, which strongly suggests the risk and exposure occurred there. However, you should view the two outliers, patient No. 16 and patient No. 52, with some skepticism simply because their onsets are so different from the rest.

In terms of *person* characteristics, the age and gender profiles appear normal, though age- and gender-specific attack rates might be revealing. But at this time in the investigation your attention should be focused on food exposures among the attendees.

So, with all the evidence at hand, what is your hypothesis as to what happened? Initially, always think in terms of single factors causing outbreaks: in this instance, one agent, one contaminated food, and one specific population at risk. Avoid muddying the waters with multifactorial hypotheses. In the great majority of instances you will be dealing with one agent, one specific exposure, and one well-defined group of people.

To put it in more epidemiologic terms: what do you think was the critical exposure that caused illness? Your hypothesis would be: "I think a single food or drink was contaminated with some agent, probably staphylococcal enterotoxin, that caused the illness in those who attended and ate at the church supper." In this context the word *exposure* means a food or drink eaten at the supper.

What Next?

You now should extract from the questionnaire data that will identify which possible exposures (foods, drinks) the persons might have had at the supper that made them ill. In other words, you will need to study and analyze these data in such a way as to be able to test and verify your hypothesis.

How Will the Information on the Questionnaire Help Test Your Hypothesis?

Your initial reflex might be to choose one of two approaches in hopes of finding out what item caused the outbreak. To do these analyses more easily, however, you first want to separate the supper participants into two groups: the ill and the well. Table A–3 shows a new line-listing with such a breakdown.

- *Approach 1*: Look at the food and drink list and see which one(s) were associated with the most number of ill persons. If one item was associated with more sick people than another item, then that might incriminate that item.
- *Approach 2*: Look at all the ill persons and see what they ate. Again, using similar logic as above, if more ill people ate a particular item more than other items, that might identify the contaminated food or drink.

Table A–3. Line-listing from an Investigation of an Outbreak of Gastroenteritis, Oswego, New York, 1940

ID	AGE	SEX	TIME OF MEAL	ILL	DATE OF ONSET	TIME OF ONSET	BAKED HAM	SPINACH	MASHED POTATOES	CABBAGE SALAD	JELLO	ROLLS	BROWN BREAD	MILK	COFFEE	WATER	CAKES	VAN. ICE CREAM	CHOC. ICE CREAM	FRUIT SALAD
52	8	M	11:00 PM	Y	4/18	3:00 PM	N	N	N	N	N	N	N	N	N	N	N	Y	Y	N
31	35	M	UNK	Y	4/18	9:00 PM	Y	Y	Y	N	Y	Y	Y	N	Y	N	Y	Y	N	Y
36	35	F	UNK	Y	4/18	9:15 PM	Y	Y	Y	Y	N	Y	Y	N	Y	N	N	Y	N	N
40	68	M	UNK	Y	4/18	9:30 PM	Y	N	Y	Y	N	N	Y	N	Y	N	N	Y	N	N
44	58	M	UNK	Y	4/18	9:30 PM	Y	Y	Y	N	N	Y	Y	N	Y	Y	Y	Y	?	Y
24	3	M	UNK	Y	4/18	9:45 PM	N	Y	Y	N	N	Y	N	N	N	Y	Y	Y	Y	N
26	59	F	UNK	Y	4/18	9:45 PM	N	N	Y	Y	Y	Y	Y	N	N	Y	Y	Y	Y	N
20	33	F	UNK	Y	4/18	10:00 PM	Y	Y	N	Y	N	Y	N	N	Y	N	Y	Y	N	N
18	36	M	UNK	Y	4/18	10:15 PM	Y	Y	N	Y	Y	N	Y	N	N	Y	N	Y	Y	N
6	63	F	7:30 PM	Y	4/18	10:30 PM	Y	Y	Y	Y	Y	Y	Y	N	Y	Y	N	Y	N	N
7	70	M	7:30 PM	Y	4/18	10:30 PM	Y	Y	Y	N	N	Y	N	N	Y	N	Y	Y	Y	N
49	52	F	UNK	Y	4/18	10:30 PM	Y	Y	Y	Y	Y	N	Y	N	Y	Y	Y	Y	Y	N
57	74	M	UNK	Y	4/18	10:30 PM	Y	Y	Y	N	Y	Y	Y	N	Y	N	N	Y	N	N
10	33	F	7:00PM	Y	4/18	11:00 PM	Y	N	Y	Y	N	N	Y	N	N	Y	Y	Y	Y	N
22	7	M	UNK	Y	4/18	11:00 PM	Y	Y	N	N	Y	Y	Y	N	N	N	N	Y	N	N
29	37	F	UNK	Y	4/18	11:00 PM	Y	Y	Y	N	Y	Y	Y	N	Y	Y	Y	Y	Y	N
55	25	M	UNK	Y	4/18	11:00 PM	Y	Y	Y	Y	N	Y	Y	N	N	N	Y	Y	N	N
75	45	F	UNK	Y	4/18	11:00 PM	Y	Y	N	Y	Y	Y	Y	N	Y	Y	Y	Y	Y	Y
38	57	F	UNK	Y	4/18	11:30 PM	Y	Y	Y	Y	Y	N	Y	N	Y	N	Y	y	N	N
60	53	F	7:30 PM	Y	4/18	11:30 PM	Y	Y	Y	Y	Y	N	Y	N	Y	Y	Y	Y	Y	N
72	18	F	7:30 PM	Y	4/18	12:00 MN	Y	Y	Y	Y	Y	N	N	N	N	Y	Y	Y	Y	N

(continued)

Table A–3. (*Continued*)

ID	AGE	SEX	TIME OF MEAL	ILL	DATE OF ONSET	TIME OF ONSET	BAKED HAM	SPINACH	MASHED POTATOES	CABBAGE SALAD	JELLO	ROLLS	BROWN BREAD	MILK	COFFEE	WATER	CAKES	VAN. ICE CREAM	CHOC. ICE CREAM	FRUIT SALAD
54	48	F	UNK	Y	4/18	12:00 MN	Y	Y	Y	Y	Y	Y	Y	Y	Y	N	Y	Y	Y	N
2	52	F	8:00PM	Y	4/19	12:30 AM	Y	Y	Y	N	N	Y	N	N	Y	N	N	Y	N	N
3	65	M	6:30 PM	Y	4/19	12:30 AM	Y	Y	Y	Y	N	N	N	N	Y	N	N	Y	Y	N
4	59	F	6:30 PM	Y	4/19	12:30 AM	Y	Y	N	N	N	N	N	N	Y	N	Y	Y	Y	N
17	62	F	UNK	Y	4/19	12:30 AM	N	N	N	N	N	Y	N	N	N	Y	N	Y	N	N
47	62	F	UNK	Y	4/19	12:30 AM	Y	Y	Y	Y	Y	N	N	N	N	N	N	Y	N	N
66	8	F	UNK	Y	4/19	12:30 AM	Y	N	N	Y	Y	N	N	N	N	N	Y	Y	Y	N
70	21	F	UNK	Y	4/19	12:30 AM	Y	N	N	N	N	N	N	N	N	N	N	Y	Y	N
71	60	M	7:30 PM	Y	4/19	1:00 AM	N	N	N	N	N	N	N	N	N	N	Y	Y	N	N
21	13	F	10:00 PM	Y	4/19	1:00 AM	N	N	N	N	N	N	N	N	N	N	Y	Y	N	N
27	15	F	10:00 PM	Y	4/19	1:00 AM	N	N	N	N	N	N	N	N	N	N	Y	Y	Y	N
32	15	M	10:00 PM	Y	4/19	1:00 AM	N	N	N	N	N	N	N	N	N	N	Y	Y	N	N
33	50	F	10:00 PM	Y	4/19	1:00 AM	N	N	N	N	N	N	N	N	N	N	N	Y	N	N
39	16	F	10:00 PM	Y	4/19	1:00 AM	N	N	N	N	N	N	N	N	N	N	Y	Y	Y	N
9	15	F	10:00 PM	Y	4/19	1:00 AM	N	N	N	N	N	N	N	N	N	N	Y	N	Y	N
48	20	F	7:00 PM	Y	4/19	1:00 AM	N	N	N	N	N	N	N	N	N	N	N	N	Y	N
58	12	F	10:00 PM	Y	4/19	1:00 AM	N	N	N	N	N	N	N	N	N	N	Y	Y	Y	N
65	17	F	10:00 PM	Y	4/19	1:00 AM	N	N	N	N	N	N	N	N	N	N	N	Y	Y	N
8	40	F	7:30 PM	Y	4/19	2:00 AM	N	N	N	N	N	N	N	N	N	N	Y	Y	Y	N
14	10	M	7:30 PM	Y	4/19	2:00 AM	N	N	N	N	N	N	N	N	N	N	Y	Y	Y	N
43	72	F	UNK	Y	4/19V	2:00 AM	Y	Y	Y	Y	Y	Y	Y	N	Y	N	N	Y	Y	N
74	52	M	UNK	Y	4/19	2:15 AM	Y	N	N	N	Y	Y	Y	N	Y	Y	Y	Y	Y	N
42	77	M	UNK	Y	4/19	2:30 AM	N	N	N	N	Y	N	N	N	N	N	N	N	N	Y

ID	Age	Sex	Time		Date	Time	C1	C2	C3	C4	C5	C6	C7	C8	C9	C10	C11	C12
59	44	F	7:30 PM	Y	4/19	2:30 AM	N	Y	N	Y	Y	N	N	N	Y	N	N	Y
16	32	F	UNK	Y	4/19	10:30 AM	N	Y	Y	Y	N	Y	N	N	N	N	N	Y
1	11	M	UNK	N			N	Y	N	N	N	N	N	N	N	N	N	N
5	13	F	UNK	N			N	Y	N	N	N	N	N	N	Y	N	N	N
11	65	M	UNK	N			N	N	Y	N	N	N	N	N	Y	Y	N	Y
12	38	F	UNK	N			Y	Y	Y	N	Y	Y	N	Y	Y	N	Y	Y
13	62	F	UNK	N			N	N	N	Y	Y	N	N	Y	Y	Y	Y	Y
15	25	M	UNK	N			N	N	N	Y	Y	Y	N	N	Y	Y	Y	Y
19	11	M	UNK	N			N	Y	Y	N	N	N	N	N	N	N	N	N
23	64	M	UNK	N			N	N	N	N	N	N	N	Y	Y	Y	Y	N
25	65	F	UNK	N			N	Y	Y	Y	Y	Y	N	Y	N	N	N	Y
28	62	M	UNK	N			N	Y	Y	N	Y	Y	N	Y	N	Y	Y	Y
30	17	M	10:00 PM	N			Y	Y	N	Y	Y	N	N	N	Y	N	N	N
34	40	M	UNK	N			N	N	Y	N	N	Y	N	Y	N	N	N	Y
35	35	F	UNK	N			N	Y	N	Y	Y	Y	N	Y	Y	N	N	Y
37	36	M	UNK	N			N	Y	N	Y	Y	Y	N	Y	Y	Y	Y	N
41	54	F	UNK	N			N	Y	N	N	Y	Y	N	Y	Y	N	N	Y
45	20	M	10:00 PM	N			N	Y	Y	N	Y	N	N	N	Y	N	N	Y
46	17	M	UNK	N			N	Y	Y	Y	N	N	N	N	N	N	N	N
50	9	F	UNK	N			N	Y	N	N	N	N	N	N	N	N	N	N
51	50	M	UNK	N			N	Y	Y	Y	Y	N	N	N	N	Y	Y	N
53	35	F	UNK	N			N	Y	N	N	N	N	N	Y	Y	N	N	Y
56	11	F	UNK	N			N	Y	N	Y	N	N	N	N	N	N	N	N
61	37	M	UNK	N			N	Y	N	N	N	N	Y	N	N	N	N	N
62	24	F	UNK	N			N	Y	N	Y	Y	N	N	N	Y	Y	Y	Y
63	69	M	UNK	N			N	N	N	Y	Y	N	N	N	N	N	N	N
64	7	F	UNK	N			N	Y	N	N	Y	Y	N	Y	Y	N	N	Y
67	11	F	7:30 PM	N			N	N	N	N	N	N	N	N	Y	N	N	Y
68	17	M	7:30 PM	N			N	Y	Y	N	N	N	N	N	Y	N	N	Y
69	36	F	UNK	N			N	Y	N	N	N	Y	N	N	N	N	N	N
73	14	F	10:00 PM	N			N	N	Y	Y	N	N	N	N	N	N	N	N

PROBLEMS WITH APPROACHES 1 AND 2

Approach 1

Simply because one food is associated with more illness than another food does not establish that one food is more likely to cause illness than another. Among the 46 who ate ham, 29 were ill; among the 54 who ate vanilla ice cream, 43 became ill; and 16 of 23 who ate Jell-o developed GI illness. What do these numbers really mean? How can you reconcile the fact that some persons became ill when they ate one food, but they also ate other foods too, and they became ill after eating them? Persuasive or not as the case may be, these numbers alone cannot validly explain or identify a contaminated food.

Approach 2

If you now look only at the ill persons, you will see that 29 ate the ham, 26 had spinach, and 45 had vanilla ice cream. These were quite popular foods. But do these numbers alone help you find out what item might have caused the outbreak? It is pretty clear that they do not. All the numbers tell you is what were the most popular or most frequently consumed items eaten by the ill persons. In no way can you validly implicate ham more than spinach just because more ill people ate ham than spinach. Moreover, what about those ill people who ate rolls or mashed potato? How do you explain them? In sum, there really is no logical or scientific way to incriminate a specific food or drink by this analysis either.

THE SOLUTION TO APPROACHES 1 AND 2 —THE CRITICAL ANALYSIS

You have now arrived at the most critical juncture in your investigation of the outbreak. Your hypothesis seems very defensible and reasonable, but your analysis thus far has not established much of anything—perhaps only what foods were popular at the supper. Specifically, neither of the above approaches helped you incriminate a food item.

So here is the logic behind the correct way to solve the problem. If you are thinking (hypothesizing) that a single food, among several, caused illness, then you might expect that that food would cause illness more frequently among those who ate that food than among those who did not eat it. If that makes sense, then, next, you should determine the rates of illness or attack rates among those who ate the food and those who did not. This is what Dr. Rubin did. See Table A–4.

Table A–4. Illness Rates among Church Supper Attendees According to Foods/Drinks Consumed, Oswego County, New York, April 1940

	NUMBER OF PERSONS WHO ATE SPECIFIED FOOD				NUMBER OF PERSONS WHO DID NOT EAT SPECIFIED FOOD			
FOOD ITEMS SERVED	ILL	NOT ILL	TOTAL	PERCENT ILL (ATTACK RATE)	ILL	NOT ILL	TOTAL	PERCENT ILL (ATTACK RATE)
Baked ham	29	17	46	63%	17	12	29	59%
Spinach	26	17	43	60%	20	12	32	62%
Mashed potato*	23	14	37	62%	23	14	37	62%
Cabbage salad	18	10	28	64%	28	19	47	60%
Jello	16	7	23	70%	30	22	52	58%
Rolls	21	16	37	57%	25	13	38	66%
Brown bread	18	9	27	67%	28	20	48	58%
Milk	2	2	4	50%	44	27	71	62%
Coffee	19	12	31	61%	27	17	44	61%
Water	13	11	24	54%	33	18	51	65%
Cakes	27	13	40	67%	19	16	35	54%
Ice cream, vanilla	43	11	54	80%	3	18	21	14%
Ice cream, chocolate*	25	22	47	53%	20	7	27	74%
Fruit salad	4	2	6	67%	42	27	69	61%

*Excludes 1 person with indefinite history of consumption of that food.

Here you can see attack rates for each food item among those who ate the food in one column and among those who did not eat the food in the opposite column. *If you* compare *the attack rates between the two, you are performing the quintessential operation of all epidemiologic analysis: the comparison of rates.* In this instance you are comparing attack rates between those exposed (who ate a food) and those not exposed (who did not eat a food).

Now if you "eyeball" these attack rates for each food in both columns on Table A–4, you will see that for all foods, except one, the attack rates were fairly similar. For example, the attack rate for those who ate ham was 63%, for those not eating ham it was 59%; for those who ate spinach it was 66%, for those not eating spinach it was 62%; and for mashed potatoes the percentages were 62% and 62%, respectively. These rates certainly do not implicate any of these foods.

However, for vanilla ice cream the comparison of attack rates showed a great difference: 80% for those who ate it compared to 14% who did not. This comparison is striking, so much so that you should ask yourself, "How often would we expect to see such a difference in attack rates if vanilla ice cream had nothing to do with the outbreak?" Or to put it another way," Assuming no relationship between eating vanilla ice cream and getting sick, how often would we see such a difference in attack rates simply by chance alone?" With some experience in this kind of "eyeballing" and a little statistical background you would likely say, "Not very often." And, indeed, you would be right. For if you perform some simple statistical tests, you could say that this difference in attack rates for vanilla ice cream would occur in less than 1 in 100,000 instances such as this, assuming that the ice cream had nothing to do with the illness.

What Should You Do Next?

- Unless you are quite familiar with the appropriate statistical function to perform, you should have your "eyeball" assessment verified by a trusted statistician.
- The statistician will confirm your conclusion that such a difference in attack rates would occur less than 1 out of 100,000 or more times (assuming no association between the ice cream and illness)—a statistic good enough, along with all the other data—for field epidemiologists worth their salt to look immediately for any remaining vanilla ice cream, culture it, and throw it out. Of course, if it was a commercially prepared ice cream, you should immediately notify your local health department of your findings. They, in turn, should call the local or regional Food and Drug Administration Office.
- You should now try to find out how the vanilla ice cream became contaminated with staphylococcus. This means locating those responsible for

preparing the vanilla ice cream, asking them exactly how they prepared the ice cream, examining them for any possible infections, and culturing them for staphylococci. Here, again, are Dr. Rubin's findings:

The ice cream was prepared by the Petrie sisters as follows:

On the afternoon of April 17 raw milk from the Petrie farm at Lycoming was brought to boil over a water bath, sugar and eggs were then added and a little flour to add body to the mix. The chocolate and vanilla ice cream were prepared separately. Hershey's chocolate was necessarily added to the chocolate mix. At 6 p.m. the two mixes were taken in covered containers to the church basement and allowed to stand overnight. They were presumably not touched by anyone during this period. On the morning of April 18, Mr. Coe added five ounces of vanilla and two cans of condensed milk to the vanilla mix, and three ounces of vanilla and one can of condensed milk to the chocolate mix. Then the vanilla mix was transferred to a freezing can and placed in an electrical freezer for 20 minutes, after which the vanilla ice cream was removed from the freezer can and packed into another can which had been previously washed with boiling water. Then the chocolate mix was put into the freezer can, which had been rinsed out with tap water and allowed to freeze for 20 minutes. At the conclusion of this both cans were covered and placed in large wooden receptacles which were packed with ice. As noted, the chocolate ice cream remained in the one freezer can.

All handlers of the ice cream were examined. No external lesions or upper respiratory infections were noted. Nose and throat cultures were taken from two individuals who prepared the ice cream. Bacterial examinations . . . were made on both ice creams. . . . Large numbers of *Staphylococcus aureus* and *albus* were found in the specimens of vanilla ice cream. Only a few staphylococci were demonstrated in the chocolate ice cream. . . . *Staphylococcus aureus* . . . [was] isolated from [the] nose culture and *Staphylococcus albus* from [the] throat culture of Grace Petrie. *Staphylococcus albus* was isolated from the nose culture of Marian Petrie. . . .

Discussion as to Source: The source of bacterial contamination of the vanilla ice cream is not clear. Whatever the method of the introduction of the staphylococci, it appears reasonable to assume it must have occurred between the evening of April 17 and the morning of April 18. No reason for contamination peculiar to the vanilla ice cream is known.

In dispensing the ice creams, the same scooper was used. It is therefore not unlikely to assume that some contamination to the chocolate ice cream occurred in this way. This would appear to be the most plausible explanation for the illness in the three individuals who did not eat the vanilla ice cream.

Control Measures: Later, all remaining ice cream was condemned. All other food at the church supper had been consumed.

Conclusions: An attack of gastroenteritis occurred following a church supper at Lycoming. The cause of the outbreak was contaminated vanilla ice cream. The method of contamination of ice cream is not clearly understood. Whether the positive Staphylococcus nose and throat cultures had anything to do with the contamination is a matter of conjecture.

What about the Two Outliers?

Patient No. 52 was a child who, while watching the freezing procedure, was given a dish of vanilla ice cream at 11:00 a.m. on April 18.

Patient No. 16 was a 32-year-old woman, whose time of eating is not known. Did she take the ice cream home to eat later, was this an unrelated illness, was this human error by the interviewer or transcriber, was this a secondary case (highly unlikely), or did she just have a long incubation period (also highly unlikely)?

What Are Some of the Important "Take-home" Messages of this Walk-through?

- This is a very typical outbreak and investigation.
- You were given a fair amount of information—simple time, place, and person data—that very often you will not have at the beginning of your fieldwork. You may know that there is an outbreak, but you will not know that the ill shared a meal, that they all became sick shortly thereafter, and that no one else became ill. These were all "givens," right up front. So be prepared.
- Recognize the limitations of a retrospective investigation:
  - Poor recall of study subjects
  - Study subjects may not understand the interview form or questions
  - Food handlers or those responsible for the meal may hide facts because of guilt, real or imagined
  - Well people tend to remember less well and less completely; also they may be questioned differently by the interviewer
- Avoid using the word "proof." Epidemiologic investigations like this one show only an association between vanilla ice cream and illness. True, it is a very strong association, but, nevertheless, it does not prove a causal relationship.

EPILOGUE

Some 32 years later a CDC epidemiologist visited Lycoming. The church was there, annual suppers were still being given, homemade ice cream was still the chief attraction, and the same two sisters were still helping out. "Although the installation of refrigeration in the early 1950s put an end to overnight incubation of the ice cream mix, they readily admit that their lapse in proper foodhandling continued until then. But a second epidemic did not occur."[1]

REFERENCES

1. Gross, M. (1976). Oswego revisited. *Public Health Rep* 91, 168–70.

INDEX

Page numbers followed by *f* and *t* indicate figures and tables, respectively.

Administrative Simplification Provisions of
HIPPA, 261–62
Age
  as confounder, 130
  person characteristics by, 103–5, 104*t*, 105*f*
  standardization, 104–5
Agent factors, 16, 18–20. *See also* Infectious
    agent
Airborne transmission, 20
Alpha (type I) error, 148
Alternative hypothesis, 147, 148
Ambulatory Sentinel Practice Network, 31, 50
Analysis. *See* Data analysis
Analytic epidemiology, 9. *See also*
    Epidemiologic studies
Animal vectors, surveillance, 34–35
Anthrax *(Bacillus anthracis)*, as biological
    warfare agent, 356, 357
Arithmetic scale line graph, 109
Association
  causal, 179–80
  disease-exposure, 144–47, 145*t*, 147*t*
  measurement, 142–44, 142*t*, 143*t*
    confidence intervals, 152–53
    vs. test of significance, 151
  strength, 168
ASTRO specimen, 387

Attack rate, 81–82, 82*f*, 83*t*, 121
  secondary, 82–83, 83*t*

Bacillus anthracis, as biological warfare
    agent, 356, 357
Bacterial disease, specimen collection and
    testing
  food-borne, 397*t*–398*t*
  general, 393*t*–395*t*
  sexually transmitted, 396*t*
Bar charts, 111–14
  100%, 113–14, 113*f*
  grouped (clustered), 112
  simple, 111, 112*f*
  stacked, 112–13, 113*f*
  two-category, 112
Behavioral Risk Factor Surveillance System
    (BRFSS), 35, 49
Beta (type II) error, 148
Bias
  diagnostic, 129
  information, 129–30, 167–68
  nonresponse, 129
  occupational disease and injury
      investigations, 310
  selection, 129, 167
Binomial regression, 161

Biological plausibility, 168–69
Bioterrorism, 354–63
  biological agents, 356–57
  communication skills, 237
  definition, 354
  detection at community level, 357–58, 359
  early concerns, 355
  epidemiologic clues, 358
  health care provider training program, 355
  laboratory testing, 360, 361, 385, 393t–395t
  preparedness, 354–63
  response, 354–63
    field activities, 360–61
    public health and governmental linkages,
      361–62
    public health goals, 355–56
    to threat, 359
  with salmonella-contaminated food, 357
  specimen collection and testing, 385–91,
      388t
    general instructions, 385–86, 388t
    guidelines, 387–89, 388t
    material required, 386–87
    summary instructions, 391
    urine samples, 389–91
  state public health powers, 266–67
  surveillance
    local community, 358–59
    role of, 357
    standardization, 361
Blood specimen collection, 392, 407
Body fluid specimen collection, 392
Botulism (Clostridium botulinum)
  as biological warfare agent, 356
  specimen collection and laboratory testing,
      397t
Bureau of Labor Statistics, 321

Calculators, 219
Campylobacter jejuni, specimen collection
      and laboratory testing, 397t
Case-control studies, 121–27, 128t. See also
      Control group
  control-to-case ratio, 127
  occupational disease and injury
      investigations, 317
  selection of controls, 123–27
  selection of subjects, 122–23
  vs. cohort studies, 127–28, 128t
Case count
  health-care setting investigations, 278
  international field investigations, 351
  methods, 67–68, 79–80, 80t, 421t–423t

Case definition
  child care setting outbreak investigations, 296
  epidemiologic studies, 119–20
  health-care setting investigations, 277–78
  international field investigations, 350–51
  methods, 40, 67–68
  restrictions, 119
  sensitivity and specificity, 67
  surveillance systems, 39–40
Case finding. See Case count
Case referent study, occupational disease and
      injury investigations, 317
Case reports, as data source, 33
Category matching, 126–27, 162
Causal association, 179–80
Causation, disease, triad model, 16–17
Cause-specific death rate, 86t
CDC. See Centers for Disease Control and
      Prevention (CDC)
Census data, 36
Centers for Disease Control and Prevention
      (CDC)
  Division of Laboratory Sciences, 387, 388t,
      390–91, 408–10
  Epi Info program. See Epi Info program
  health-care setting guidelines, 287
  Office of Health and Safety, 408
  outbreak assistance, 274
  publications, 328
  Rapid Response and Technology
      Laboratory (RRAT Lab), 385
  role in state and local field investigations, 327
  website, 50
Chain of infection, 18–21
Charts, 111–14
  bar, 111–14, 112f–113f
  design and use, 114–15
  pie, 114
  principles, 108
Chemical toxicants
  specimen collection and testing, 385–91, 388t
    general instructions, 385–86, 388t
    guidelines, 387–89, 388t
    material required, 386–87
    summary instructions, 391
    urine samples, 389–91
  specimen shipping protocol, 407–10
  state public health powers, 266–67
Chi square table, 171
Chi square test, 149–50, 151, 152
Child care setting
  outbreak investigations. See Child care
      setting outbreak investigations

public health aspects, 290–91
reporting requirements, 293–94
surveillance, 291–94
  direct reporting, 293–94
  indirect reporting, 292–93
  interview script, 304–5
  post-intervention, 300
  uses, 291–92
Child care setting outbreak investigations,
  294–303
cohort process, 301–2
common diseases, 294–95
education and training, 301
information dissemination, 301
preparation, 295–96
reasons for, 294
steps
  case definition, 296
  confirmation of diagnosis, 296–97
  control and prevention measures, 300–
   302, 305
  data orientation by time, place, and
   person, 297–98
  determining existence of outbreak, 296
  hypothesis comparison with facts, 299–
   300
  hypothesis development and testing,
   299
  planning systematic study, 300
  reports, 303
  risk determination, 299
Cholera
  outbreak investigations, 330*t*, 339–41
  specimen collection and laboratory testing,
   398*t*
Choropleth maps, 100, 101*f*
Clinic field investigations. *See* Health-care
  setting investigations
Clostridium botulinum, 356, 397*t*
Cluster, definition, 22
Cluster sampling, 204, 205–6, 370–71
Cohort studies, 118, 120–21
child care setting outbreak investigations,
  301–2
occupational disease and injury
  investigations, 316–17
prospective, 121
retrospective, 121, 128*t*
vs. case-control studies, 127–28, 128*t*
Common source outbreak, 23, 91, 91*f*
Communicable Disease Center. *See* Centers
  for Disease Control and Prevention
  (CDC)

Communication
child care setting outbreak investigations,
  301, 303
computers for, 230–32
epidemiologic findings, 183–95
international field investigations, 352
natural disaster investigations, 376–77
occupational disease and injury
  investigations, 309–10
public. *See* Media coverage; News
  interview
skills, 183–84, 237
Community health, 10
Compulsory measures, public health statutes,
  264–67
Computers, 217–34. *See also* Data,
  computerized; Internet
communication using, 230–32
field use, 220–21
future, 234
hardware, 218
legal issues, 233–34
obtaining information with, 231–32
portable, 218
questionnaire design for use with, 221–26.
  See also Questionnaires
selection, 218
software, 219–20
technical assistance, 232
viruses, 232
word processing, 221
Concordant pairs, 163
Confidence intervals
interpretation, 153
for measures of association, 152–53
sample size and, 130
Confidentiality
of computerized data, 233
health-care setting investigations, 286
of investigational records, 258–60
of personal health information, 261–62
state and local field epidemiology
  programs, 325
of state public health records, 262–63
surveillance systems, 37, 331
"Confidentiality of Individually Identifiable
  Health Information," 262
Confounding, 168
definition, 157
epidemiologic studies, 130
stratified analysis and, 157–59
Consumer Product Safety Commission
  (CPSC), 36

Contact transmission, 19–20
Continuing common source outbreak, 91, 91*f*
Control group
  definition, 119–20
  selection
    health-care setting investigations, 281
    principles, 123–25
    sampling methods, 125–27
  size, 127
Control measures, 180. *See also* Interventions
  child care setting outbreak investigations,
      300–302, 305
  field investigations, 76
  surveillance, 45, 46*f*
Convenience sampling, 203
Council of State and Territorial
      Epidemiologists, 50, 262–63
Counts. *See* Case count
Coverage error, surveys, 212–13
Cox proportional hazard model, 161
Cross-product ratio, 143–44, 143*t*
Cross-sectional studies, occupational disease
      and injury investigations, 316
Crude death rate, 86*t*
Cultural considerations, international field
      investigations, 348–49, 351, 353
Cultures, specimen collection, 407
Cyclical time patterns, 97, 97*f*–98*f*
Cyclones, medical and public health effects,
      379–80

Data. *See also* Data analysis; Data sources;
      Databases
  collection
    legal issues, 258–63
    natural disaster investigations, 371, 372*t*
    occupational disease and injury
        investigations, 310
  computerized
    backup, 232–33
    confidentiality, 233
    obtaining and using, 230
  description. *See* Descriptive epidemiology
  entry and validation, 133–35, 210–11, 226–
      27
  interpretation, 166–71
    biological plausibility, 168–69
    confounding, 168
    consistency, 169
    dose-response effect, 169
    exposure-disease sequence, 169
    information bias, 167–68
    investigator error, 168

    selection bias, 167
    strength of association, 168
  legal issues, 233–34, 258–63
  orientation by time, place, and person
    child care setting outbreak investigations,
        297–98
    field investigation, 68–71, 69*f*–70*f*
    health-care settings, 278–81, 279*f*, 280*f*
  quality, 107
  software programs, 219
Data analysis, 132–66, 227–29
  confidence intervals, 152–53
  confounding, 157–59
  dose response, 160, 161*t*
  effect modification, 159
  matching, 162–66, 164*t*–166*t*
  measures of association, 142–44, 142*t*, 143*t*
  measures of public health impact, 142*t*,
      144–47, 147*t*
  methods, 142–66, 227–29
  modeling, 160–61
  planning, 132–42, 134*f*
  steps, 134*f*
  strategy development, 135–41, 136*t*, 141*f*
  stratified, 154–59, 155*t*–157*t*. *See also*
      Stratified analysis
  summary exposure tables, 153–54, 154*t*
  surveillance data, 43–44
  survey data, 211–12
  table shells, 136–40
  tests of statistical significance, 147–52,
      150*t*
  two-by-two table, 141–42, 141*t*–143*t*, 145*t*,
      147*t*
Data sources, 5
  animal vector studies, 34–35
  case reports, 33
  databases, 35–36
  demographic data, 36–37
  disease surveillance, 29–37
  environmental data, 37
  epidemic reporting, 33–34
  health care providers, 331
  health surveys, 35–36
  laboratory data, 32–33
  morbidity data, 31–32
  mortality data, 29–30
  sentinel systems, 34
  state and local field epidemiology, 327–29
Databases
  design, for questionnaires, 222
  for state and local field epidemiology, 327–
      29

for surveillance, 35–36
  pitfalls, 330*t*, 339–41
Day care setting outbreaks. *See* Child care
  setting outbreak investigations
Death certificate data, 30
Death rate, 86*t*
Death-to-case ratio, 86*t*
Demographic data, 36–37
Descriptive epidemiology, 9, 14, 78–115. *See
  also* Data
  case count, 79–80, 80*t*, 421*t*–423*t*
  charts, 111–14, 112*f*–113*f*, 115
  data quality, 107
  dimensions, 78
  frequency distributions, 109, 110–14
  graphs, 108–9, 114–15
  histograms, 109, 110–11
  maps, 98–100, 99*f*, 101*f*, 108
  person characteristics, 100, 102–5, 103*f*,
    104*t*, 105*f*, 106*f*
  place patterns, 97–100, 99*f*
  population-level characteristics, 107
  purposes, 79
  rates, 80–85, 83*t*
  tables, 111
  time patterns, 85, 87–97, 88*f*–98*f*
Diagnosis, confirmation
  child care setting outbreak investigations,
    296–97
  field investigations, 66
  health-care setting investigations, 277
Diagnostic bias, 129
Direct transmission, 19–20
Directional hypothesis, 148
Discordant pairs, 163
Disease. *See also* Infectious disease
  agent factors, 16, 18–20
  baseline level, 21–22
  causation, triad model, 16–17
  chain of infection, 18–21
  clinical, 18
  endemic, 22
  environmental factors, 17
  host factors, 17, 20
  hyperendemic, 22
  levels, 21–22
  natural history and spectrum, 17–18, 44, 45*f*
  occupational. *See* Occupational disease and
    injury investigations
  outbreak. *See* Outbreak(s); Outbreak
    investigations
  rapidly emerging, state field investigations,
    332–34

rare, epidemiologic studies, 128, 144
reporting
  physicians vs. clinical laboratories, 331
  requirements, 31, 260, 274, 293–94
specimen collection and testing, 393*t*–404*t*
sporadic, 22
subclinical, 17–18
surveillance. *See* Surveillance
Disease-exposure association, 144–47, 145*t*,
  147*t*, 169
Dissemination of findings, 43–44
Division of Laboratory Sciences (DLS), 387,
  388*t*, 390–91, 408–10
Dose-response effect, 169
  analysis, 160, 161*t*
  occupational disease and injury
    investigations, 320–21
Droplet spread transmission, 20
"Dummy table," 136

E. coli
  specimen collection and laboratory testing,
    397*t*
  subtyping system, 341–42, 342*f*–343*f*
Eastern equine encephalitis, surveillance
  system, 34–35
Effect modification, 155, 159
Emergency Public Health Powers Act,
  266–67
Emerging Infectious Disease, 328
Endemic disease, 22
Environmental data, 37
Environmental factors, in disease, 17
Environmental Protection Agency, as data
  source, 36
Environmental toxicants
  inorganic, 388*t*, 389
  organic, 388–89, 388*t*
  specimen collection and testing, 385–91, 388*t*
    general instructions, 385–86, 388*t*
    guidelines, 387–89, 388*t*
    material required, 386–87
    summary instructions, 391
    urine samples, 389–91
Epi Info program
  analysis module, 141, 141*f*, 227–29
  availability, 219, 231
  file format, 230
  Fisher exact test, 228
  geographic variables, 229–30
  graphs, 229
  histograms, 228
  two-by-two tables, 141, 141*f*, 228

Epi Info program (*continued*)
  using, 221–27
  website, 231–32
Epidemic. *See also* Outbreak(s)
  causes
    artifactual, 66
    probable, 22
  definition, 22, 415
  determining existence of
    field investigations, 65–66
    health-care setting investigations, 276–77
  intermittent, 23
  media coverage, 248–49
  mixed, 23
  patterns, 22–24
  reporting, as data source, 33–34
Epidemic curve, 23, 88–96, 89*f*
  biologic factors in, 94
  continuing common source, 91, 91*f*
  environmental factors in, 93, 93*f*
  field investigations, 68–69, 69*f*
  health-care setting investigations, 278–79,
    279*f*–280*f*
  histograms as, 110
  Oswego problem, 420, 424, 424*f*
  point source, 89–90, 90*f*
  point source with secondary transmission,
    90, 91*f*
  propagated, 92, 92*f*
  seasonal, 98*f*, 110–11
  stratification, 95–96, 96*f*
  vector-borne disease, 94, 95*f*
  zoonotic disease, 93–94, 94*f*
Epidemic Intelligence Service (EIS), 13, 355
Epidemic investigations. *See* Field
    investigations; Outbreak
    investigations
Epidemiologic field investigations. *See* Field
    investigations
Epidemiologic paper. *See also* Reports
  basic structure, 184–88
  guidelines, 188–89
  method and materials, 184–85
  order of writing, 188
  presenting, 190–95
  problems, 189–90
  results, 185–87
  writing, 184–90
Epidemiologic studies, 117–31
  case-control, 121–27. *See also* Case-control
    studies
  cohort, 120–21. *See also* Cohort studies
  defining exposure groups, 118–19

defining outcomes (case definition), 119–20
  information bias, 129–30
  objectives, 13–14
  operations performed in, 15–16
  pitfalls, 128–31
  rare exposure, 127–28
  risk measurement, 127
  sample size, 130–31
  selection bias, 129
  types, 118
Epidemiologic surveillance. *See* Surveillance
Epidemiologic triad, 16–17
Epidemiologists
  communication skills, 183–84
  core competencies, 12
  litigation issues, 263–64, 286
  operations performed by, 15–16
  state, authority of, 53–54
  web sites for, 49–50
Epidemiology
  analytic, 9
  core functions, 12–15
  definition, 8, 183–84
  descriptive. *See* Descriptive epidemiology
  field
    definition, 3–4
    state and local. *See* State and local field
        epidemiology
  framework, 325–26
  laboratory support, 384–411
  occupational. *See* Occupational disease and
      injury investigations
  principles, 8–10
  public acceptance, 179
  publications, 328–29
  uses, 10–12
Epidemiology Monitor Newsletter, 329
Error
  in hypothesis testing, 148
  investigator, 168
  in surveys, 212–14
Experimental study, 117
Exposure-disease association, 144–47, 145*t*,
    147*t*, 169
  occupational disease and injury
      investigations, 315–18
Exposure groups, defining, 118–19
Exposure of interest, 153–54, 154*t*
Exposure tables, 153–54, 154*t*

Face-to-face surveys, 198, 208–10
Fatality Analysis Reporting System (FARS),
    36, 50

Field investigations, 13–14, 62–77. *See also*
    Outbreak investigations;
    Surveillance
analytic studies. *See* Data analysis;
    Epidemiologic studies
bioterrorism-related. *See* Bioterrorism
causation and, 179–80
child care settings. *See* Child care setting
    outbreak investigations
communicating findings. *See*
    Communication; Epidemiologic
    paper; Reports
computers. *See* Computers
critical steps, 413–14
data sources, 5, 29–37
departure meeting, 60–61
description of findings. *See* Descriptive
    epidemiology
disasters. *See* Natural disaster investigations
dissemination of findings, 43–44
follow-up activities, 60–61
future directions, 180
initiation, 57–58
international settings. *See* International
    field investigations
interventions, 176–79, 180
invitation to perform
    evaluation, 53–54
    response, 54–55
laboratory support, 55–56, 384–411
legal considerations, 255–67, 325–26. *See
    also* Legal authority; Legal issues
local coordination, 55
local health department. *See* State and local
    field investigations
management framework, 58–60
media coverage. *See* Media coverage; News
    interview
natural disasters. *See* Natural disaster
    investigations
objectives, 13, 180
occupational disease and injury. *See*
    Occupational disease and injury
    investigations
operational aspects, 53–61, 414
overall purposes and methods, 62–63
pace and commitment, 63–64
preparation
    administrative instructions and
        notification, 56–57
    collaboration and consultation, 55–56
reasons for, 54–55, 174–76
reluctance to participate, 6

responsibilities, 54–55
retrospective aspects, 64–65
sample size, 5
specimen collection. *See* Specimen
    collection
standards, 6–7
state health department. *See* State and local
    field investigations
steps, 64–76, 65*t*
    case count, 67–68
    case definition, 67
    confirm diagnosis, 66
    control and prevention measures, 76
    data orientation by time, place, and
        person, 68–71, 69*f*–70*f*
    determine existence of epidemic, 65–66
    epidemic curve construction, 68–69, 69*f*
    hypothesis comparison with facts, 72–74
    hypothesis development and testing, 71–
        72
    plan systematic study, 74–75
    prepare report, 61, 75–76
    risk determination, 71
team selection, 56
unique challenges, 4–6
vs. planned epidemiologic studies, 4
walk-through exercise, 413–34
Fisher exact test, 148–49, 150, 170
Floods, medical and public health effects,
    378–79
Follow-up study. *See* Cohort studies
Food and Drug Administration (FDA)
    contact information, 274
    outbreak reporting requirements, 274
Food-borne disease, specimen collection and
    testing, 397*t*–398*t*
Food contamination
    gastroenteritis caused by, 419*t*
    with salmonella, as bioterrorism, 357
Foodborne Disease Handbook, 328
Francisella tularensis, 356, 395*t*
Freedom of Information Act, 259–60
Frequency, definition, 9
Frequency distributions, 109, 110–14
Frequency matching, case-control studies,
    126–27, 162
Frequency polygon, 109, 110
Frost, W. H., 183–84

Gastroenteritis
    agents causing, 417–18, 419*t*
    shellfish-associated, state and local field
        investigations, 334–35

Generation period, 90
Genotyping, health-care setting investigations, 273–74, 274t
Geocoding, definition, 229
GIS (Geographic Information Systems), 229–30
GPS (Geographic Position Sensor), 229
Graphs
    arithmetic scale, 109
    design and use, 114–15
    principles, 108
semilogarithmic scale, 109

Health, public. See Public health
Health and Human Services Administration, website, 262
Health care providers, as data source, 331
Health-care setting investigations, 268–87
    background, 268–71, 269t
    collaboration and consultation, 273–75
    infections in, characteristics, 268–70
    medico-legal aspects, 285
    overall purposes, 270
    pace and commitment, 270–71
    preparation, 273–75
    recognition and response, 271–73
    report of possible outbreak, 271–72
    request for assistance, 272
    response and responsibilities, 272–73
    steps, 275–85
        case count, 278
        case definition, 277–78
        confirmation of diagnosis, 277
        data orientation by time, place, and person, 278–81, 279f–280f
        determining existence of epidemic, 276–77
        epidemic curve construction, 278–79, 279f–280f
        hypothesis comparison with facts, 282, 284
        hypothesis development and testing, 281–82
        planning systematic study, 284–85
        reports, 285
        risk determination, 281, 283t
Health care system databases, for state and local field epidemiology, 327–28
Health departments, state and local. See State and local field epidemiology
Health information, privacy standards, 261–62
Health Insurance Portability and Accountability Act (HIPPA), 261–62

Health jurisdictions, nature of, 54
Health maintenance organizations, morbidity data, 32
Health practices, surveillance, 47
Health surveys, as data source, 35–36
Healthy worker effect, 129, 320
Hepatitis A outbreak, state and local field investigations, 337–39, 338f
Histogram, 88, 110–11, 228
Hospital settings
    field investigations in. See Health-care setting investigations
    infections in, characteristics, 268–70
Host factors, in disease, 17, 20
"Human element," 40–41
Human subjects research, legal issues, 260–61
Hurricanes, medical and public health effects, 379–80
Hypothesis
    alternative, 147, 148
    comparison with facts
        child-care setting investigations, 299–300
        field investigations, 72–74
        health-care setting investigations, 282, 284
    development and testing
        child-care setting investigations, 299
        field investigations, 71–72
        health-care setting investigations, 281–82
        surveillance data and, 44, 46f
    directional, 148
    nondirectional, 148
    null, 147–48

Immunization practices
    impact of field studies, 176
    international field investigations, 346
    natural disaster investigations, 378–79, 382
    vaccine efficacy studies, 146–47, 147t
Incidence rates, 81, 83t
    cumulative, 81–82, 82f
    person-time, 84
Incident cases, 79, 80, 82f, 121
Incident rate, 121
Indirect transmission, 20
Industrial hygienist, 314, 318
Infant mortality rate, 86t
Infection
    chain of, 18–21
    transmission, 19–20. See also Transmission
Infection control professionals (ICPs), 271–72, 274–75

Infectious agent, 18
  cultures, 407
  identification, 391–92, 393*t*–406*t*, 407
  infectivity, 18
  modes of transmission, 19–20
  pathogenicity, 18
  relationship to host, 20
  reservoir, 18–19
  specimen collection and testing, 391–92,
      393*t*–406*t*, 407
  specimen shipment, 392, 407–10
  surveillance, 45, 47, 47*f*
  virulence, 18
Infectious disease
  agent factors, 16, 18–20. *See also* Infectious
      agent
  child care–associated, 294–95. *See also*
      Child care setting outbreak
      investigations
  data networks, 31–32
  hospital-aquired vs. community setting,
      268–70. *See also* Health-care setting
      investigations
  outbreak. *See* Outbreak(s); Outbreak
      investigations
  surveillance. *See* Surveillance
Infectivity, 18
Influenza
  specimen collection and laboratory testing,
      393*t*
  surveillance data, 30
Information bias, 129–30, 167–68
Informed consent, 261
  child care setting outbreak investigations, 297
  state and local field epidemiology
      programs, 325–26
International field investigations, 345–53
  case count, 351
  case definition, 350–51
  changing dynamics, 349
  communicating and reporting, 352
  cultural considerations, 348–49, 351, 353
  logistical concerns, 350
  preparation, 346–49
    administrative instructions and
        notification, 347
    introduction to local authorities, 350
    protocol meeting, 349–50
  publication, 352–53
  self-care during, 351–52
  steps, 349–53
  travel health guidelines, 347
  types of outbreaks, 346

Internet, 49–50, 230–32. *See also* Computers
Interventions
  bioterrorism-related, 266–67. *See also*
      Bioterrorism
  child care setting outbreak investigations,
      300–302
  community involvement, 180
  compulsory measures, 264
  control measures, 178
  determinants, 176–79, 177*f*
  isolation and quarantine, 264–65
  legal issues, 264–66
  occupational settings, 318, 319–20
Interviewer training, 208–10
Investigator error, 168
Isolation activities, surveillance, 47
Isolation authority, 264–66

Jacobson v. Massachusetts, 256, 265
Joint Commission on Accreditation of
    Healthcare Organizations (JCAHO),
    271
Judgment sampling, 203

Laboratory data, 32–33
Laboratory Response Network, for
    bioterrorism, 361
Laboratory support
  field investigations, 55–56, 384–411
  list of abbreviations, 410–11
  National Center for Environmental Health,
      385, 387, 388*t*, 390–91, 408–10
  National Center of Infectious Diseases, 391,
      409–10
  specimen collection, 385–97. *See also*
      Specimen collection
  specimen shipping, 407–10
Laboratory testing
  bacterial disease
    food-borne, 397*t*–398*t*
    general, 393*t*–395*t*
    sexually transmitted, 396*t*
  bioterrorism, 360, 361, 385, 393*t*–395*t*
  mycotic infection, 404*t*
  natural disaster investigations, 376
  parasitic infection, 405*t*–406*t*
  rickettsial disease, 404*t*
  viral disease
    general, 399*t*–401*t*
    vector-borne, 402*t*–403*t*
Langmuir, A. D., 27
"Least restrictive alternative" principle,
    265

Legal authority
    for bioterrorism emergency response, 266–
        67, 356
    for occupational disease and injury
        investigations, 307–8
    for public health protection. *See* Public
        health powers
Legal issues
    computerized data, 233–34
    confidentiality. *See* Confidentiality
    data collection, 258–63
    disease reporting, 260
    field investigations, 255–67, 325–26
    health-care setting investigations, 285
    public health interventions, 264–67
    research involving human subjects, 260–61
    surveillance, 37–38, 330
Legionnaires' disease, 3, 12, 178, 393*t*
Line-listing
    definition, 420
    format, 79, 80*t*, 421*t*–423*t*, 427*t*–429*t*
Listeriosis
    field investigations, 73–74
    specimen collection and laboratory testing,
        394*t*
Litigation, role of epidemiologist, 263–64, 286
Local health department. *See* State and local
        field epidemiology
Logistic regression, 160–61
Long-term care facilities, field investigations
    in. *See* Health-care setting
    investigations

Mail surveys, 198
Mantel-Haenszel chi-square, 149–50, 151,
        219, 228
Maps, 98–100
    area, 100, 101*f*
    choropleth, 100, 101*f*
    principles, 108
    spot, 70, 70*f*, 98–99, 99*f*
Matched pairs, 125–26, 162, 163–64, 164*t*
Matched sets, 165
Matched triplets, 165, 165*t*, 166*t*
Matching
    advantages and disadvantages, 162–63
    case-control studies, 162–66, 164*t*–166*t*
    category (frequency), 126–27, 162
    definition, 162
    goal, 162
    schemes, 162
    variable, 165
Material Safety Data Sheet, 321

Maternal mortality rate, 86*t*
McNemar chi-square test, 164
Measurement error, surveys, 213
Media coverage, 5–6, 236–51. *See also* News
        interview
    background, 236–39
    deadlines, 238–39
    epidemic management, 248–49
    health-care setting investigations, 275
    news business, 239
    news process, 238
    outbreaks in day care, 303
    press conference, 249–50
    press embargo, 250
    public information personnel, 240
    special situations, 250–51
    state and local field investigations, 330
MEDLARS database, 231
Mercury, urine specimen collection, 390
Metals, urine specimen collection, 389–90
Microbial agent. *See* Infectious agent
Microcomputers, 218. *See also* Computers
Minnesota Department of Health, *E. coli*
        subtyping system, 341–42, 342*f*–
        343*f*
Mixed epidemics, 23
MMWR Recommendations and Reports, 328
Model State Emergency Public Health Powers
        Act, 266–67
Modeling, 160–61
Morbidity
    data, 31–32
    measures, 81, 83*t*
Morbidity and Mortality Weekly Report
        (MMWR), 41, 44, 50, 328
Mortality
    data, 29–30
    measures, 81, 86*t*
Multiple strata display, 95–96, 96*f*
Multistage sampling, 206
Mycotic infection, specimen collection and
        testing, 404*t*

National Ambulatory Medical Care Survey
        (NAMCS), 31, 49
National Automotive Sampling System
        (NASS), 36, 50
National Birth Defects Prevention Network,
        32, 50
National Center for Environmental Health
        (NCEH), Division of Laboratory
        Sciences, 385, 387, 388*t*, 390–91,
        408–10

National Center for Health Statistics (NCHS), 32
National Center of Infectious Diseases (NCID), 391, 409–10
National Drug and Therapeutic Index, 31
National Electronic Injury Surveillance System (NEISS), 36, 50
National Fire Incident Reporting System, 36, 50
National Health and Nutrition Examination Survey 49,(NHANES), 35
National Health Interview Survey, 35, 50
National Highway Traffic Safety Administration (NHTSA), 36
National Hospital Ambulatory Medical Care Survey, 32, 49
National Hospital Discharge Survey, 32, 50
National Influenza Surveillance System, 30
National Institute of Occupational Safety and Health (NIOSH), 322
National Library of Medicine, MEDLARS database, 231
National Mortality Follow-back Survey, 30, 49
National Nosocomial Infection Surveillance System, 32, 50
National Weather Service, 50
Natural disaster investigations, 365–82
  coordination, 377
  determination of rates, 368–69
  of earthquakes, 381–82
  field problems, 366–69
  of floods, 378–79
  general considerations, 366–67
  historical development, 366
  information management, 377–78
  laboratory testing, 376
  logistics, 367–68
  medical and public health effects, 378–82
  methodologic issues, 367, 368t
  rapid assessment, 369–71
    data collection, 371, 372t
    methods, 370–71
    objectives, 369
    timeliness, 369
  reporting, 376–77
  of rumors, 375–76
  surveillance, 371, 373–75
    active, 374
    communicating data, 376–77
    general considerations, 371, 373
    sentinel, 374–75
  of tornadoes, 380

of tropical cyclones, 379–80
of volcanic eruptions, 380–81
Neonatal mortality rate, 86t
Nesting approach, case-control studies, occupational disease and injury investigations, 317
New York State Department of Health, shellfish-associated gastroenteritis investigation, 334–35
News interview, 239–47. See also Media coverage
  bridging technique, 242
  difficult, 243
  flagging statements, 242–43
  language, 241–42
  objective, 240–41
  planning, 243–45
  print, 245
  radio, 245–46
  rules of thumb, 241
  techniques, 242–43
  TV, 246–47
News media. See Media coverage
Nondirectional hypothesis, 148
Nonprobability sampling, 203
Nonresponse bias, 129
Nonresponse error, surveys, 213–14
North American Primary Care Research Group, 31
Null hypothesis, 147–48, 153, 167
Nursing homes, field investigations in. See Health-care setting investigations
Nutritional surveillance, disaster situations, 366

Observational study, 117
Occupational and Environmental Medicine List Service, 322
Occupational disease and injury investigations, 306–22
  bias, 310
  communication about consequences, 309–10
  contracts, 308
  data collection, 310
  dose-effect relationship, 320–21
  exposure-disease relationship, 315–18
  general concerns, 319–21
  healthy worker effect, 129
  hierarchy of prevention, 312–13
  industrial hygienist in, 314, 318
  information sources, 321–22
  of intervention effectiveness, 318–19

Occupational disease and injury investigations (*continued*)
of known occupational etiology, 311–13
new areas of focus, 319–20
notification of results, 310–11
preparations, 307–11
request for assistance, 307
right of entry, 307–8
risk assessment, 315–16
safety considerations, 317–18
of sentinel health events, 312, 313
special considerations, 319–21
study designs, 121, 316–17
trade secrets, 308
tripartite relationship, 308–9
types, 311
of unknown etiology, 313–14
years of potential life lost considerations, 320
Occupational Safety and Health Administration (OSHA)
mandates for health-care settings, 287
OSHA 200 logs, 321
Odds ratio, 143–44, 143*t*
formula, 165
prevalence, 144, 145*t*
"One-tailed" test, 148
OSHA 200 logs, 321
Oswego problem, 413–34
Outbreak(s). *See also* Epidemic
after natural disasters, 376
common source, 23, 91, 91*f*
community vs. hospital-based, 268–70
definition, 22, 415
determining existence of, child care setting outbreak investigations, 296
health-care settings. *See* Health-care setting investigations
international field investigations, 346
point source, 23
propagated, 23
Outbreak investigations. *See also* Field investigations
case definition, 40
child-care settings. *See* Child care setting outbreak investigations
health-care settings. *See* Health-care setting investigations
state and local
cholera, 330*t*, 339–41
hepatitis A, 337–39, 338*f*
with public health laboratory collaboration, 341–42, 342*f*–343*f*

shellfish-associated gastroenteritis, 334–35
typhoid fever, 335–37
Outcomes, defining, epidemiologic studies, 119–20
"Overmatching," 125

Pair matching, case-control studies, 125–26, 162, 163–64, 164*t*
Pandemic, 22
Parasitic infection, specimen collection and testing, 405*t*–406*t*
Passive surveillance, 28
Pathogenicity, 18
Pattern, 9
Pearson uncorrected chi-square, 149
Person characteristics, 100, 102–5
by age, 103–5, 104*t*, 105*f*
child care setting outbreak investigations, 297–98
comparative representations, 105, 107
field investigations, 70–71
health-care setting investigations, 280–81
by personal contact and network groups, 102, 103*f*
Pesticides, urine specimen collection, 389–90
Physicians, disease reporting by, 331
Pie charts, 114
Place patterns, 97–100, 99*f*, 101f. *See also* Maps
child care setting outbreak investigations, 297–98
comparative representations, 105, 107
field investigations, 69–70
health-care setting investigations, 279–80
Plague *(Yersinia pestis)*
as biological warfare agent, 356
specimen collection and laboratory testing, 395*t*
Point prevalence, 83*t*, 84
Point source outbreak, 89–91, 90*f*
with secondary transmission, 90, 91*f*
Poisson regression, 161
Police power, state-level
bioterrorism-related, 266–67
compulsory measures, 264–66
isolation and quarantine, 264–66
to protect public health, 256–57
Policy development, role of epidemiology, 14
Population health, 10
Postneonatal mortality rate, 86*t*
Presentation, scientific paper, 190–95
Press conference, 249–50. *See also* News interview

Press embargo, 250
Prevalence odds ratio, 144, 145t
Prevalence rates, 82f, 83t, 84
Prevalence ratio, 144, 145t
Prevalent cases, 79, 80, 82f
Prevented fraction in exposed group, 146–47, 147t
Prevention measures
    child care setting outbreak investigations, 301
    field investigations, 76
    occupational disease and injury investigations, 312–13
Print interview, 245
Privacy. See Confidentiality
Privacy Act, 261
Probability sampling, 203–6
Probability (P) value, in tests of statistical significance, 147–48, 149, 150
Promed, 328
Propagated outbreak, 92, 92f
Proportional mortality, 86t
Protection of Human Subjects, 45 C.F.R. Part 46, 260–61
Public health
    bioterrorism threats. See Bioterrorism
    child care settings. See Child care setting outbreak investigations
    interventions. See Interventions
    measures of impact, 142t, 143t, 144–47, 147t
    natural disaster threats. See Natural disaster investigations
Public health epidemiologist, interactions with child care providers, 291
Public health laboratory
    collaboration with, 341–42, 342f–343f
    as data source, 329
Public health powers
    bioterrorism, 266–67, 356
    compulsory procedures, 264–66
    federal level, 255–56
    under Freedom of Information Act, 259–60
    for gaining access, 257–58
    limitations, 256–57, 265–66
    local level, 325–26
    under Model State Emergency Public Health Powers Act, 266–67
    under Privacy Act, 261
    under Public Health Service Act, 255, 257–58
    state level, 256–57, 264–67, 325–26
    surveillance, 37–38, 330

Public health records, privacy of, 262–63
Public Health Service (PHS), 255–56
Public Health Service Act, 255, 257–58
Public information personnel, 240
Public relations. See Media coverage; News interview
Purposive sampling, 203

Quakstick, 366
Quarantine authority, 264–66
Questionnaires, 221–29. See also Surveys
    analysis. See Data analysis
    computer formats, 223–24
    data base design, 222
    Epi Info, 222–29
    format, 200–201
    multiple-choice questions, 225–26
    outline, 221–22
    pretesting, 201–2
    for state and local field epidemiology, 328
    symptom question, 226
    validation, 227
    writing questions, 199–200

Radio interview, 245–46
Random sampling, 125, 203–4
Rapid Response and Technology Laboratory (RRAT Lab), 385
Rapidly emerging disease, state field investigations, 332–34
Rare disease, epidemiologic studies, 128, 144
Rare exposure, epidemiologic studies, 127–28
Rates, 80–85
    area maps, 100, 101f
    attack, 81, 82f, 83t
    incidence, 81, 83t
        person-time, 84
    prevalence, 82f, 84
    secondary attack, 82–83, 83t
    secular trend, 96–97
    time patterns, 96, 110
Ratios, 84–85, 86t, 87f
    geographic display, 100
    odds, 143–44, 143t
    prevalence, 144, 145t
    risk, 142t, 143
Records protection, 258–60
Regression models, 160–61
Relative odds, 143–44, 143t
Relative risk, 142t, 143
Reporting requirements, disease, 31, 260, 274, 293–94

Reports. *See also* Epidemiologic paper
  child care setting outbreak investigations,
    303
  field investigations, 61, 75–76
  health-care setting investigations, 285
  international field investigations, 352
  natural disaster investigations, 376–77
Research
  definition, 260
  human subjects, 260–61
Reservoir, infectious agent, 18–19
Response rate, surveys, 210
Reynolds v. McNichols, 265
Rickettsial disease, specimen collection and
    testing, 404*t*
Risk
  attributable risk percentage, 143*t*, 145
  measurement, epidemiologic studies, 127
  population attributable risk percentage, 146
  relative, 142*t*, 143
Risk determination, 71, 81
  age categories, 103–4
  child care setting outbreak investigations,
    299
  field investigations, 71
  health-care setting investigations, 281, 283*t*
  occupational disease and injury
    investigations, 315–16
  small populations, 102
Rumors, natural disaster investigations, 375–
    76

Safety considerations, occupational disease
    and injury investigations, 317–18
Salmonellosis
  field investigations, 74, 357
  specimen collection and laboratory testing,
    397*t*
Sample designs, 204–6
Sample size, 5
  formulas, 207
  small, epidemiologic studies, 130–31
  statistical significance and, 130
  surveys, 206–8
Sampling
  case-control studies, 125–27
  cluster, 204, 205–6, 370–71
  convenience (chunk), 203
  judgment (purposive), 203
  multistage, 206
  nonprobability, 203
  probability, 203–6
  random, 125, 203–4

stratified, 162, 205
  survey, 202–8
  frame, 204
  size, 206–8
  types, 203
  systematic, 125, 204–5
Sampling error, 213
Sampling frame, 204
Scientific paper. *See* Epidemiologic paper
Seasonal curve, 98*f*, 110
Seasonal time patterns, 97, 98*f*
Secondary attack rate, 82–83, 83*t*
Secondary transmission, point source outbreak
    with, 90, 91*f*
Secular trend, 96–97
SEER (Surveillance Epidemiology and End
    Results) system, 36, 50
Selection bias, 129, 167
Semilogarithmic scale line graph, 109
Sentinel Health Event (Occupational),
    SHE(O), 312, 313
Sentinel surveillance, disaster situations, 374–
    75
Sentinel systems, 34
Sexually transmitted disease, specimen
    collection and testing, 396*t*
Shellfish-associated gastroenteritis, state and
    local field investigations, 334–35
Shigellosis, specimen collection and
    laboratory testing, 398*t*
Shipping. *See* Specimen shipping
"Shoeleather epidemiology," 13
Simple random sampling, 204
Single Overriding Communication Objective
    (SOCO), 241
SLACK OFF mnemonic, 59–60
Smallpox *(Variola major)*, as biological
    warfare agent, 356
Software, 219–20
Specimen collection, 5, 385–90
  bacterial disease
    food-borne, 397*t*–398*t*
    general, 393*t*–395*t*
    sexually transmitted, 396*t*
  blood, 392, 407
  for chemical/environmental toxicants, 385–
    91, 388*t*
  general instructions, 385–86, 388*t*
  guidelines, 387–89, 388*t*
  material required, 386–87
  summary instructions, 391
  urine samples, 389–91
  cultures, 407

for microbial identification, 391–92, 393*t*–
    406*t*, 407
  general instructions, 391–92, 407
  universal precautions, 392
  mycotic infection, 404*t*
  parasitic infection, 405*t*–406*t*
  rickettsial disease, 404*t*
  serum, 392, 407
  slides, 407
  universal precautions statement, 392
  urine
    chemical/environmental toxicants, 388*t*
    metals and pesticide analysis, 389–90
  viral disease
    general, 399*t*–401*t*
    vector-borne, 402*t*–403*t*
Specimen shipping, 407–10
  frozen specimens, 409
  materials needed, 408–9
  refrigerated specimens, 410
  temperature requirements, 408
  urine samples of chemical toxicants, 390–91
Sphere Project, natural disaster investigations,
    376
Spot maps, 70, 70*f*, 98–99, 99*f*
State and local field epidemiology, 324–43
  data sources and technologies, 327–29
  effectiveness of collaboration, 326–27
  federal role, 329
  funding, 326
  goals, 332
  information sharing, 327
  information transfer, 327–29
  media, 330
  networking, 327
  personnel, 326
  political issues, 329
  sample investigations, 332–42
  statutes, regulations, codes, and ordinances,
    325–26
  success markers, 332
  surveillance issues, 330–31
State and local field investigations
  of disease outbreak
    hepatitis A, 337–39, 338*f*
    with public health laboratory
      collaboration, 341–42, 342*f*–343*f*
    shellfish-associated gastroenteritis, 334–35
    typhoid fever, 335–37
  of pseudo-outbreak (cholera), 330*t*, 339–41
  of rapidly emerging disease (toxic shock
    syndrome), 332–34
  role of CDC, 327

State epidemiologist, authority of, 53–54
State health department. *See* State and local
    field epidemiology
Statistical Analysis System (SAS), 212, 219
Statistical Programs for the Social Sciences
    (SPSS), 212, 219
Statistical significance tests, 147–52, 150*t*
Stratification, epidemic curve, 95–96, 96*f*
Stratified analysis, 154–59, 155*t*–157*t*, 228–29
  confounding and, 157–59
  effect modification and, 159
  Mantel-Haenszel formula, 149–50, 219
  two-by-four table, 156–57, 156*t*–157*t*
Stratified sampling, 162, 205
Strength of association, 168
Streptococcus infection, specimen collection
    and laboratory testing, 395*t*
Study design. *See also* Epidemiologic studies
  occupational disease and injury
    investigations, 121
Summary exposure tables, 153–54, 154*t*
Surveillance, 26–48. *See also* Surveillance
    systems
  active, 28, 374
  background, 27–28
  bioterrorism situations, 357, 358–59, 361
  child care settings, 291–94
    direct reporting, 293–94
    indirect reporting, 292–93, 304–5
    post-intervention, 300
    uses, 291–92
  data analysis, 43–44
  data sources, 29–37. *See also* Data sources
  disaster situations, 374
Surveillance Epidemiology and End Results
    (SEER) system, 36, 50
Surveillance systems
  case definition, 39–40
  confidentiality, 37, 331
  conflicts of interest, 37–38
  establishment, 38–43
  evaluation, 48
  goals, 38–39
  initiating, 41–43
  ongoing (long-term), dissemination of
    findings, 44
  personnel, 39
  sentinel, 34
Survey Data Analysis (SUDAAN), 212
Surveys, 196–215. *See also* Questionnaires;
    Sampling
  classification, 196
  cluster-sampling, 370–71

Surveys (*continued*)
  data analysis, 211–12
  data entry and editing, 210–11
  definition, 196
  error sources, 212–14
  face-to-face, 198
  interviewer supplies, 210
  interviewer training, 208–9
  mail, 197–98
  modes, 197–99
  natural disaster investigations, 370–71,
    372*t*
  preparing for fieldwork, 208–10
  protocol, 197
  questionnaire development, 199–202
  rapid
    bioterrorism investigations, 361
    natural disaster investigations, 370–71
  reporting results, 212
  response rate, 210
  sample selection, 202–8
  shortcuts to avoid, 214–15
  steps, 197
  telephone, 198
Systematic sampling, 125, 204–5

Table shells, 136–40
Tables, 111, 114–15
Telephone surveys, 198
Television interview, 246–47
Terrorism. *See* Bioterrorism; Chemical
    toxicants
Tests of statistical significance, 147–52, 150*t*
Time line, 87–88, 88*f*
Time patterns
  child care setting outbreak investigations,
    297–98
  comparative representations, 105, 107
  cyclical, 97, 97*f*–98*f*
  description, 80*t*, 85, 87–97, 88*f*–98*f*
  epidemic curve as, 88–96. *See also*
    Epidemic curve
  field investigations, 68–69
  health-care setting investigations, 278–79,
    279*f*, 280*f*
  for rates, 96, 110
  seasonal, 97, 98*f*
  secular trends, 96–97
  time line as, 87–88, 88*f*
Tornadoes, medical and public health effects,
    380
Toxic shock syndrome, state field
    investigations, 332–34

Toxicants, environmental. *See* Environmental
    toxicants
Trade secrets, occupational disease and injury
    investigations, 308
Training, state and local field epidemiology,
    325
Transmission
  airborne, 20
  contact, 19–20
  direct, 19–20
  droplet spread, 20
  indirect, 20
  modes, 19–20
  vector-borne, 20
  vehicle-borne, 20
Travel health guidelines, international field
    investigations, 347
Tropical cyclones, medical and public health
    effects, 379–80
Tularemia (*Francisella tularensis*)
  as biological warfare agent, 356
  specimen collection and laboratory testing,
    395*t*
Two-by-four table, 156–57, 156*t*–157*t*
Two-by-two table, 141–42, 141*t*–143*t*, 145*t*,
    147, 147*t*
  statistical tests, 148–51
"Two-tailed" test, 148
Type I error (alpha error), 148
Type II error (beta error), 148
Typhoid fever outbreak, state and local field
    investigations, 335–37
Typhoons, medical and public health effects,
    379–80
Typing methods, 274, 274*t*

Urine specimen collection, 388*t*, 389–91
U.S. Census Bureau, as data source, 36
U.S. Constitution, welfare clause, 255–57
U.S. Public Health Service, 255–56

Vaccine efficacy, 146–47, 147*t*
Variable matching, 165
Variola major, as biological warfare agent, 356
Vector-borne disease, 94, 95*f*
  viral, specimen collection and testing,
    402t–403*t*
Vector-borne transmission, 20
Vector species, surveillance, 34–35
Vehicle-borne transmission, 20
Viral disease, specimen collection and testing
  general, 399t–401*t*
  vector-borne, 402*t*–403*t*

Virulence, 18
Virus, computer, 232
Volcanic eruptions, medical and public health
        effects, 380–81

Water contamination, gastroenteritis caused
        by, 419*t*
Websites, 49–50, 230–32
West Nile virus
    field investigation, 38–43, 362
    specimen collection and laboratory testing,
        403*t*

Word processing, 221
Written reports. *See* Reports

Yates corrected chi-square, 149
Yates corrected formula, 151
Years of potential life lost (YPLL),
        occupational disease and injury
        investigations, 320
Yersinia pestis, 356, 395*t*

Zoonosis, 19
Zoonotic disease, epidemic curve, 93–94, 94*f*